Psycho-Oncology for the Clinician

Shulamith Kreitler

Psycho-Oncology for the Clinician

The Patient Behind the Disease

Springer

Shulamith Kreitler
Professor of Psychology
School of Psychological Sciences
Tel-Aviv University
Tel Aviv
Israel

ISBN 978-3-030-06124-1 ISBN 978-3-030-06126-5 (eBook)
https://doi.org/10.1007/978-3-030-06126-5

Library of Congress Control Number: 2019931836

This Springer imprint is published by the registered company Springer Nature Switzerland AG
The registered company address is: Gewerbestrasse 11, 6330 Cham, Switzerland

The book is dedicated to Jimmie C. Holland (1928–2017), a pioneer in Psycho-Oncology

Preface

The appearance at the present time of a book with the title *Psycho-Oncology for the Clinician: The Patient Behind the Disease* requires some kind of explanation. One could wonder why is a book about Psycho-Oncology written at a time when cancer care is becoming increasingly complex as is and, on top of it, expensive at a barely imaginable degree. Neither national institutions nor private patients can cover all expenses. Do we need another target of expenses? Furthermore, one may wonder why deal with Psycho-Oncology at a time when breakthroughs in medicine loom large, spotlighting genetics and immunology, which are indeed expensive but promise recovery, while Psycho-Oncology – what does it actually promise?

The answer is simple – it promises and enables better medicine. There is a long list of potential results. Here is a sample of some of its benefits: better adherence of the patients with the medications, better cooperation of the patients with the treatments, higher satisfaction of the patients with the care they get, easier communication between the clinicians and the patients, lower levels of stress and especially of empathic fatigue in the health carers, better quality of life for patients and family members during treatment and in the survival period, and lower levels of anxiety and of depression in patients especially during crisis phases. In addition, there are no negative side effects to the service of Psycho-Oncology, and it is a cheap service which requires no drugs or mechanical devices, only skilled and trained practitioners.

Yet, Psycho-Oncology is not a fully accepted and legitimate component of cancer care. Even though it is already available in most hospitals and clinics, patients do not always address this service, and, in general, it is not considered as an essential component of cancer care.

So, this is where the message of this book comes in. The book is designed to clarify two main points. One is that Psycho-Oncology is an essential component of cancer treatment and not just a luxury which one may or may not use, at will. As such, it is a major constituent that should be integrated into personalized medicine. It fits in perfectly with what personalized medicine is expected to be, namely, an approach that strives to improve the outcomes and use of medicine by tailoring it to the relevant needs and characteristics of the individual patient. The book is designed to show that psychological needs of the patient are an important aspect that should be considered for optimizing the effects of cancer treatment, no less than genetic, immunological, physiological, and other medical features that are often considered as necessary components of personalized medicine.

The second point is that Psycho-Oncology has become a real science. It has started as a human support-based approach designed to help cancer patients and has evolved into a full-fledged flourishing and dynamic scientific discipline, which has carved for itself a specific space, affiliated with both medicine and psychology yet autonomous in regard to both. However, this scientific breakthrough has not brought in its wake a loss of the human support component of Psycho-Oncology. Quite on the contrary, it has enhanced it.

The audience for which the book is designed is quite broad. The book is intended for clinicians, so that they become updated concerning the benefits and scientific bases of Psycho-Oncology. As a result, they are expected to consider it in treatment and encourage patients to use it. It is intended for patients so that they do not avoid it but rather carve a space for it in the course of their journey through cancer, because a patient who has been exposed to Psycho-Oncology has an easier life and less suffering than a patient who was not. It is intended for clinical researchers in oncology so that they become aware of potential interactions between physiological parameters and psychological variables which they could consider. It is intended for policymakers to become convinced that Psycho-Oncology is important enough to provide some financial resources for its development and availability. It is intended also for psycho-oncologists so that they have a chance to become fully aware of the treasure they have at hand to offer the patients and clinicians.

The information presented in the book is based on scientific studies and on the personal experience of the author who has been working continuously with cancer patients and their families for about 40 years, has developed two Psycho-Oncology centers in two major hospitals in Israel, has done research work in Psycho-Oncology, and has taught Psycho-Oncology to healthcare professionals of all kinds. Thus, the style is readable, and the contents is grounded in scientific sources enlightened and clarified by personal experience.

The author's hope is that the book will contribute to the further scientific development of Psycho-Oncology, to expanding its use as a treatment modality, to strengthening its status as an essential component of cancer care, and to promoting the acceptance of Psycho-Oncology as the new evidence-based constituent of personalized medicine in oncology.

My heartfelt thanks are due to all the doctors, nurses, health professionals of all kinds and primarily the patients of all ages and diagnoses and in so many countries who have taught me and let me learn about cancer and about how to live with it and despite it.

Tel Aviv, Israel
October, 2018

Shulamith Kreitler

Contents

Chapter 1
The History of Psycho-Oncology

Introduction

One may wonder about the meaning of history in regard to Psycho-Oncology. Why examine the history of Psycho-Oncology when it is evident that Psycho-Oncology has always existed, actually from early times when one individual approached a cancer patient with a smile or a gentle touch. Yet, it is no less evident that nowadays Psycho-Oncology includes much more and has a completely different status. History is designed to bridge the gap between the early times and the astounding situation at present, when – at least in the Western world – it is hardly conceivable that a cancer patient does not get psychooncological treatment as part of the overall medical handling of his or her case.

But if Psycho-Oncology has always existed, why is it that it has taken such a long time for it to get recognized formally?

Reasons for the Delay in the Development of Psycho-Oncology

With the best of intentions, it would be possible to identify the mid-1970s as the time when Psycho-Oncology came to life in a formal sense. There are reasons of different kinds that have contributed to the difficulties in the formation of Psycho-Oncology.

The Status of Medical Oncology One major set of reasons has to do with the status of medicine in regard to cancer. The speciality of medical oncology is relatively young [1]. It is only in the 1900s that successful removal of early tumors was carried out and radiation introduced as an oncological treatment modality. The 1940s witnessed the advance in the treatment of lymphoma (with nitrogen mustards) and of acute leukemia (with aminopterin). The big breakthrough came with the advent of chemotherapy in the early 1950s [2, 3]. These are just glimpses into

S. Kreitler, *Psycho-Oncology for the Clinician*,
https://doi.org/10.1007/978-3-030-06126-5_1

the slow and hard development of medical oncology that have given rise to the first National Cancer Plan in the USA in 1972. It is understandable that prior to the development in medical oncology, there was no possibility, space, or option for Psycho-Oncology. The beginnings of Psycho-Oncology took shape in those same years in the form of studies of quality of life of cancer patients (European Organization for Research and Treatment of Cancer [EORTC], founded in 1962) and the establishment of full time psychiatry service at the Memorial Sloan Kettering Cancer Service (1977). These early projects and the many others heralded by them could barely take place without weakening of the taboo characterizing cancer, the initiation of large-scale clinical trials in oncology, the beginning evidence for successful cures with chemotherapy, and development of different medical modalities and drugs for treating cancer patients, followed by the developments in immunology, molecular biology, and genetics that enabled spectacular breakthroughs in medical oncology [4].

The Taboos Regarding Cancer Another important set of reasons for the delay in the development of Psycho-Oncology are the various taboos connected with cancer. All diseases are probably unpleasant concepts, but some are considered as outright taboos. Mental disorders, sexually transmitted diseases, and notably cancer are major items on this list. Cancer has been viewed as taboo primarily in the long periods when there was no treatment for it, no hope, and no respite from the pain and other associated symptoms. In addition to the suffering, cancer patients were burdened with guilt, shame, and the pressure to hide their disease and the unsightly lesions that sometimes appeared. Cancer was not something to be spoken about, by the patient or the family. Only about the 1950s there began the debate about whether cancer diagnoses can at all be revealed to patients. As long as the barriers of denial and silencing prevailed, there was barely a chance to approach patients psychologically, not to mention the possibility of studying the psychological correlates of cancer. It is possible that the stigma accompanying cancer may be grounded also, at least to some extent, in the association of cancer with death. Actually, the stigma overshadowing cancer is still not completely deleted or overcome in the case of all patients and families in all countries. The taboo was replaced by suspicions that discussing cancer openly may harm patients. These attitudes, shared by lay individuals as well as by health professionals, formed a difficult barrier against the development of Psycho-Oncology [5].

The Scientific Status of Psycho-Oncology That is where a third set of reasons that delayed the development of Psycho-Oncology comes in. This is the limited amount of evidence-based information that existed in regard to Psycho-Oncology. This issue should not be considered as constituting a particularly difficult barrier. However, it turned out not to be easily surmountable. Evidence-based information requires empirical research, and this kind of scientific activity requires among other things getting information about different aspects of cancer from patients and their families by means, such as administered questionnaires, observations, and interviewing, performed only with the patients' full legally established informed consent. Limitations concerning addressing the issue of cancer directly or indirectly render empirical research difficult and slow due to the reluctance of the patients and families to participate in the studies. The reluctance was enhanced, particularly in the early stages, by the lack of experience of patients and families to discuss openly the emotional and other personal aspects of cancer [6].

Negative Attitudes Toward the Relations of Psychology with Cancer A fourth set of reasons that slowed down the development of Psycho-Oncology has to do with the negative attitude of patients toward the involvement of psychology in cancer. Considering psychology as a means for understanding or treating cancer evokes the association of mental disorders or illness. Mental disorders have been feared and avoided by people for generations [7, 8]. Individuals with mental problems were no less stigmatized than cancer patients and have often been blamed, punished, and ostracized because of their problem. Even nowadays, individuals who may have mental problems are avoided and often treated differently [9]. Hence, cancer patients would be reluctant to admit that possibly they have psychological problems in addition to their cancer.

Moreover, psychological issues tend to be interpreted as signs of weakness, portending the inability of the patient to handle one's problems. Since cancer is often related to quite serious difficulties of coping, cancer patients are afraid that admitting to psychological problems would weaken their coping ability and would make others consider them as helpless and dependent.

Underlying these negative attitudes to psychology, there is another more general problem which may be described as the unclarity of the relations between psychology and physical disorders in general, or in simpler terms: What does psychology have to do with cancer at all? It is really quite surprising that this issue is still alive and seems relevant.

The issue is a manifestation of basic theoretical shortcomings in the conception of the image of the human being, reflecting on science in general and on medicine and psychology specifically. Basically the problem arises from lack of conceptual clarity about the relations between the constructs of body and mind. Tracing the changes in the conceptualization of *body-mind relations* in the behavioral sciences reveals five major phases [10]. They will be mentioned here because they may shed light on understanding the status and history of Psycho-Oncology.

The *first phase* of the body-mind relations is characterized by the view that there is nothing but the body. This approach describes the status of oncology prior to the beginnings of Psycho-Oncology. Even at present it seems to be shared by medical oncologists and probably also by an undefined number of cancer patients. It is apparently a simple approach that relieves both doctors and patients of the need to deal with psychological issues that probably seem to them controversial, unsupported by any objective evidence, and possibly harmful for patients. The major shortcoming of this approach is that it denies patients the possibility of getting the psychological support which they may need and which could help them. A possible result of this approach is that cancer patients turn for support to alternative treatments and sometimes to various highly doubtful methods without consulting with their doctors and often without informing them. It cannot be ruled out that the results could be harmful for the patients.

The *second phase* is marked by the conception that the mind is the only relevant factor. Although this approach seems to be favorable for Psycho-Oncology, it does not do good service to Psycho-Oncology because it is based often on unfounded beliefs, such as that recovering from cancer can be attained by the mere desire to be healthy or by adhering to a certain cult or a certain healer. Another danger associated with this approach is that patients would refuse to get medical treatment either because they view it as superfluous or useless or because it would indicate the incompleteness of their faith in the nonmedical treatments they endorse. This approach is strongly rejected by oncologists and is probably espoused only by a minority of cancer patients.

The *third phase* in conceptualizing the body-mind relations is that both body and mind exist and are operative, but they function in parallel tracks. It seems that many oncologists as well as patients have chosen to support this conception. It seems to be a comfortable conception because it consists in a liberal acceptance of the major entities – the medical and the psychological – without however bothering about their possible interactions or mutual influences. The implication is that what happens in the body, including even serious physical disorders, does not have much to do with the psychological plane of functioning. And the psychological phenomena, however emotional and important they may seem to observers and to the patients themselves, do not have anything to do with the physical phenomena. Hence, the impact or manifestations of the physical level on the psychological one as well as those of the psychological level on the physical one may be safely disregarded regardless of how impressive or convincing the mutual effects may seem or be experienced by the individual or by observers. This approach enables proceeding with research and therapy on the purely medical level as well as on the psychological level, without considering the implications of the empirical or therapeutic results on one level in regard to the other level. Hence, in the framework of the third phase approach, it is difficult to identify a right niche or space or field for examining the interactions between body and mind or, for that matter, the possible effects of psychological factors on one's physical health and state and of the physical phenomena on one's psychological status. This conclusion is of particular importance for research in Psycho-Oncology because it limits the theoretical space of psychooncological variables only to the sphere of psychology or at best it allows to consider them as correlates of physical variables or phenomena, but not as causes or results.

The *fourth phase* of body-mind relations is based on the assumption that both body and mind exist and that they function in interaction, namely, the phenomena on each level may be considered as affected by those on the other level and as affecting them. Adopting this approach is definitely less comfortable theoretically and practically than the approach of parallelism of the third phase. The reason is that it requires considering – both in research and therapy – the mutual effects of the medical and psychological levels. This provides a new opening and challenge particularly for Psycho-Oncology. The challenge consists primarily in the need to create theoretical models for identifying and defining the intervening constructs and mediating variables through which the psychological effects get translated or transferred from the psychological to physical phenomena relevant for disease and health in general and for cancer in particular. The potential routes include biological factors, such as molecular reactions and cellular responses in the immunological and genetic frameworks. The new approach gave rise to new theoretical frameworks enabling the exploration of the psycho-physical interactions, mainly psychoneuroimmunology [11, 12] and biopsychosocial models [13–16], or examining the contribution of psychological factors, e.g., cognitive to physical disorders, as identifying psychological risk factors for cancer [17] or examining the impact of physical phenomena on psychological and emotional reactions, as identifying tumor characteristics evoking depression [18] or the impact of chemotherapy on cognitive impairment [19]. Contributions from health psychology [20], psychosomatics [21], cognitive-behavioral approaches [22], and psychopharmacology [23] have been particularly productive. Exploring the connections between the physical and psychological phenomena sometimes provides initial support for the view that body and mind are actually identical and under certain conditions constitute merely different manifestations of the same core energy or material.

The interactional view of body-mind is favorable for scientific research in each of the spheres of medicine and Psycho-Oncology. It encourages exploring the psychological effects of physical phenomena, such as the impact of the occurrence of cancer and of different oncologic treatments on the patients' quality of life [24, 25]. It also enabled developing and applying various psychological interventions for helping cancer patients.

Development of Psycho-Oncology

The foregoing introductory section highlighted some of the major reasons that delayed the development of Psycho-Oncology. In addition, it clarified that the development of Psycho-Oncology has to be traced along three different intertwined tracks: the scientific track, the applied track, and the organizational track.

The Scientific Track of Development

As noted, there have been various difficulties that limited the availability of cancer patients as subjects in research. Some had to do with the reluctance of the patients themselves, due to suspicions about incomplete privacy, or no desire to devote time during their disease to something that does not seem to them to be of equal importance to medicine. A painful situation arises not infrequently when patients agree to participate but leave the questionnaires incomplete or withdraw too soon from the studies. Other difficulties of recruiting patients for studies may have had to do with regulations in clinics and hospitals based on requirements of ethics committees that made it sometimes overly difficult to recruit patients for studies that involved no more than validating a simple questionnaire. Further, the elaborated models of experimental research that have been developed in psychology proper could not be transferred without changes to the field of Psycho-Oncology, because of the special characteristics of patients with chronic diseases in general and of cancer patients in particular. Psychosomatic research could not provide much help because the research models it has developed up to the 1970s in regard to other illnesses, particularly asthma, rheumatoid arthritis, gastric ulcer, and hypertension, were either too crude or inapplicable to cancer. Hence, it is evident that psychooncologists had to elaborate new research models for their scientific studies, and this task sounds simpler than it actually is.

In reality devising adequate research models in Psycho-Oncology required several methodological decisions. One of these referred to defining *research groups*. This involves deciding whether it is possible to combine in one sample patients with different cancer diagnoses, or patients in different disease stages, or patients in different phases of treatment (e.g., pretreatment, after the first or second cycle of treatment, patients in remission). A related issue concerns the definition of *control groups* in studies with cancer patients. Healthy control subjects may not always provide ideal comparison for subjects with cancer when the goal is to identify characteristics of the cancer patients. Additionally, blinding is particularly difficult to achieve because consent procedures require participants to understand differences in treatments, which in Psycho-Oncology may often have obvious implications. Another important methodological issue concerns the *control variables* that need to be considered, ranging from kinds of treatments to duration of treatments, stages of disease, comorbidities, lifestyle factors, and the various demographic characteristics. A fourth research issue concerns the selection of adequate, available, and relevant *medical correlates* that are sometimes required or advisable for psychological variables. The need arises for identifying and assessing physiological variables especially when the psychological ones are not as unambiguous as desired, for example, one may wonder whether cognitive impairment following chemotherapy is a manifestation of lack of concentration or interest or a brain-grounded phenomenon. A fifth methodological issue concerns the preparation of relevant as well as valid and reliable *research tools* for Psycho-Oncology. Very early it became clear that psychosocial research with cancer patients requires devising adequate tools for cancer patients. Since the standard tools in psychology are mostly inadequate for Psycho-Oncology, new tools for assessment and for intervention have to be developed for specific needs or issues concerning cancer patients, such as doctor-patient communication or attitudes toward dying. Major developments in this field included the measures of quality of life questionnaires by the European Organization of Research and Treatment of Cancer (EORTC) [26], the Functional Assessment of Cancer Therapy Scale [27], the Memorial Symptom Assessment Scale [28], the Distress Thermometer [29], McCorkle's Symptom Distress Scale [30], the Brief Symptom Inventory (BSI) [31], Fear of Recurrence Inventory [32], Decisional Conflict scale [33], the play-performance scale for pediatric patients [27], and tools for assessing various psychological phenomena in children with cancer patients [34, 35]. Meaning-centered psychotherapy [36], dignity therapy [37] for advanced and palliative cancer patients, and psychoeducational interventions for melanoma patients [38] are examples of interventions developed specifically for cancer patients.

Despite all these theoretical, methodological, and practical difficulties, Psycho-Oncology investigators proceeded courageously on the track of development, trying as best as possible to explore new territories and adhere to the strict criteria applied to evaluating studies considered as potential candidates for inclusion in Cochrane reviews.

Clinical Application

Clinical applications in Psycho-Oncology constituted originally a new unknown and unexplored territory. It was not even evident that cancer patients need psychooncological help or, for that matter, that there may be a psychological aspect to any medical patients with chronic diseases. It seems that until the 1900s, physicians were unaware that chronic medical patients may suffer from emotional difficulties, including depression, stress, and adjustment problems. One of the pioneers in this domain was Adolf Meyer who encouraged medical colleagues and students to consider "the whole person," thereby facilitating the integration of psychology into medical practice. The first psychiatric ward for patients with chronic physical diseases opened in Albany, New York, in 1902 [4].

In the 1930s psychiatric consultation began to be introduced into medical wards. At the same time psychosomatic conceptions were being developed in the framework of psychoanalysis by investigators such as F. Alexander, E. Simmel, E. Witkower, and others who started treating with psychoanalytic tools individuals with different somatic disorders, mainly bronchial asthma, essential hypertension, peptic ulcer, ulcerative colitis, rheumatoid arthritis, and neurodermatitis [21]. Although the results were not always impressive, and cancer was not one of the disorders treated psychotherapeutically, there was enough evidence in the procedures to provide impetus for attention to the suffering of cancer patients. One of the early most impressive ventures was done by Loma Feigenberg who started treating psychotherapeutically patients with advanced cancer [39]. He also promoted psychological support for the dying, which constituted part of the emerging interest in providing psychological help to dying cancer patients in the framework of palliative care in hospitals and hospices [40, 41].

Nurses filled an all-important role in the development of the trend to supply psychosocial support to cancer patients. Their personal, empathic, and professional support for cancer patients on an almost daily basis formed an important source of help to patients and inspired other healthcare professionals.

A completely different source of inspiration for developing psychooncological help for cancer patients consisted of the sporadic self-help groups organized initially informally by cancer patients, outside the formal frameworks. The interest and enthusiasm these attempts evoked sent a clear message to those who could take care of organizing psychooncological help top-down.

The awareness of the need for psychooncological services was further enhanced by different advocacy groups and especially by publication of studies and surveys of specific issues concerning cancer patients, such as responses of patients to radical surgery, reactions to truth telling to patients and families, and side effects of chemotherapy, which resulted from developments in medical oncology.

A further factor that enhanced the need for psychooncological clinical work was the development of palliative care in hospitals and in hospices. Taking care of the dying required professional devoted work of many health professionals, including psychosocial experts.

Integrating psychooncological treatment into the formal regular medical treatment of cancer was not an easy process. The barriers consisted partly of the explicit but more often implicit resistance of doctors to let nonmedical specialists invade the formal frameworks of medical practice. An anecdote that may illustrate how difficult the situation was is provided by the fact that the first position confirmed for a clinical psychologist in a medical hospital occurred as late as 1938 in Vienna (the psychologist was the late Hans Kreitler). In addition, there were difficulties related to absence of locations, funding, and procedures. It is only slowly that the so-called consultation-liaison psychiatry experts were replaced by providers of psychooncological support. When the barriers were gradually set aside, there began a trickle of helpers that consisted of psychologists, social workers, reinforced in time by spiritual experts, art therapists, play therapists, experts in mindfulness meditation and yoga, as well as volunteers of all kinds. Alternative practitioners joined in but only later in the formal frameworks as departments in the hospitals, clinics, and sick funds.

Concerning psychologists there was a problem of professional education. Psychotherapeutically educated psychologists were primarily schooled in regard to patients and problems of personality disorders and mental health. This professional background was not only inadequate for treating cancer patients but actually limited the responsiveness of cancer patients to psychologists. Contact with psychologists was considered initially as suggesting that the cancer patients were mentally deranged. This attitude subsided only when psychologists began to be trained in the framework of the newly formed discipline of health psychology.

Clinical work by increasingly psychosocially trained professionals led to devising special interventions and psychotherapeutically oriented programs. The *Handbook of Psychotherapy in Cancer Care* [42] presents some extraordinary contributions in this domain. The text *Pediatric Psycho-Oncology* [43] presents some interventions designed specifically for pediatric cancer patients. Most of the interventions are modifications of programs and procedures standard in psychology, such as cognitive-behavioral therapy. But some are particularly targeted for cancer patients, such as dignity therapy. The different intervention programs are based on the basic psychotherapeutic principles, such as empathy and acceptance, but manifest as well adaptations to the specific issues of cancer, often including flexibility in approach, and involvement of family members, as well as focusing on problems that may concern cancer patients, such as meaningfulness of life or adjustment to life under different or uncertain conditions [36–38].

Organizational Development

The scientific and clinical development of Psycho-Oncology required a parallel organizational development on which it partly depended. Organizational developments consisted of several major steps that are necessary for defining and promoting Psycho-Oncology. These included mainly mobilizing and training professional healthcare workers and gaining for Psycho-Oncology the formal status and the means that would ensure the possibilities for providing cancer patients the needed and best Psycho-Oncology services. The following steps are all necessary and important and have all been done, although not necessarily in the cited sequence and often in interaction and collaboration with each other.

One major task was promoting and establishing formal professional societies for defining standards of practice, promoting the activities and status of Psycho-Oncology, and mobilizing professionals for the cause. Another step consisted in establishing research units or centers for promoting investigations and experiments in Psycho-Oncology. An important step focused on promoting the dissemination of information about Psycho-Oncology in the form of publications, journals, scientific conferences, seminars, and workshops. This led to the development of a curriculum for Psycho-Oncology representing major findings, approaches, conceptions, and practices, enjoying the support of the majority of Psycho-Oncology practitioners and investigators. A further important goal referred to getting formal recognition on the national levels and then from international organizations as well (e.g., the WHO or the UN). It was also necessary to obtain recognition and raise the status and development of Psycho-Oncology as a profession by promoting the establishment of units, programs, and departments in universities and in other institutions of higher learning devoted to researching and teaching of Psycho-Oncology in academic frameworks. All these means are necessary in regard to each discipline but have been mandatory especially in regard to Psycho-Oncology which has not been identified as a profession, and there has been no formal framework within which it could be placed and thrive.

Since the 1900s there has been a slow development of Psycho-Oncology in the organizational sense, which has become faster and also more noticeable after the 1950s. In the 1970s there have been large important Psycho-Oncology-inspired projects in different countries, such as smoking cessation and sunscreen protection in Australia. At the same time small groups of researchers of Psycho-Oncology formed in the UK, Belgium, Sweden, Australia, and Canada. Thus, a psychosocial research unit devoted to breast cancer was established by psychosocial investigators at the King's College Medical School in the UK in 1971; the multidisciplinary Cancer and Leukemia Group B (CALGB) supported by the NCI national clinical trials group was formed in 1976 in the USA; a psychosocial research unit, established in Amsterdam by Fritz van Dam in 1976, dealt with developing quality of life assessment tools (EORTC) that contributed to the assessment of outcomes in clinical trials [4].

An important development was the confirmation in 1972 of the War on Cancer Act by President Nixon which established the Division of Cancer Control and

Rehabilitation (DCCR) that provided the possibility of applying for grants for supportive care for cancer. At the same time period, different palliative care projects and units were formed, for example, the Omega Project by Weisman and Warden in the MASS General Hospital in the USA [40] and the end-of-life care by Cicely Saunders in the UK [41], who is credited with establishing the St Christopher's Hospice [44].

Organizing psychosocial oncology societies constituted a further step toward promoting the accreditation of Psycho-Oncology. Thus, the British Psychosocial Oncology Society was formed in 1982, the American Psychosocial Oncology Society in 1986, the Canadian Association of Psychosocial Oncology in 1985, the French Society of Psycho-Oncology in 1982, and the Dutch Society of Psychosocial Oncology in 1993. Societies were formed also in other parts of the world, for example, in Brazil in 1992, in China in 2006, in Japan in 1987, in Israel in 1992, and in South Korea in 2006. Most societies welcome members from across the disciplines, ranging from oncologists and psychiatrists to nurses or from psychologists to social workers and pastors, all who are involved in education, research, and caring for cancer patients and those who care for them.

Very early the International Psycho-Oncology Society (IPOS) was established. At present it includes as members 28 national societies from all over the globe and about 6000 professionals in over 40 countries. In September 2007, the IPOS Board of Directors and participants in the meeting of national societies voted to establish an IPOS Federation of Psycho-Oncology Societies which includes 26 member countries. IPOS is a member organization of the Union for International Cancer Control (UICC) and a partner of the World Health Organization (WHO) [45].

The psychosocial oncology societies promote the interest of psychooncologists and of Psycho-Oncology. They organize national meetings and international congresses since 1992 in different countries, thereby encouraging and promoting the presentation and dissemination of scientific – theoretical and applied – information and contacts between psychooncologists [46]. Training was promoted, for example, in the form of IPOS-sponsored online lecture series delivered by experts and in the framework of the Psychosocial Academy by workshops offered about themes, such as Research Methods in Psychosocial Oncology, Integrating Hypnotic Approaches in Cancer and Palliative Care, Communication Skills: Concepts and Teaching, and Screening for Distress: The 6th Vital Sign.

The societies promote also the development of guidelines and implementation of standards of care in Psycho-Oncology [47–49]. In 2010 IPOS defined the following standards of care in Psycho-Oncology which function as a kind of manifest for Psycho-Oncology: "Psychosocial cancer care should be recognised as a universal human right; Quality cancer care must integrate the psychosocial domain into routine care; and Distress should be measured as the 6th Vital Sign after temperature, blood pressure, pulse, respiratory rate and pain."

Societies, organizations, or speciality units devoted to Psycho-Oncology were formed also in the framework of some of the disciplines of health carers dealing with cancer patients. Most notable are the Association of Oncology Social Work, the Oncology Nursing Society, and the European Health Psychology Society.

An additional track of development concerned education in Psycho-Oncology. When the amount of studies relating to Psycho-Oncology increased, the evidence-based information began to accumulate. *Psycho-Oncology*, the first international journal in the field, was published in 1992. The *Handbook of Psycho-Oncology*, the first reliable and comprehensive text in the field, was published in 1989 [50]. The updated editions followed later and were joined by other important handbooks [51, 52]. A standard curriculum for Psycho-Oncology was formed, and the basics of this new profession were taught in teaching rounds, web seminars, workshops, national conferences, and numerous publications.

The recent stage of development in regard to education concerns the inclusion of Psycho-Oncology in university programs. The first department of psychiatry and behavioral sciences that had an institutional academic status was established at the Memorial Sloan Kettering Cancer Center in 1995. Over the years more than 350 professionals in Psycho-Oncology were trained in that center. At present there are research units devoted to Psycho-Oncology research in many universities, for example, the Psycho-Oncology Research Unit at Aarhus University; Psycho-Oncology and Subjective Health Measures Research Group that unites French-speaking researchers (oncologists, epidemiologists, psychiatrists, psychologists, psychometricians, social scientists, health economists, and statisticians) from France, Switzerland, Italy, Germany, and Belgium; the National Research Center for Hematology in Moscow, Russia, dealing with Psycho-Oncology in regard to hematological patients; and the Department of Medical Decision Making at Leiden University in the Netherlands. The organization of Psycho-Oncology Research Centers in Europe (PoCoG) includes research centers in 11 countries in which research in Psycho-Oncology is being conducted. Additionally, there are a fair number of universities that offer graduate and postgraduate studies in Psycho-Oncology on the master's or doctoral levels, e.g., University of Dublin, Bristol, McGill, and Colorado.

Some Concluding Notes

If one considers that in the early 1900s modern medical oncology barely started to appear and that there was yet no sign of awareness for the psychological needs of cancer patients, the change that has occurred in regard to Psycho-Oncology is nothing less than miraculous. When professionals in the field started to refer openly to the psychological aspects of cancer, there was as yet nothing: no conception, no constructs, no findings, no framework, no procedures, no profession, and not even a definition of a profession. At present, it is undeniable that there is a firm scientific basis for Psycho-Oncology, there is a research methodology, there are guidelines for psychooncological care and interventions, and there are a great many professionals from different disciplines devoted to application, research, and education of Psycho-Oncology in most countries of the world. Considering the staggering numbers – all running in the millions – of cancer patients at present, of the survivors, of those who die, and of the newly diagnosed cases per year in all countries worldwide, it is barely possible to imagine the load of suffering caused by this disease which is a major cause for death at present. Psycho-Oncology is one discipline devoted to, targeted for, and applied in regard to this kind of problem and suffering. It has proceeded along the multiple tracks of development, being guided and responding to bottom-up and top-down influences, discovering on the way the variety of needs of cancer patients, ranging from emotional to instrumental, from social to spiritual. On the basis of its remarkable development in the scientific sense, in clinical applications, and in terms of organization, it has become a major focus of assistance and hope. As long as cancer is not yet completely cured or eliminated, Psycho-Oncology is one venue or tool for proceeding toward attainment of the commonly shared goal of providing adequate psychosocial care to every person affected directly or indirectly by cancer in any corner of the planet.

References

1. Kennedy, B. J. (1999). Medical oncology: Its origin, evolution, current status, and future. *Cancer, 85*(1), 1–8.
2. Band, P. R. (2014). *Therapeutic revolution: The history of medical oncology from early days to the creation of the subspecialty*. Sharjah: Bentham Science.
3. Wagener, T. (2009). *The history of oncology*. Houten: Springer Uitgeverij.
4. Holland, J. C., & Wiesel, T. W. (2015). Introduction: History of psycho-oncology. In J. C. Holland, W. S. Breitbart, P. N. Butow, P. B. Jacobsen, M. J. Loscalzo, & R. McCorkle (Eds.), *Psycho-oncology* (3rd ed., pp. xxiv–xxxv). New York: Oxford University Press.
5. Holland, J. C. (2002). History of psycho-oncology: Overcoming attitudinal and conceptual barriers. *Psychosomatic Medicine, 64*(2), 206–221.
6. Holland, J. C. (2004). IPOS Sutherland memorial lecture: An international perspective on the development of psychosocial oncology: Overcoming cultural and attitudinal barriers to improve psychosocial care. *Psycho-Oncology, 13*(7), 445–459.
7. Fabrega, H., Jr. (1990). Psychiatric stigma in the classical and medieval period: A review of the literature. *Comprehensive Psychiatry, 31*, 289–306.
8. Fabrega, H., Jr. (1991). The culture and history of psychiatric stigma in early modern and modern western societies: A review of recent literature. *Comprehensive Psychiatry, 32*, 97–119.
9. Moses, T. (2010). Being treated differently: Stigma experiences with family, peers, and school staff among adolescents with mental health disorders. *Social Science and Medicine, 70*(7), 985–993.
10. Kreitler, S. (2018). The mind-body problem: The perspective of psychology. *Open Journal of Philosophy, 8*(1), 82765, 16 pages. https://doi.org/10.4236/ojpp.2018.81006.
11. Segerstrom, S. C. (2012). *The Oxford handbook of psychoneuroimmunology*. New York: Oxford University Press.
12. Andersen, B. L., Kiecolt-Glaser, J. K., & Glaser, R. (1994). A biobehavioral model of cancer stress and disease course. *American Psychologist, 49*(5), 389–404.
13. Engel, G. L. (1980). The clinical application of the biopsychosocial model. *American Journal of Psychiatry, 137*(5), 535–544.
14. Alonso, Y. (2004). The biopsychosocial model in medical research: The evolution of the health concept over the last two decades. *Patient Education and Couseling, 53*, 239–244.
15. Suls, J., & Rothman, A. (2004). Evolution of the biopsychosocial model: Prospects and challenges for health psychology. *Health Psychology, 23*(1), 119–125.

16. Schwartz, G. (1982). Testing the biopsychosocial model: The ultimate challenge facing behavioral medicine? *Journal of Consulting and Clinical Psychology, 50*, 1040–1053.
17. Kreitler, S., Kreitler, M. M., Len, A., Alkalay, Y., & Barak, F. (2008). Psychological risk factors for colorectal cancer? *Psycho-Oncologie, 2*, 131–145.
18. Pyter, L. M., Pineros, V., Galang, J. A., McClintock, M. K., & Prendergast, B. J. (2009). Peripheral tumors induce depressive-like behaviors and cytokine production and alter hypothalamic-pituitary-adrenal axis regulation. *Proceedings of the National Academy of Sciences, 106*(22), 9069–9674.
19. Briones, T. L., & Woods, J. (2011). Chemotherapy-induced cognitive impairment is associated with decreases in cell proliferation and histone modifications. *BMC Neuroscience, 12*, 124.
20. Ogden, J. (2012). *Health psychology: A biopsychosocial approach*. Berkshire: The Open University, McGraw-Hill Education.
21. Levenson, J. L., & Wulsin, L. (2006). *Textbook of psychosomatic medicine: Psychiatric care of the medically ill* (2nd ed.). Arlington: The American Psychiatric Publishing.
22. Beck, J. S. (2011). *Cognitive-behavior therapy: Basics and beyond* (2nd ed.). New York: Guilford Press.
23. Meyer, J. S., & Quenzer, L. F. (2018). *Psychopharmacology: Drugs, the brain, and behavior* (3rd ed.). New York: Oxford University Press.
24. Boini, S., Briancon, S., Guillemin, F., Galan, P., & Hercberg, S. (2004). Impact of cancer occurrence on health-related quality of life: A longitudinal pre-post assessment. *Health and Quality of Life Outcomes, 2*, 4.
25. Bottomley, A. (2002). The cancer patient and quality of life (EORTC data center). *The Oncologist, 7*, 120–125.
26. Aronson, N. K., Ahmedzai, S., Bergman, B., et al. (1993). The European Organization for Research and Treatment of Cancer QLQ-C30: A quality-of-life instrument for use in international clinical trials in oncology. *Journal of the National Cancer Institute, 85*(5), 365–376.
27. Cella, D. F., Tulsky, D. S., Gray, G., Sarafian, B., Linn, E., Bonomi, A., Silberman, M., Yellen, S. B., Winicour, B., Brannon, J., et al. (1993). The functional assessment of cancer therapy scale: Development and validation of the general measure. *Journal of Clinical Oncology, 11*(3), 570–579.
28. Portenoy, R. K., Thaler, H. T., Konblith, J., McCarthy, L., Friedlander-Klar, H., Kiyasu, E., Sobel, K., Coyle, N., Kemeny, N., Norton, L., & Scher, H. (1994). The memorial symptom assessment scale: An instrument for the evaluation of symptom prevalence, characteristics and distress. *European Journal of Cancer, 30A*(9), 1326–1336.
29. Mitchell, A. J. (2007). Pooled results from 38 analyses of the accuracy of distress thermometer and other ultra-short methods of detecting cancer-related mood disorders Alex J. Mitchell. *Journal of Clinical Oncology, 25*, 4670–4681.
30. McCorkle, R., & Young, K. (1978). Development of a symptom distress scale. *Cancer Nursing, 15*, 373–378.
31. Derogatis, L. R. (2000). *BSI-18: Brief symptom inventory 18 – administration, scoring, and procedures manual*. Minneapolis: NCS Pearson.
32. Simard, S., & Savard, J. (2009). Fear of cancer recurrence inventory: Development and initial validation of a multidimensional measure of fear of cancer recurrence. *Supportive Care in Cancer, 17*(3), 241–251.
33. O'Connor, A. M. (1995). Validation of a decisional conflict scale. *Medical Decision Making, 15*, 25–30.
34. Lansky, S. B., List, M. A., Lansky, L. L., Ritter-Sterr, C., & Miller, D. R. (1987). The measurement of performance in childhood cancer patients. *Cancer, 60*(7), 1651–1656.
35. Munitz-Shenkar, D., Kreitler, M. M., & Kreitler, S. (2012). Assessment tools in pediatric psycho-oncology. In S. Kreitler, M. W. Ben-Arush, & A. Martin (Eds.), *Pediatric psycho-oncology: Psychosocial aspects and clinical interventions* (2nd ed., pp. 271–297). Chichester: Wiley-Blackwell.

36. Breitbart, W., & Poppito, S. (2014). *Individual meaning centered psychotherapy treatment manual*. New York: Oxford University Press.
37. Chochinov, H. M., Hack, T., Hassard, T., Kristjanson, L. J., McClement, S., & Harlos, M. (2005). Dignity therapy: A novel psychotherapeutic intervention for patients near the end of life. *Journal of Clinical Oncology, 23*(24), 5520–5525.
38. Fawzy, F. I., Canada, A. L., & Fawzy, N. W. (2003). Malignant melanoma: Effects of a brief, structured psychiatric intervention on survival and recurrence at 10-year follow-up. *Archives of General Psychiatry, 60*(1), 100–103.
39. Feigenberg, L. (1980). *Terminal care: Friendship contracts with dying cancer patients*. New York: Brunner/Mazel.
40. Weisman, A. D., & Worden, J. W. (1975). *Psychosocial analysis of cancer deaths*. Boston: Omega Project, Department of Psychiatry, Harvard Medical School.
41. Saunders, C. (2001). The evolution of palliative care. *Journal of the Royal Society of Medicine, 94*(9), 430–432.
42. Watson, M., & Kissane, D. W. (Eds.). *Handbook of psychotherapy in cancer care*. Hoboken: Wiley-Blackwell.
43. Kreitler, S., Ben-Arush, M. W., & Martin, A. (Eds.). *Pediatric psycho-oncology: Psychosocial aspects and clinical interventions* (2nd ed.). Chichester: Wiley-Blackwell.
44. Clark, D. (2007). From margins to centre: A review of the history of palliative care in cancer. *Lancet Oncology, 8*(5), 430–438.
45. Dunn, J., Bultz, B. D., & Watson, M. (2015). Emerging international directions for psychosocial care. In J. Holland, W. S. Breitbart, P. N. Butow, P. B. Jacobsen, M. J. Loscalzo, & R. McCorkle (Eds.), *Psycho-oncology* (3rd ed., pp. 739–743). New York: Oxford University Press.
46. Grassi, L., Watson, M., On behalf of the IPOS Federation of Psycho-Oncology Societies', et al. (2012). Psychosocial care in cancer: An overview of psychosocial programmes and national cancer plans of countries within the International Federation of Psycho-Oncology Societies. *Psycho-Oncology, 21*(10), 1027–1033.
47. Holland, J., Watson, M., & Dunn, J. (2011). The IPOS new international standard of quality cancer care: Integrating the psychosocial domain into routine care [editorial]. *Psycho-Oncology, 20*(7), 677–680.
48. Breitbart, W., Bultz, B. D., Dunn, J., Grassi, L., & Watson, M. (2013). 2012 President's plenary international psycho-oncology society: Future directions in psycho-oncology [editorial]. *Psycho-Oncology, 22*(7), 1439–1443.
49. Bultz, B. D., Cummings, G. G., Grassi, L., Travado, L., Hoekstra-Weebers, J., & Watson, M. (2014). 2013 President's plenary international psycho-oncology society: Embracing the IPOS standards as a means of enhancing comprehensive cancer care. *Psycho-Oncology, 23*(9), 1073–1078.
50. Holland, J. C., & Rowland, J. H. (Eds.). (1989). *Handbook of psychooncology: Psychological care of the patient with cancer*. New York: Oxford University Press.
51. Grassi, L., & Riba, M. (2012). *Clinical psycho-oncology: An international perspective*. Chichester: Wiley-Blackwell.
52. Mehnert, A., & Koch, U. (Eds.). (2017). *Handbuch psychoonkologie*. Boston: Hogrefe.

Chapter 2
The Special Characteristics of Oncology and Psycho-Oncology

Psycho-Oncology is one of the first domains of health psychology that have developed at the borderline of medicine and psychology. In order to understand the reasons it is first necessary to consider the special characteristics of cancer, especially from the point of view of the common person in general and of patients in particular.

What Do Patients Know in General About Cancer?

In order to understand the approach, decisions, and behavior of patients, it is important to learn about what they think or assume about cancer. Cancer is a prominent theme in the media and is often discussed by people in different social occasions. Information about cancer is shared quite freely precisely because it is a scary subject and getting information may provide some sense of mastery or protection.

What do patients usually know about cancer? Here is a list of some of the most salient and common characteristics of cancer mentioned by patients [1].

Difficulty Many of the beliefs and assumptions about cancer focus on difficulty. Majority if not all people know that cancer is a very difficult disease, in all respects and for every person. There is a kind of belief that even though the disease may subside or respond well to some treatment, it still deserves to be called "difficult." Notably, even though there are other difficult diseases, the reputation of cancer is relatively worse than that of the others. The mere name of the disease is already indicative of its problematic character. Whereas diseases are mostly named after the main affected organ (e.g., headache), major symptom (e.g., whooping cough), or responsible agent (e.g., typhoid named after *Salmonella Typhi*), cancer is named after an animal that causes harm but is not the cause of cancer. Notably the word "cancer" has turned into a metaphor for a malicious agent that penetrates insidiously some bigger system causing harm and disorder [2].

S. Kreitler, *Psycho-Oncology for the Clinician*,
https://doi.org/10.1007/978-3-030-06126-5_2

Prevalence A second most salient aspect of information about cancer is its prevalence. Most people know that it is a highly prevalent disease. No one is immune: young children, teenagers, young adults, midlife adults, and the elderly – anyone can get cancer. Almost every person knows someone in the family or circle of acquaintances or neighborhood or from the media who is a cancer patient or died from cancer. Many people have had personal contact with a cancer patient. These personal experiences contribute to the feeling or illusion of many people that cancer is everywhere. Experiments in cognitive psychology have shown that the evaluation of the frequency of cancer may be subject to at least two so-called cognitive biases. One is known by the name "availability heuristic," and it consists in the tendency to overestimate information that is easy to recall. The other is the "confirmation bias" which is the tendency to seek information that confirms and prioritizes information and conclusions that one already has.

Indeed, it is often difficult to pinpoint exactly the frequency or incidence of cancer, but it is evident for everyone who tries to get hold of the numbers that the incidence runs in the millions – millions of new cases, millions of death cases, and millions of survivors. But all these numbers boil down to a frightening mass of cancer events. Indeed, the numbers are somewhat confusing for anyone who tries to understand the situation. On the one hand the declaration is that the incidence of cancer does not increase, but on the other hand the news proclaim a higher number of projected cancer cases reflecting presumably better or finer diagnosis and probably an increase of certain types of cancer. Hence, the impression one may get is that not only is cancer a highly prevalent disease, but its incidence seems to be on the increase, and the age of its occurrence tends to get lower. Patients often mention the fact that a disease such as breast cancer that in former generations was known to be a disease of elderly or mostly postmenopausal women appears increasingly in young women, even as young as 30 years old. Patients often hear in the media about the discussions concerning lowering of the age of mandatory breast screening for women. They also refer often to information about breast cancer occurring in men, which creates the impression that the disease is spreading. Similarly, screening for colorectal cancer is increasingly undertaken as a standard measure for young men and women, such as those enlisting for the army.

Dangerous Further, most patients know that cancer is a very dangerous disease. In regard to cancer, danger means most often death. Indeed, death is the first association that patients have when they or someone close to them gets the diagnosis of cancer. Although there are undoubtedly many other fatal diseases, the connotation of cancer as a mortal or fatal disease is superior and highly dominant. Actually, it seems that cardiological diseases cause more deaths than all forms of cancer together [3]. Nevertheless, cancer is more closely reminiscent of death than heart diseases. This belief is further nurtured by the common publications about cancer statistics. Almost every publication about cancer statistics includes not only the number of cancer patients at a given time but also the number of deaths during that period as well as the number of cancer survivors, whereby even the mere use of the word survivor clearly denotes someone who has been close to death and somehow escaped that fate.

The dangerous character of cancer is enhanced especially because of the treatments for cancer which are notoriously known to be both difficult and not always useful. Cancer is known to be one of the most ancient diseases and yet does not have any reliable treatment. The short remark about a case of cancer found in an old Egyptian papyrus from the second millennium B.C. "there is no treatment" still applies in the view of many patients.

Chronic Disease When a patient gets the diagnosis of cancer, it is evident to him or her that if the verdict is not for death, then "this is for life," namely, there is no recovery. Cancer is conceived as a one-way disease: once you are in it, there is no way out. The diagnosis of cancer stays forever. Patients often remark about the extraordinary situation of staying bound to the label, or rather the stigma of cancer forever, for as long as one lives. One often hears patients complaining about cancer as a set of unbreakable handcuffs placed on a person forever. The nagging question is, Why is it that one can be released from any disease, ranging from heart disease to syphilis, but not from cancer?

Elusiveness Elusiveness is one of the most salient negative aspects of cancer that render it difficult to deal with. All too often it turns out that the cancer has been in the patient's body for a long time prior to its detection by accident, in the course of standard diagnostic procedures or on the basis of manifest symptoms. Furthermore, when it is finally detected, it may indeed be too late for full recovery or even for treatment. These facts are very scary because they give the patient the feeling that the cancer is hiding somewhere in the body, lurking in the darkness, as a kind of thief or some other evil creature that may leap out of nowhere unexpectedly with full force. Many patients tend to describe cancer as a hidden enemy which may be anywhere and everywhere without being detected. How can one fight a powerful enemy that resides in oneself without producing any signs of his or her existence? This conception of cancer is surprising because actually the same claims can be made about other diseases, including cardiological diseases, celiac disease, or multiple sclerosis, that develop slowly in the body over years without producing any specific symptoms that could lead to their detection on time. Diseases of this kind resemble cancer also in that for a long time they may produce fuzzy nonspecific symptoms which may be confusing and render it hard to identify the underlying cause. However, it is mainly cancer that gets the bad reputation of being elusive and non-detectable.

Moreover, the diagnosis of cancer is far from straightforward. It is often based on a series of medical tests which may take time to decipher. Sometimes even after some time, the diagnosis is not always conclusive, and different experts may have different opinions about it. Further, there are over 100 different cancers, and some of them have distinct pathologies and manifestations. Actually, patients are aware of the more recent conceptualization of cancer as a family of diseases.

And then, there is the issue of metastases about which every patient knows. This aspect of cancer is highly disconcerting. Metastases may mean two things to a regular patient: one is that although the main tumor or nodule of cancer has been overcome by treatment, there may still be components of the cancer in the body that may be too elusive or tiny for detection at that time. The other implication is that one may never know whether one is healthy or free of cancer or not. This is particularly upsetting for patients because upon diagnosis, they have learned that for months or even years, the cancer may have been developing in their body without them being aware of this in any way.

A similar situation exists in regard to biomarkers. Biomarkers are considered by physicians and patients as indicators of malignancy but not always, that is, not in regard to every cancer and not in regard to every patient and not in regard to any phase of the disease. Thus, if the patient gets information about biomarkers that clearly supports the existence of malignancy, there is some clarity in the meaning of that information. If, however, there is no indication for biomarkers, the patient still remains in limbo. The nagging question "Do I have cancer or am I healthy" persists without answer.

Physical Suffering The conception of many patients concerning cancer and its treatments may be summarized under the heading of suffering. Many patients have recollection of their relatives, sometimes parents, in former generations or other acquaintances who have gone through the process and have complained of a lot of physical suffering. This may be one source of information for most patients. For many people cancer is related to pain, harm to the body, loss of body organs or limbs due to surgery, physical deformation, fatigue, physical wasting, loss of weight, swelling of body or body parts, loss of appetite, nausea, and weakness.

Psychological Suffering Many patients may be more scared of the psychological suffering than of the physical suffering they envisage for cancer. Patients expect that cancer would bring about many changes in their routine and daily life and that they would not be able to do most of the things they are used to doing and that bring them joy and make them happy. They are doubtful about the possibility of going on with their work, and some of them are conflicted about whether they would like to go on working. At least some may have financial worries due to difficulties with work and treatment expenses. They also expect changes in their social life, mainly because they assume that their friends and acquaintances may not like to continue the relationship with them or may withdraw because of the stigma connected with cancer. They know this about others because maybe they themselves have experienced similar emotions when friends or acquaintance got cancer. They felt then they did not want to have anything to do with the cancer. Hence, they also know that it is difficult to talk with others about one's cancer. Doing so may cause others to pity you or withdraw. The patients assume that getting cancer means sadness and loneliness.

Patients also know that no one stays the same after getting cancer. There are changes in role at home and at work, there is loss of mastery and independence, and there may be a need for help from others which may impact one's self image and self-confidence.

And then, on top of everything, there are the emotional reactions of fear, anxiety, depression, and even anger that are often related to cancer in different forms and which the patients expect and worry about.

Information Cancer is a disease about which it is difficult to get information. In the Western world in former generations, cancer was a taboo disease about which people did not talk in public and doctors preferred to keep silent. The probable reason was that cancer was considered as a bad and untreatable disease terminating always in death. Nowadays the taboo has been lifted, and in many countries the diagnosis of cancer has to be communicated to the patient by law. As such the law which dictates medical communication is an exceptional practice insofar as diseases are concerned. Still there are many countries in which this is not the case. Be it as it may, patients are still doubtful about whether they get all the relevant information and are highly suspicious in regard to communication with their physicians (see also Chap. 12). Cancer patients are particularly concerned with getting information about their disease and its treatments that is updated, adequate, and comprehensive. They and their family members and acquaintances spend a lot of energy and time to get this information. In this respect too, cancer patients differ from patients with other diseases.

Decisions and More Decisions Having cancer involves the patient in a series of many decisions concerning the disease and the treatments. Some of these are simple, some commonplace, and some of high importance. They may involve choice of doctor and of treatment or treatments, site of treatment, and time at which one begins the treatment, as well as many other decisions, such as whom to tell, what to share, etc. (see Chaps. 3 and 7). One patient quoted to me recently the following statement by C.S. Lewis [4]: "Crying is all right in its way while it lasts. But you have to stop sooner or later, and then you still have to decide what to do." Even in a highly ordered setup, there is no way for the patient to escape completely the need to make decisions. The difficulty of the situation is that the patient needs to make decisions in an area in which he or she have very little experience and even less information. Decisions in regard to medical issues are particularly difficult because most people lack the relevant background information, even if they happen to be health professionals. Pressuring patients to undertake such decisions is part of the widespread tendency for empowering patients by involving them in the process of the treatment. Even if patients resist and choose to adopt the simpler venue of letting others decide, they are pressured by family and friends who believe the patient needs to be involved in order to enhance the chances of recovery. Some decisions are simply unavoidable, such as those that concern relations with family, friends, fellow workers, and even neighbors. Patients need to decide whom to tell about their plight, how much to tell, when to tell, or whether to tell at all. The mentioned decisions are merely examples, actually only the peak of the iceberg, most of which is not evident in the beginning and gets uncovered only slowly in the course of the unfolding of the disease.

Unclarity about Causes (or Am I to Blame for My Cancer?) The fact that it is still unclear what the causes of cancer are is in itself very disturbing. The unclarity creates the feeling that the causes could be anywhere although one would not know how to protect oneself against it. The commonly mentioned information about the genetic impact adds to the anxiety because there is nothing one can do about the genetic contribution one got perhaps from relatives and which one may be transmitting to one's children. However, what causes most anxiety in patients is the direct and often indirect information about cancer determinants that place the patient himself or herself in the role of the possibly responsible agent. There are a great many factors that have been connected to the incidence of cancer which depend at least to some extent on the patient. These include smoking, obesity, exposure to the sun, living or working in polluted environments, eating unhealthy food, no exercising and other lifestyle factors that seem to the patient as if they depend exclusively on him or her (about these and other determinants, see Chap. 4; about the dependence on the patient, see Chap. 8). Learning about these commonly mentioned factors evokes in most patients – indeed in most people – more than a slight uneasiness and a nagging sense of guilt.

However, things turn much worse when we get to the psychological factors. Two major terms keep recurring in this regard: stress and positive thinking. The direct implication for the patient is that one can reduce the chances for cancer if one avoids stress and if one maintains constantly a positive thinking approach. These requirements are really harmful for the patient for several reasons. Firstly, it is evident that it is impossible to keep them. One cannot possibly avoid stress or control one's stress reactions simply by deciding to do so. Furthermore, positive thinking means not to become irritated, not to be angry or sad, to be always in a good mood, and to overlook frustrations and other unwelcome situations. It is evident that stress avoidance and positive thinking are impossible to implement, especially without preparatory training by psychosocial health professionals. Secondly, it is far from clear that keeping these requirements would have any impact on the chances of getting cancer or would result in positive outcomes for the patient in general. Thirdly, since failure to keep the stated requirements is unavoidable, the patient is thereby exposed to frustration and is kept in a constant state of guilt, attributing to himself/herself at least some of the blame for the cancer. As will be seen later, this situation affects negatively also the patient's readiness to get psychological help (see Chaps. 7 and 8).

What Does Research Tell Us About the Psychological State of Cancer Patients?

There is a lot of research about the psychological state of cancer patients. Most of the studies deal with phenomenological characteristics, without necessarily delving into the causes and deeper determinants of the psychological reactions. There is a large body of data indicating that the patients tend to suffer from anxiety and depression in the different stages of the disease and the treatments (e.g., [5–10]). The evidence relates to all kinds of cancer, to patients in all ages, and in all countries in which studies of this kind have been conducted. Stress and distress are the main psychological characteristics of the situation for many months. There is evidence that even after termination of the treatments, and even in the state of remission after 5 years, there are still signs of distress although of lower intensity. As may be expected, the distress characterizes also caretakers and family members of the patients [11].

The reports about anxiety, depression, and stress of the patients are in accord with what the patients believe or know about cancer. Although the information is almost self-evident, it is of importance to keep it in mind without depreciating its importance for understanding out patients already in the preliminary encounters (see Chap. 3).

What About Psycho-Oncology?

Hesitation About Addressing Psychologists Considering the state of the patients and the issues that worry them, it would be natural to suggest to the patients to get psychological help in the very least in order to mitigate their suffering, anxiety, and distress in the difficult situation of getting the diagnosis and treatments for cancer. The service of Psycho-Oncology is available, most often freely. Experts in this domain usually perform reaching out so that the patients do not have to worry about creating the contact. However, patients are reluctant to address the service and to use it.

The point is illustrated clearly in a recent publication based on 53 studies that assessed the rate of uptake or adherence psychosocial interventions for 12,323 cancer patients [12]. On the whole, the rate of uptake and adherence was only 60.1%. Notably, patients identified in screening as distressed were less likely to accept the suggestion for therapy than unselected patients (50.3% versus 66.3%), and uptake was higher for therapy delivered by telephone rather than face-to-face (71.2% versus 53.8%) or by nurses rather than by other health professionals (68.3% versus 50.5%).

The described findings indicate that 40% of patients to whom supportive intervention is offered decline the offer, especially when they have been identified as distressed, when the therapy is designed to be face-to-face, and when the therapists are professionals. This situation may seem bizarre, but it is understandable. There are some reasons patients cite as explanations for avoiding psychooncological help.

One major reason is that Psycho-Oncology is identified as psychological help and hence as possibly indicating a mental health problem. The patient wonders whether the cancer has affected negatively one's mind and turned him or her into a psychiatric case. The reasoning goes "Isn't it enough that I have cancer, now it seems I am also crazy?"

Another reason is that many patients are wary to get help because this might indicate that they are weak and cannot cope on their own. The reasoning goes "In order to win the battle against cancer I need to be strong, very strong and not admit to any weakness; getting psychological help is the last thing I need in the state in which I am; if I am going to overcome cancer, I must prove to myself and to my body that I am really OK."

A third reason may be related to the abovementioned issue of experiencing some responsibility for having contracted cancer. The strategy is based on converting the guilt into a powerful weapon against the enemy, viz., the cancer. The reasoning goes "If I am kind of responsible for the cancer because of my life style and because I have not controlled sufficiently my stress and have not maintained persistently positive thinking, then I can certainly change my behavior and attitude now and overcome the cancer. I can do it on my own because I know where I failed and what I did wrong."

Finally, it needs to be mentioned that most patients have very little experience with psychological treatments and psychological reasoning. On the one hand, it may seem to many of them to be a simplistic procedure based exclusively on "conversations" and talking, so that anyone can apparently practice it without requiring any particular expertise. Many assume that psychological help is not any different from what takes place in their daily encounters with friends and acquaintances. On the other hand, psychological therapy may seem to many of them to be a kind of mysterious delving into the unconscious mind, extracting hidden memories and secrets about acts and events they would rather hide or deny. Psychological help may thus seem frightening because it may imply loss of control over oneself and one's hidden inner life. Be it as it may, both approaches would lead one to avoid psychological interventions.

Alternatives for Moderating Anxiety and Depression Nevertheless, the mental suffering and the distress are hard to overlook. Many patients – probably around 50% – reach the conclusion that possibly at some point some kind of help would be needed. So what do they know about the alternatives for controlling their expected anxiety, depression, and stress?

Surveys show that patients assume that they could use medication for moderating anxiety or depression but do not expect that they would need to use them. The reasons are first, because they consider themselves as mentally healthy, and secondly because they expect the anticancer treatments would involve enough chemical stuff introduced into the body.

Another commonly considered approach is focused on alternative or complementary medicine. This is considered by patients as a respectable set of methods that mostly does not involve any potentially harmful medication, is supposedly based on culturally validated healing secrets that have been developed over hundreds of years, does not require contact with expert health professionals, and does not require talking and telling about oneself, as in the framework of psychology.

A third common approach is turning to religion or spirituality that may be manifested by "contacting" privately the higher powers, getting guidance from a religious leader (priest or rabbi or kadi), or joining some religious community for social support. Notably, patients relying on religious support tend also to use more alternative medicine methods [13].

Many patients consider using one or more of the mentioned methods, sometimes concurrently with Psycho-Oncology and encouraged by Psycho-Oncology (for these and other methods, see Chaps. 7 and 8). Notably, the three methods mentioned in this context as preferred by patients share at least three major characteristics. The first important one is that they are not specific for cancer patients. Cancer patients assume rightly that many people who may or may not be sick use medication against anxiety or depression, so much so that either the drugs may be bought over the counter or the prescriptions are provided by the family doctor rather than by a psychiatrist, similarly complementary medicine. Many people turn to the alternative therapists for stress reduction or for getting relief. There is nothing in complementary medicine especially geared for cancer patients. Addressing a complementary therapist does not require identifying oneself as a cancer patient. Evidently, religion is also here for everyone. Religious leaders and communities treat all human being alike providing help and support to whoever approaches them or is in need. This characteristic helps the patients to consider themselves as regular human beings rather than special or unique because of their health situation.

The second characteristic shared by the three preferred methods is that the practitioners do not need to be specialists in regard to cancer or even specialists in any formal sense. A pharmacist can sell an OTC antianxiety medication, a practitioner of complementary medicine with or without formal training may apply a whole set of methods, and any person can use religion or pray alone or with others. This characteristic helps patients reduce the seriousness of their health situation.

The third characteristic shared by the preferred methods is that they do not require activity on the part of the patients. They may be practiced or applied by the patient without doing any special activity which means that the expected effect of the method consists in the impact of something external, such as an ingested medication, a treatment like Reiki or acupuncture or massage done by the alternative therapist, or the beneficial contact with the spiritual powers or religion. The patients do not need to do any mental labor or talk about themselves or disclose their inner conflicts or personal life as they expect to do in psychological therapy.

In sum, cancer patients tend to feel as potentially separated from others, being placed by their disease and problems in a unique location from which they expect to be delivered by methods that do not capitalize on their distinct situation. Beliefs, attitudes, and expectations of this kind are a heavy load with which clinicians, psychooncologists, and other health professionals devoted to helping cancer patients need to cope so as to provide cancer patients the optimal help they need and can apply.

References

1. Yennurajalingan, S., Rodrigues, L. F., Shamieh, O., & Bruera, E. (2018). Perception of curability among advanced cancer patients. An international collaborative study. *The Oncologist, 23*(4), 501–506.
2. Penson, R. T., Schapira, L., Daniels, K. J., Chabner, B. A., & Lynch, T. J., Jr. (2004). Cancer as metaphor. *Oncologist, 9*(6), 708–716.
3. American Heart Association 2016. Heart diseases and stroke statistics at-a-glance, 2016.
4. Lewis, C., & Lewis, S. (1953). *The silver chair*. New York: Geoffrey Bles.
5. Neilson, K., Pollard, A., Boonzaier, A., Corry, J., Castle, D., Smith, D., Trauer, T., & Couper, J. (2013). A longitudinal study of distress (depression and anxiety) up to 18 months after radiotherapy for head and neck cancer. *Psychooncology, 22*(8), 1843–1848. PMID: 23239423.
6. Watts, S., Leydon, G., Eyles, C., Moore, C. M., Richardson, A., Birch, B., Prescott, P., Powell, C., & Lewith, G. (2015). A quantitative analysis of the prevalence of clinical depression and anxiety in patients with prostate cancer undergoing active surveillance. *BMJ Open, 5*(5), e006674. ISSN: 2044-6055. PMID: 26002689.
7. Stafford, L., Judd, F., Gibson, P., Komiti, A., Mann, G. B., & Quinn, M. (2015). Anxiety and depression symptoms in the 2 years following diagnosis of breast or gynaecologic cancer: Prevalence, course and determinants of outcome. *Supportive Care in Cancer: Official Journal of the Multinational Association of Supportive Care in Cancer, 23*(8), 2215–2224. ISSN: 1433-7339. PMID: 25559036.
8. Cardoso, G., Graca, J., Klut, C., Trancas, B., & Papoila, A. (2016). Depression and anxiety symptoms following cancer diagnosis: A cross-sectional study. *Psychology, Health & Medicine, 21*(5), 562–570. ISSN: 1465-3966. PMID: 26683266.
9. Li, M., & Wang, L. (2016). The associations of psychological stress with depressive and anxiety symptoms among Chinese bladder and renal cancer patients: The mediating role of resilience. *Plos One, 11*(4), e0154729. ISSN: 1932-6203. PMID: 27128438.
10. Gheihman, G., Zimmermann, C., Deckert, A., Fitzgerald, P., Mischitelle, A., Rydall, A., Schimmer, A., Gagliese, L., Lo, C., & Rodin, G. (2016). Depression and hopelessness in patients with acute leukemia: The psychological impact of an acute and life-threatening disorder. *Psychooncology, 25*, 979–989.
11. Tomarken, A., Holland, J., Schachter, S., Vanderwerker, L., Zuckerman, E., Nelson, C., Coups, E., Ramirez, P. M., & Prigerson, H. (2008). Factors of complicated grief pre-death in caregivers of cancer patients. *Psychooncology, 17*(2), 105–111. ISSN: 1057-9249. PMID: 17443644.
12. Brebach, R., Sharper, L., Costa, D. S. J., Phodes, P., & Butow, P. (2016). Psychological intervention targeting distress for cancer patients: A meta-analytic study investigating uptake and adherence. *Psychooncology, 25*, 882–890.
13. Silvestri, G. A., Knittig, S., Zoller, J. S., & Nietert, P. J. (2003). Importance of faith on medical decisions regarding cancer care. *Journal of Clinical Oncology, 21*, 1379–1382.

Chapter 3
The Phases of the Confrontation with Cancer

Cancer is not only a disease. It is a whole narrative which often turns into a life narrative. It consists of an unfolding story with phases and dramas, studded with conflicts and decisions, with failures and victories, threaded with a lot of pain and suffering. No one knows ahead of time how the story will be written.

Phase 1: Getting Tested for Cancer

Screening Getting tested for cancer is a process, and it starts somewhere in the past, prior to facing the tests or the diagnosis. What are the usual tracks by which one gets to be tested for cancer? One major venue for cancer detection is screening. It is natural to expect that most cancer cases would be detected through screening. Indeed, many individuals undergo screening on a regular basis for specific kinds of cancer (usually breast and colorectal) or general whole-body screening for cancer on private initiative or as part of a health insurance. Screening is presented as the best way for detecting cancer and for doing so early enough while it is still treatable. However, despite the great efforts invested by governments and health agencies in promoting screening, many individuals do not follow the instructions and do not get screened. Even if they get screened once, they often do not repeat the experience and do not adopt screening as a routine [1, 2]. Some of those who undergo screening do so under the pressure of their doctors or families, or because they are at risk (due to genetic background or exposure to harmful conditions, such as asbestos or radiation). Other frequent triggers for screening may be a case of cancer in the family or among one's friends or a celebrity that is diagnosed with cancer.

There are several reasons why screening is not regularly practiced by many individuals. The issue is of particular importance in regard to individuals for whom screening is available. Some of the reasons are of a more objective nature, others of a more subjective or psychological nature. Both kinds interact, whereby the objective reasons enhance the psychological ones. Thus, on the more objective level, it is

S. Kreitler, *Psycho-Oncology for the Clinician*,
https://doi.org/10.1007/978-3-030-06126-5_3

well-known that there are various unclarities concerning screening. Generally promoted screening that is presented as reliable and recommended or required for all includes screening for only a few cancers (bowel, breast, cervical). There are other screening tests that are performed, but their reliability is doubtful (e.g., for prostate cancer or skin cancer). Further, some of the recommendations for screening are unclear or change or depend on the recommending source [3]. Individuals are also aware of the fact that the doctors themselves are not always decided about whether screening is indeed necessary or whether screening is recommended in specific cases, considering the risks and costs of screening in view of factors, such as the kind of cancer, the screening procedure, or the age of the individual [4–6]. In addition, patients are wary of inconclusive or unreliable results that may take the form of false negative or false positive results [7] not to mention the ambiguous findings (e.g., "the lung scan does not tell us exactly what the dark spot in the right lung is and we need a biopsy" or "mammography ruled out the existence of cancer in your breast but a finer-tuned technique such as perhaps MRI or high definition breast tomosynthesis would have provided a clearer answer"). And then only few patients forget to mention the unpleasantness involved in different screening procedures (e.g., mammography with squeezing of the breast or preparation for colonoscopy) or the potential harm that could be caused through the screening procedure, ranging from inflammations, or perforation of the bowel, to exposure to excess radiation in the breast or lung. Thus, it needs to be considered that concepts such as false negatives, overdiagnosis, or lead time bias have turned into household terms.

All these details gain importance in view of the serious hesitation that many individuals have concerning screening for cancer. The hesitation is rooted primarily in the fear from cancer which is so strong that it may lead many to complete denial of the whole domain including anything that may be reminiscent of cancer. Actually, we are dealing with a characteristic and highly frequent behavior pattern of screening avoidance. Studies showed that individuals who undergo regular screening for breast cancer or colorectal cancer are characterized by a special profile of beliefs about specific themes, such as emotional control, projecting good impression, realism, and readiness to face problems, which constitute the underlying motivation for screening. This profile of beliefs enables predicting who will undergo screening and to implement an intervention procedure for encouraging individuals to undergo the recommended screening [2, 8, 9].

Other Ways of Getting There If it is not screening so how do individuals arrive to get tested or detect cancer? First, there are the alternative replacements of screening which many people prefer and apply, such a self-examination of the breast or examination by a surgeon, an oncologist, or gynecologist, depending on the kind of cancer. These alternatives may not be as good as actual screening but are less scary and sometimes have the advantage of being more thorough or complete [10–12].

Another track of entering the phase of testing for cancer may start with sharing with one's family doctor one's fears or doubts about having cancer, or presenting openly some specific complaint about a wound or lump or simply protracted flu or fatigue. A doctor attuned to the patient may hear overtones that may alert him or her to the potential risk of cancer that justify referring the patient to a series of relevant tests.

In a fair number of cases, the cancer seems to get detected as it were by chance, accidentally. For example, a mother may go with her child to the doctor for some minor ailment of the child and may as if by chance mention to the doctor that she has noticed a lump in her neck or breast and asks for the doctor's advice, or she bares her shoulder as if accidentally so that the doctor has the chance of noticing a suspicious skin lesion. Such cases are not as rare as one would assume.

There are also still other possibilities that it is of interest to note. Some people just know somewhere at the back of their minds that they are about to be get cancer. This awareness, which is sometimes called "perceived cancer risk" [13], may be dormant for many years while they go about their life and wait for the opportunity of disclosure. They keep the information inside as a kind of secret which they do not share with anyone until the right moment comes, which resembles a kind of revelation. Sometimes they are so convinced that the right moment has come that they prepare themselves for dealing with the disease by closing up a business, finalizing different arrangements so as to be free to devote the time and attention to the disease. Individuals of this kind are not necessarily at genetic risk and are certainly not hypochondriac. When these people undergo screening, they are not really surprised when cancer is actually detected.

Undergoing Tests for Cancer When a person reaches the stage at which he or she is referred to tests for detecting cancer, one's world changes as if with a thunderbolt. At this point the patient understands that all his or her doubts and fears and thoughts may actually be real and that at least someone considers seriously the possibility that he or she may really be a cancer case. The fact that this someone is an expert, a doctor, only makes things worse. Patients who have some suspicious symptom often address a non-expert for diagnosis or treatment just in order to convince themselves that their case is not really serious, for example, they would address a cosmetician when they have some suspicious skin lesion or an alternative therapist when they suffer from hoarseness for many months.

The tests for detecting cancer may involve a whole series of medical examinations, sometimes presented to the patient in one package all at once, at other times presented one at a time, with more tests being added in view of the results of former tests. In the course of this period, which may last a month or even more, the patient's life is as if on hold. Nothing seems real or actual, everything is happening as if behind a wall of glass. The only real thing is the suspension, the waiting, which often may not even be suffused with tension because even feelings are suppressed to a certain extent so as not to become the victim of overwhelming fear [14, 15]. Notably, some physicians are aware of the fact that it is beneficial to let the patients participate actively in the administrative tasks of organizing the medical tests and getting permissions for them because it keeps them busy and maintains anxiety on a tolerable level.

Undergoing the medical tests is difficult for the patient for several reasons. Sometimes the tests are painful, and biopsies may involve anesthetics, which is scary because it reminds the patient of surgery. The patient mostly gets no information about what exactly is being tested in each test and what the results of every specific test are. The patient is in contact only with technicians or physicians who perform the tests but are not allowed to give the patient the results. During this period there is yet no contact with one main physician with whom the patient can communicate so as to learn how things proceed. The patient is waiting for the data to come in although he or she does not even get the results and their meaning as long as the whole process is not completed. Thus, the patient is left alone free to scare oneself to death with different imaginary or non-imaginary conceptions about possible developments with nothing to curb or stop the imaginative process. The patient keeps running in one's mind the worst scenarios and gets little or no support from family or friends because at this stage, one is not considered as a cancer patient that needs or deserves to get support. One patient aptly compared the period of undergoing the tests for cancer to the Kafkaesque situation of being on trial without knowing yet for what and what the result would be [16].

Waiting for Diagnosis When the period of testing gets closer to its end, the patient's level of anxiety starts rising. The prospect of getting finally the diagnosis infuses in the patient more courage because the impending moment of decision holds to equal degrees the prospects of both yes cancer, no cancer. It is in this period that the patient sometimes enters some kind of negotiation with fate or the other powers that may be involved. The negotiation takes usually the familiar form of "if it turns out that I don't have cancer, I will henceforth be a good person, I will forgive X and Y, I will control my temper, I will maintain a healthy lifestyle, I will volunteer for Z, I will do A and B which I have decided to do already 20 years ago and never did it, etc.…" Notably, the contents of the promises one makes refers partly to obligations in regard to others, including humanity at large, and partly to obligations toward oneself. A patient's wife who is herself an oncologist wrote aptly "waiting for bad news is actually worse than receiving bad news" [17].

Getting the News Getting the diagnosis is one of the most crucial moments in the personal narrative of cancer for the patient. It is important and highly meaningful even if the news is "you are free of cancer," but it is of much deeper and more meaningful nature when the news indicate the diagnosis of cancer. The manner in which the patient handles the information in either case has long-term impacts on his or her life in later years too. Regardless of whether the news is "good" or "bad," the patient has undergone a psychologically upsetting experience through the encounter with the idea or possibility of death.

There are many studies dealing with the manner of delivering the bad news and its effects. The absolute majority of these studies deal with the physicians, namely, with the skills necessary for delivering the news, the structuring of the session in which this takes place, and so on. There are hundreds of workshops designed to teach physicians of all levels and experience how to deliver the bad news to the patient without being themselves affected too much by the procedure (e.g., [18, 19]). However, there are only few studies about the impact of bad news on the patient [20]. The following statement made in a medical paper published in 1959 about disclosure of cancer diagnosis seems to be as true today as it was then: "The patient's own views are seldom heard" [21, p. 208]. The scarcity of studies about the patients' reactions seems to be based on the assumption that physicians or health professionals in general know what the patients feel or want to know. Unfortunately this is mostly not the case. Studies show that there is an impressive gap between what the health professionals think about the patients and what the patients actually think, feel, and want to know [22, 23]. The situation is deplorable especially since it has been shown that the style of communication affects the patients' trust and hope [24], whereas inadequate communication of the medical information is associated with poorer clinical and psychosocial results, lower adherence to treatment, and worse pain control. Patients who got adequate information have a better quality of life [25], while those who did not get sufficient information suffer from unclarity over prognosis and resent not being involved in decision-making [26].

There are several occasions in the course of the patient's cancer narrative when getting medical information becomes the issue, for example, when the disease recurs or prior to the transition from active treatment to the phase of palliative care. However, in these other cases, the patient is in a completely different situation than in the first encounter with the diagnosis (see section "Phase 4: Disease Recurrence"). It is hardly possible to overrate the importance of the experience for the patient of getting a cancer diagnosis. Getting the diagnosis is an event that changes the patient's life completely. The effect may range from a world-shattering experience to a highly upsetting event but is never negligible.

What information does the patient get? The issue of whether the patient should be told the truth about his or her diagnosis of cancer is still being discussed in medical journals, but more often concerning patients in non-Western countries than in countries in the Western hemisphere [e.g. 27–29]. In most Western countries, it seems to be evident that the physician should tell the patient the truth. In some countries (e.g., Israel), it is even supported legally. Difficulties may arise if the family resists the communication but the relatives are mostly convinced sooner or later to cooperate [30]. Research findings indicate that nondisclosure of the diagnosis is related to lower adherence on the part of the patients, shorter treatment duration, and worse medical results [31], whereas disclosure leads to better medical and treatment results [32]. However, in other cultures it is still not evident that the diagnosis should be disclosed to the patient. This is partly due to cultural habits and medical traditions in other countries [33, 34] and partly to the attitude of doctors who believe that disclosing the diagnosis may cause the patients too much suffering and moreover that not all patients want to know the truth [35, 36].

Yet, it needs to be kept in mind that even if the diagnosis is not disclosed to the patient, patients who are interested or suspicious can find out and mostly do find out in indirect ways, such as overhearing conversations of others, setting tricky questions to their doctors, and interviewing nurses or other patients on the ward.

The situation is further complicated by considerations that concern the doctors and the patients. From the point of view of the doctors, the delivery of bad news which includes of course disclosure of a cancer diagnosis is considered to be a very unpleasant task [37], because it involves exposure to the emotional suffering of the patient who gets the news and no less because the doctor may feel helpless as a professional expert to enable the patient to recover from the cancer.

From the point of view of the patient, the issue of getting information about the diagnosis may be highly complicated. First, it is necessary to keep in mind that actually not all patients desire to get full information and many do not consider it their right or a factor that may contribute to their well-being. Further, what many patients understand by the term "information about diagnosis" is not the title of the disease or its code number, grade, and stage but rather whether the disease is fatal, whether there is a chance of survival, and whether there is any treatment for the disease [38]. Secondly, many patients consider it best to accept simply what the doctor says without trying to understand it or its implications, assuming that "the doctor knows best what I should be told or what I should know." Moreover, there are not a few patients who would skip the whole act of getting the information about the diagnosis if it were not for the pressure of their family and friends who consider getting the information as an essential component of patient empowerment, which they view as important for recovery.

Getting the diagnosis may mean different things to the physician and to the patient. For the physicians the crux of the communication consists in formulating the diagnosis in medical terms that are habitual for them. In their desire to be sincere and communicate authentically all the relevant information, they may use medical terms which seem to them quite commonplace. However, patients are quite ignorant of medical language concerning malignancy, especially at the phase of getting the initial diagnosis. Even those who have prepared themselves through the Internet or other sources understand very little of the medical lingo and barely differentiate between correct information and a lot of myths and false or misleading references about cancer to which they are exposed. Thus, they are liable to fall into the trap of misunderstandings, both by way of exaggerating the bad news or not grasping the optimistic or good news or not even getting simply the message that they have cancer. The danger of misunderstandings is further enhanced by the emotional state of the patient who is upset and anxious on that occasion and by the tendency for denial that dominates the situation at the time of the encounter with the doctor and even more so later [39].

Misunderstanding of the information delivered by the doctor is not a black-and-white issue, just as denial is not a binary phenomenon either. Patients may understand part of the message (e.g., the diagnosis but not the prognosis) or may distort the message (e.g., combine a word like cancer with a word like small and decide that they have a small cancer).

Be it as it may, the percentage of those who have been given the medical information about their diagnosis and admit that they have it is about 50% [23, 28]. Notably, even special instructions and explanations do not raise the percentage of awareness above 55% [40]. These figures indicate that accepting the diagnosis of cancer is a psychologically difficult act, for which only about a half of the patients are ready. The responses of the other 50% of the patients reflect partly misunderstandings on their part of what they have been told and partly outright denial.

Denial of diagnosis may take many forms. In addition to forgetting the diagnosis or distorting it, patients may get into a state of consciousness in which they can repeat the diagnosis but do not believe that it is part of reality. The dominating thought may be "It is not real," "It has not happened," "The doctor did not say it," and "It is simply a bad dream from which I will soon wake up."

Sometimes the patient turns to another physician or medical center to get a second opinion on one's diagnosis. This may indeed reflect some degree of distrust in the physician, but not necessarily so. The reason for seeking a second opinion may be a need for absolute certainty or surrender to the pressure of one's family to address a "greater expert" or a barely expressed hope against hope that there may be a mistake in the information imparted to him or her.

Suicidal thoughts and even suicidal attempts are not uncommon during the period following the getting of information about the diagnosis. The rate of reported suicides in this phase is higher than in other phases of coping with cancer, as shown by many studies in different countries [e.g., 41–44]. These findings should be considered with caution because it is possible that suicidal acts in later phases of cancer are produced by more sophisticated means, such as drugs, which are used by patients who are more experienced and know more about different medical means and procedures which they may use if they want to conceal their suicidal attempt. In contrast the early suicides are based on more crude and commonplace means so that they get more noticed and reported. Be that as it may, it is evident that it is mandatory to guard patients after they get their diagnosis and provide them with all the psychosocial and family support possible so as to help them cope in this highly difficult period.

Phase 2: Getting Treated for Cancer

Deciding About the Treatments Discussing treatments with the doctor is a relatively easier phase for both doctor and the patient. The obvious reason is that the doctor can start acting within the familiar context of his or her expertise, providing the patient the means for overcoming the disease. For the patient it is also a relief to move away from the scary hopelessness domain of information about a diagnosis that is never too far from the connotation of death. Treatments are practical means, concrete procedures for apparent solution of an apparently insoluble problem.

The discussion of treatments may get complicated, for the patient even more than for the physician. From the point of view of the physician, in the first phase after diagnosis, the recommended treatments for most cancers involve basically decisions about the mode of treatment (e.g., surgery, radiotherapy, chemotherapy, other medications), sometimes a choice of a particular protocol, considering in addition mainly the phase of the disease, the overall state of the patient, and genetic information if available.

From the point of view of the patient, the issues are very different. Primarily it is necessary to consider that the situation is completely new and unknown for most patients, actually for all patients even if they are doctors but not oncologists. Studies show that the majority of patients base their treatment decisions on information sources additional to their physician (up to 70% according to [45]). These include the Internet, information provided by other patients and acquaintances, as well as direct-to-consumer advertisements [e.g., 46]. Thus, many patients are faced with the task of understanding, evaluating, and integrating information from diverse sources, some of which may not be as reliable as desired.

Most patients accept the need for treatments, and they are concerned with issues, such as whether they are getting the best possible or the most modern/updated treatment, whether the choice of treatment has not been determined by limited financial budget, and whether they have received all the relevant information concerning available treatments anywhere in the world. Patients of this kind may still be required sometimes to make actual decisions about treatment options, for example, in the case of prostate cancer [47]. In their desire to have the best and most complete treatments available, at least some patients strive to combine standard medical treatments with complementary treatments, not always daring or choosing to inform their doctors of this decision (e.g., 40% as reported by [48]). Sometimes patients are faced with the difficult decision to participate in a clinical trial (see Chap. 7). In their decisions about treatments, patients are often conflicted in regard to the desired balance between likely positive medical effects and possible negative effects on quality of life. At least some patients are seriously worried and bothered by this issue [48].

A smaller group of patients is reluctant or undecided about whether they should at all get treatments against cancer. The size of this group varies in different periods, depending on information in the media and other sources, including fashion trends. The reasons may be that the patients believe that the treatments have no benefit at all or there is no certainty that they will be helpful or are useless because anyway they cannot provide perfect recovery or may cause too much physical harm and psychological suffering [49]. In addition, some patients may refuse treatments because they prefer complementary or alternative treatments [50, 51] or rely on some specific therapeutic medium, based on so-called spiritual, natural, mystical, ethnic, or even extraterrestrial means which, needless to mention, are not evidence-based. A minority of patients may choose not to undergo any treatments at all, relying on faith in God or accepting their fate ("what should be will anyway happen") without intervening in the natural course of events, enjoying their life as long as possible.

Who decides about the treatments? In recent years the answer to this issue is far from clear. Whereas in former decades it was evident that the major if not the single decision-maker was the doctor, sometimes supported by the family, at present the patients have become important associates in the process. Twenty years ago [52], 59% of the patients said they wanted their physician to make the decision. The present situation is somewhat more complex. Many patients feel that they want or should or are expected by the system or their family and friends to assume a more decisive role in regard to treatment choice. A large number of patients were found to have information and preferences about treatments concerning their disease [53, 54]. However, a recent study [55] shows that 38.9% of treatment decisions were patient controlled (especially when the evidence for the treatment was uncertain), 43.6%

were shared (especially when the treatment was supported by good evidence), and 17.5% were physician controlled (especially when there was no evidence for or against the treatment). The implicit implication of these findings is that the physician is still dominantly involved in decisions concerning treatments. Moreover, studies confirm this impression by showing that most patients still prefer to play a passive role in treatment decisions [53, 54]. The evident contradictions reflect conflicts that characterize the experience of many patients.

Preparing for the Treatments Selecting the treatments does not conclude the stage of decisions preceding the treatments. In order to get a comprehensive picture of the experience of patients in this phase, it is necessary to mention further salient issues that require decisions. One such issue concerns the doctor or sometimes even the medical center that the patients choose for their treatment. It is possible that patients feel a need to make choices of this kind in order to preserve some kind of control over a situation in which they feel increasingly helpless. A special set of issues concerns preserving fertility despite the treatments. Taking care of fertility may involve quite stressful decisions and more or less complicated medical procedures (see Chaps. 6 and 7).

Some patients decide to undergo complementary or alternative treatments. In that case the patient needs to decide which interventions to select and which therapist to choose. A highly delicate issue consists in the decision whether and how to share this information with one's physician.

In the pretreatment period patients are in a state of anxiety, nurtured by fear of the unknown that faces them. Often they waver between two extremes: sometimes thinking that they would be able to continue their life as at present and that there would be no changes, at other time expecting that everything will change completely when they start treatments and that they would not be able to continue doing any of the things they have always done. Actually they don't know what to expect and are very scared especially of the pain and physical suffering that may be caused by the treatments. One bothering question is "will I be able to withstand it?"

There are further decisions surrounding the issue of the treatments. One of them may be when to begin the treatments and how to prepare for them physically (e.g., taking care of one's other diseases), psychologically (e.g., making a nice trip so as to reduce stress and store good memories prior to the difficult period), and in terms of daily life arrangements (e.g., asking someone to accompany one to the medical center for the treatment, arranging for help in the household management and for taking care of partners, children, and one's parents). However, many patients are seriously conflicted about getting help or support of any kind because they often feel that this is an admission of weakness that may contribute to reducing their chances of recovery.

Above all the pretreatment period is dominated by the two following questions patients have. One concerns work and revolves around considerations, such as "will I be able to go on working?" and "now that my life span is limited, should I spend so much time working?" The other issue may be labeled "whom to tell about my cancer" which involves questions about one's image, relations, strength, coping, and sharing (see also Chap. 7).

Undergoing the Treatments Undergoing the treatments in the first phase of the disease is a unique experience that does not resemble treatments in later phases. It is unique physically as well as psychologically. Physically the patient undergoes unusual experiences including changes in body volume, in sensations, in strength, and in vitality, due, for example, to chemotherapy or radiotherapy. Psychologically, the patient may feel weak, anxious, depressed, sometimes confused, and very often estranged from oneself. There is nothing to which one can compare these changes that are unpleasant and scary, constituting part of the suffering patients undergo during this period. If however the treatments are experienced less negatively, the patients may wonder whether the treatment is at all working or whether they have been given the right medication.

When patients have undergone surgery, there may be further experiences related to the loss of a limb or organ, depending on the kind of cancer and the performed surgery. Externally visible scars or losses tend to be more distressful than other scars and losses although the patient is aware more or less continuously of both kinds, sometimes interpreting them as the price that is required as payment for life. The latter interpretation may be enhanced if the patient participated in the selection of the kind of surgery.

Depending on the kind of treatment protocol, the patients may suffer from side effects of the treatments affecting all their bodily systems, including the gastrointestinal (e.g., nausea, bloating, diarrhea, constipation, lack of appetite), neurological, skin, kidneys, the senses (vision, taste, smell, hearing), sleep, movement, sex, fertility, mood, and cognition. Some blood components are affected too, which may necessitate blood transfusions and taking special care not to be exposed to possible infections when in contact with other people. Most disturbing for many patients are the cognitive changes, mainly in memory and problem-solving [56], and the emotional changes that are often identified as anxiety and depression but sometimes resemble some kind of toxic, melancholic state of demoralization [57] (see Chap. 6). However, not only the treatments and the side effects are new to the patient. Also the environment in which all this occurs is new to many patients. Patients have to learn to function and find help if needed in an unfamiliar setting of the hospital or clinic in which they are treated, to find out the roles of the different health professionals and how best to contact them.

The first phase of treatments is also marked by the procedures of tests often made in order to check whether or to what extent the treatment is useful. This includes undergoing the tests, waiting for the results, and comprehending the findings which are not always clear and may need interpretation.

The treatments are prolonged and may last months. Sometimes there are complications that require further delays, for example, until certain blood counts are corrected or an infection is taken care of. The patient learns slowly what he or she is allowed to do in the course of the treatments and what kind of actions or locations are better avoided, which kind of symptoms justify or require contacting the doctor or the clinic, and which ones can be tolerated without risk.

Patients also learn how best to use the time periods between courses of treatment and what to expect from each set of treatments. One thing that is most difficult for many patients is to get used to the fact that the effect of each course of treatments may be different so that even if the last course was difficult, the side effects of the next one may be quite tolerable. The unexpected changes and differences between the treatment courses lead many patients to adopt the "one day at a time" strategy. Due to the frequent unexpected changes, most patients need to learn not to plan too far ahead in time and when they do to be prepared to change the plan or adapt it to the prevailing circumstances.

Phase 3: Remission and Survivorship

From Patient to Survivor: Health Issues The road from patient to survivor is marked by several steps that may contribute to paving a road which is not necessarily smooth. The first step consists in simply completing the final course of treatment. Patients may expect to feel relief, but it is still not there. In the first few days the patients do not feel any different than they felt after the previous courses of treatment. To their surprise even after the first few days, the situation does not revert to the original state because their blood or body is still saturated with the different medications. And then it is still necessary to get the legitimation that all is OK from the final medical tests, which may be performed 6–12 weeks after termination of the last course of treatment.

The contact of survivors with the medical system is not over with the completion of the first phase of treatments [58]. Survivors are expected to undergo follow-up at specific times, such as every 3 months in the beginning and later only once a year, unless they have specific complaints. In addition, most survivors are required to undergo surveillance, which may involve screening and imaging (e.g., colonoscopy, mammography) because of treatments they have undergone or the risk of cancer recurrence or the occurrence of other late effect that may include malignancies or other disorders (e.g., cardiovascular after chest radiation). In the case of some cancers, patients are required to take medications for several more years (e.g., breast cancer) and after bone marrow transplantations to treat different persistent symptoms of guest-versus-host disease. Regardless of the time that has elapsed since the termination of treatments, cancer patients experience a lot of anxiety prior to and following each follow-up or surveillance exam.

The follow-up meetings with the doctor provide the patients the opportunity to pose their questions and present their fears and doubts. This aspect of the follow-up is very important because it gives the patient relief from anxiety and offers some security for patients who may feel quite lost and scared without the constant contact with the hospital or clinic which they have had for so many months [59]. However, it also reminds them that they are not healthy and cannot be considered as such, because – as they often complain – "who has seen a healthy person who comes to the doctor in the hospital every three months?" It is an open secret, only rarely discussed openly, that an unspecified number of cancer patients after 2 or more years stop taking the medications they are required to take after treatment termination (e.g., tamoxifen) in order to avoid their side effects and start feeling "healthy." They do this of their own accord, sometimes without telling their doctor, although they know it may be risky [60].

The follow-up procedure creates further problems for many patients who may find it hard to identify the right kind of doctor for the follow-up (e.g., the family doctor, the oncologist, a second opinion oncologist, the surgeon?). In addition, it may be difficult for some patients to decide what exactly to report to the doctor, which symptoms or bodily manifestations are at all relevant. Many patients are seriously confused about this issue and report either too many symptoms (e.g., what they felt and what happened every single day starting from the last follow-up meeting) or too few symptoms (e.g., "it was OK"). This kind of uncertainty is to be expected in patients who have lost their trust in their body due to the disease and the treatments they have undergone.

In addition, there are different late effects of the treatments that persist for weeks or months following the termination of the treatments. For example, patients may continue to feel nausea, fatigue and lack of energy and muscular weakness, or have cardiovascular symptoms, most of which need special care [60].

After having undergone months of medical treatments, it is not surprising that many patients worry in general about their physical state and look for different means that could contribute to enhancing their health. Many of them turn at this stage to means such as healthy food, different kinds of diet, massage, and physical fitness.

Most survivors share the persistent concern about disease recurrence. This concern may be manifested in the form of repeated bouts of anxiety, recurrent thoughts about the cancer that may prop up unexpectedly any time, a tendency to interpret any common physical symptoms as a sign of cancer, and increased interest in information about cancer and late effects of treatments [60].

Being a Survivor: Psychosocial Aspects Taking care of psychosocial needs is a central concern for survivors. A large survey of survivors who had been diagnosed at least 5 years earlier showed that 30.2% had at least one unmet need in the emotional, social, or spiritual domains and most often the need of help in reducing stress [61].

There are many reasons for the stress that so many survivors experience, sometimes admitting it openly, but often not. Entering the phase of survivorship brings with it a flood of questions, such as Am I now healthy or not? Will the cancer recur or not? How will I know whether I am sick or not, since in the past the cancer has been growing in my body without my awareness? Can I trust my body? Should I go on with my previous life routine or should I change? Should I go on working or not? Should I change my work? Should I change my apartment so as to get away from the "bad luck" that has overcome me there? Why did I get this disease? How long will I live? What should I do with my life and with myself? Should I avoid all feelings of anger? Should I cultivate the "positive thinking" approach? Can I go one with my marriage? This is just a sample of the questions that arise in the survivor's mind after terminating treatments.

What these and similar questions demonstrate is that survivors may have lost contact with their life due to the cancer diagnosis and the long period of treatments [62]. What they face when they become officially survivors is the uncertainty about the future and the present and the need or even pressure to undertake serious decisions about their life. Even reinstituting their familiar routine and continuing their previous life constitutes a problem because it requires a decision to adopt anew their own life, which has lost its familiarity.

These and similar questions revolve around the following major foci: regaining existential security, reestablishing one's future time perspective, reconstructing one's personal identity, and elaborating one's meaningfulness of life. Patients handle these problems in different ways, mostly by looking for spiritual support and psychological help. It is the special expertise of psychooncologists to help patients precisely in regard to these concerns (see Chaps. 6 and 8).

Phase 4: Disease Recurrence

Disease Recurrence Disease recurrence is one of the most dreaded and stressful junctures in the narrative of cancer [63]. All through survivorship, patients deal with the possibility of recurrence so that if and when it arrives, many of them are not really surprised, but they are nevertheless deeply shocked and traumatized. It is like a prophecy (a bad one) come true. When cancer recurs patients admit for the first time that they start considering seriously the possibility of death. Indeed, they have thought of death when they first got the diagnosis, but at that phase it could be mostly set aside by diverting one's attention to the treatment possibilities and the optimism communicated by physicians and the other health professionals with whom the patient has been in contact. At present, death becomes a reality that needs to be faced and dealt with. The fear of death assumes a concrete form [64].

Some of the issues previously experienced in the initial phase of cancer diagnosis including the decision about treatments recur now but in a highly different form. First, the diagnosis about the medical situation and the progression of the disease is dealt with by the doctor and mostly by the patient too in a matter of fact manner. The problems of disclosure are mostly not of central concern anymore. The patient is already much more experienced in dealing with the doctor, the hospital environment, and the medical terms too. Paradoxically, now that the patients can comprehend much better the medical terminology and style of expression, they ask much less, partly because they can understand by themselves and partly because they may not want to understand that much.

The discussion concerning treatment options also takes a different form than in the former phase. The selection of treatments is mostly based on a more extended discussion. Often the patients address also other medical experts in order to get a second and sometimes a third opinion. The issue of accepting or being accepted in a clinical trial becomes highly relevant and is seriously considered by both patients and doctors. At this phase the emphasis is more on saving life and stopping the progression of the disease than on maintaining quality of life. Since the patients and their families have already undergone the initial phases of the treatments together, they have evolved a strategy of interaction that provides for a closer involvement of the family in the process of decisions about treatments.

Additional Phases of Treatment The treatments at the phase of disease recurrence are mostly more difficult physically. There are often more complications with the need for recurrent hospitalization. The physical suffering is often not mitigated by an overly optimistic attitude but is embedded in a more realistic coping strategy. The patients are aware that the treatment options are becoming limited, simply because not too many are available. Some of the patients know that doctors do not recommend more than two or three additional cycles of treatment courses. In these circumstances, patients often assume the attitude that even if the specific treatment they get does not really solve the medical problem, the main point is to gain time so that eventually maybe somewhere in the world someone would devise a new treatment.

Psychosocial Needs At this phase patients are highly stressed and often complain of anxiety. They are sad and distressed but tend to be scared to admit their sadness because they believe depression may affect the disease negatively [65]. The distress may be alleviated somewhat by medication but is not overcome. Patients feel lonely and in need for support – emotional, spiritual, social – from any available source.

Phase 5: Palliative Care and Confronting Dying

Transition to Palliative Care Palliative care addresses the needs of the patient on many levels, emphasizing the patient's quality of life as the prime goal. Palliative care is often introduced already in former phases of the disease, and some claim it should be part of the treatment from the very beginning. However, transition to palliative care means that the curative goal has been given up and has been replaced by the palliative goal.

The transition to the palliative phase is mostly based on decisions shared by the doctor, the family, and the patient. The adoption of this option implies that medicine as such has little more to offer the patient by way of cure or recovery. The treatment options have been largely exhausted. It is often the family that pressures both the doctor and the patient to still try some further treatment, although the benefit in terms of life prolongation may be minimal or doubtful and the cost in terms of deteriorated quality of life may be large. At this stage many patients tend to accept the option of palliative care and may even experience a kind of relief by being spared the highly unpleasant side effects of the treatments. Sometimes the choice of this option is brought up precisely by the patients who prefer to enjoy the last period of their life in greater peace and less stress than previously.

At this phase patients may worry about whether they have disappointed their doctor by not responding better to the various treatments they have undergone. They may consider the transition to palliative care not always as a salvage from suffering but as a "failure."

Palliative care requires often a continuous contact with health professionals, including a doctor and nurses. The major focus of the provided medical support is alleviation of pain and of other bodily symptoms that may cause suffering. Nutrition is an important issue because many patients find it difficult to ingest and digest food due to previous side effects of treatments or current metastases. Hence, cachexia is a common symptom [66]. Helping the patient to accept nutrition may contribute a lot to keeping him or her in a better physical state.

Emotional Reactions There is a great variety of emotional responses characterizing patients at this phase. Depression is one of them but often not the major one. It is sometimes manifested as demoralization which is more akin to indifference than to outright depression. The patient may be responsive to external stimuli but manifests little or no initiative. Some patients develop spiritual interests and emotions, thinking about their life, their achievements, and what they have failed to achieve. Others concentrate evidently on the present situation, focusing in a kind of mindfulness approach on present sensory experiences and events, cultivating relief and peace of mind. Some are openly angry, expressing their discontent at the injustice of this disease and its progression. Psychooncological help is greatly appreciated at this phase.

Where Do Patients Go? Sometimes patients who need a hospital may stay in the regular hospital which usually keeps a room or several beds for patients who may need transfer to the hospice but insist on avoiding this choice. The hospice is a common option, in case it exists. It may be a ward in the general hospital or a separate institution. The decision whether to leave home and go to a hospice is a major issue which often bothers many patients and their families. Indeed, in some cases staying at home is not an option if there is no home in which the patient can stay or the patient is too sick and requires the kind of nursing which the family cannot afford to provide. Some patients avoid staying at home in order to facilitate the situation for their family or because they do not desire this option. Be it as it may, the transition to the hospice is extremely stressful for most patients because it indicates stepping into the last phase of life. The hospice is a place where only palliative care is applied, without any vestiges of curative procedures. Although in some rare cases patients can leave the hospice, more often than not, they do not come back home.

A fair number of patients spend the last months or weeks of their life in nursing homes that are specifically targeted for cancer patients or not.

In some countries the health service provides a kind of in-between option which is called "home hospice." The patient stays at home but gets palliative care through regular visits of a doctor or a nurse. When necessary the patient is transferred to a hospital where he or she are treated and if possible are transferred back home. Sometimes psychological help is also available through a psychooncologist, a social worker, or someone who provides spiritual guidance and help, if the patient desires. Home hospices are an intermediate solution bridging the home and the hospice.

According to most surveys, the majority of patients would like to die at home [67]. Yet most of them do not die at home but in some other institution, which is mostly the hospital or a nursing home. Studies show that even when patients stay at home during the palliative care period, they mostly die in the hospital where they are brought by family members who are at a loss with how to deal with certain medical crises. Yet staying at home during the final period of life provides the patient a better quality of life and more opportunities to enjoy relations with one's family than most other locations (see Chap. 12).

References

1. Henry, K. A., McDonald, K., Sherman, R., Kinney, A. Y., & Stroup, A. M. (2002). Association between individual and geographic factors and nonadherence to mammography screening guidelines. *Journal of Women's Health, 23*(8), 664–674.
2. Kreitler, S., Chaitchik, S., Kreitler, H., & Weissler, K. (1994). Who will attend tests for the early detection of breast cancer? *Psychology and Health, 9*, 463–483.
3. Smith, R. A., Andrews, K., Brooks, D., DeSantis, C. E., Fedewa, S. A., Lortet-Tieulent, J., Manassaram-Baptiste, D., Brawley, O. W., & Wender, R. C. (2016). Cancer screening in the United States, 2016: A review of current American Cancer Society guidelines and current issues in cancer screening. (English). *CA: A Cancer Journal for Clinicians, 66*(2), 96–114.
4. McCunney, R. J., & Li, J. (2014). Radiation risks in lung cancer screening programs: A comparison with nuclear industry workers and atomic bomb survivors. *Chest, 145*(3), 618–624.
5. Freund, M., Lueftner, D., & Wilhelm, M. (2014). Benefits and risks of cancer screening. *Oncology Research and Treatment, 37*(Suppl 3), 1.
6. Riemann, J. F., Schröder, C., Kallenbach, M., Giersiepen, K., & Schmoll, H. J. (2014). Benefits and risks of colorectal cancer screening. *Oncology Research and Treatment, 37*(Suppl 3), 11–20.
7. Gøtzsche, P. C., & Nielsen, M. (2013). Screening for breast cancer with mammography. *Cochrane Database of Systematic Reviews*, Issue 6, Art. No.: CD001877. https://doi.org/10.1002/14651858.CD001877.pub5.
8. Kreitler, S., Chaitchik, S., & Kreitler, H. (1990). The psychological profile of women attending breast-screening tests. *Social Science and Medicine, 31*, 1177–1185.
9. Chaitchik, S., & Kreitler, S. (1991). Induced versus spontaneous attendance of breast-screening tests by women. *Journal of Cancer Education, 6*, 43–53.
10. Kreitler, S., & Chaitchik, S. (1995). The paradox of the self-diagnosed lump in the breast. *Psychooncology Letters, 6*, 39–52.
11. Kreitler, S., & Chaitchik, S. (1996). Self diagnosis through breast self-examination. Is it a solution? *Journal of Cancer Education, 11*(Suppl), 22.
12. Thomas, D. B., Gao, D. L., Ray, R. M., Wang, W. W., Allison, C. J., Chen, F. L., Porter, P., Hu, Y. W., Zhao, G. L., Pan, L. D., Li, W., Wu, C., Coriaty, Z., Evans, I., Lin, M. G., Stalsberg, H., & Self, S. G. (2002). Randomized trial of breast self-examination in in Shanghai: Final results. *Journal of the National Cancer Institute, 94*, 1445–1457.
13. Peipins, L. A., McCarty, F., Hawkins, N. A., Rodriguez, J. L., Scholl, L. E., & Leadbetter, S. (2015). Cognitive and affective influences on perceived risk of ovarian cancer. *Psychooncology, 24*(3), 279–286.
14. Pineault, P. (2007). Breast cancer screening: Women's experiences of waiting for further testing. *Oncology Nursing Forum, 34*(4), 847–853.

15. Wiener, R. S., Gould, M. K., Woloshin, S., Schwartz, L. M., & Clark, J. A. (2015). "The thing is not knowing": Patients' perspectives on surveillance of an indeterminate pulmonary nodule. *Health Expectations, 18*(3), 355–365.
16. Putora, P. M., & Oldenburg, J. (2014). The Kafkaesque process of cancer diagnosis. *Journal of Clinical Oncology, 32*, 1087–1088.
17. Roberts, T. K. (2016). The other side of bad news. *The Oncologist, 21*, 506–507.
18. Fujimori, M., Shirai, Y., Asai, M., Akizuki, N., Katsumata, N., Kubota, K., & Uchitomi, Y. (2014). Development and preliminary evaluation of communication skills training program for oncologists based on patient preferences for communicating bad news. *Palliative & Supportive Care, 12*(5), 379–386.
19. Sweeny, K., Shepperd, J. A., & Han, P. K. (2013). The goals of communicating bad news in health care: Do physicians and patients agree? *Health Expectations, 16*(3), 230–238.
20. Munoz Sastre, M. T., Sorum, P. C., & Mullet, E. (2011). Breaking bad news: The patient's viewpoint. *Health Communication, 26*(7), 649–655.
21. Aitken-Swan, J., & Easson, E. C. (1959). Reactions of cancer patients on being told their diagnosis. *British Medical Journal, 1*, 288.
22. Kreitler, S., Chaitchik, S., Rapoport, Y., & Algor, R. (1995). Psychosocial effects of level of information and severity of disease on head-and-neck cancer patients. *Journal of Cancer Education, 10*(3), 144–154.
23. Seifart, C., Hofmann, M., Bär, T., Riera Knorrenschild, J., Seifart, U., & Rief, W. (2014). Breaking bad news-what patients want and what they get: Evaluating the SPIKES protocol in Germany. *Annals of Oncology, 25*(3), 707–711.
24. Cao, W., Qi, X., Yao, T., Han, X., & Feng, X. (2017). How doctors communicate the initial diagnosis of cancer matters: Cancer disclosure and its relationship with patients' hope and trust. *Psycho-Oncology, 26*, 640–648.
25. Annunziata, M. A., Foladore, S., Magri, M. D., Crivellari, D., Feltrin, A., Bidoli, E., & Veronesi, A. (1998). Does the information level of cancer patients correlate with quality of life? A prospective study. *Tumori, 84*, 619–623.
26. Kiesler, D. J., & Auerbach, S. M. (2006). Optimal matches of patient preferences for information, decision-making and interpersonal behavior: Evidence, models and interventions. *Patient Education and Counseling, 61*(3), 319–341.
27. Al-Amri, A. M. (2009). Cancer patients' desire for information: A study in a teaching hospital in Saudi Arabia. *Eastern Mediterranean Health Journal, 15*(1), 19–24.
28. Motlagh, A., Yaraei, N., Mafi, A. R., Hosseini Kamal, F., Yaseri, M., Hemati, S., Shahbazian, H., Sedighi, A. A., Khodabakhshi, R., Taghizadeh, A., Ansari, J., Seyednejad, F., Khanduzi, R., Mojir Sheibani, K., Azadeh, P., Emranpour, M. H., Mosalei, A., Vojdani, S., Nazari, A. M., Nazarimenesh, L., Fazl-Alizadeh, A., & Akbari, M. E. (2014). Attitude of cancer patients toward diagnosis disclosure and their preference for clinical decision-making: A national survey. *Archives of Iranian Medicine, 17*(4), 232–240.
29. Narita, Y., Miyakita, Y., Momota, H., Miyahara, R., Shibui, S., & Geka, N. S. (2009). A survey of neurosurgeons' policies and attitudes regarding the disclosure of a diagnosis of glioma and the decision to pursue end-of-life care in glioma patients. (Japanese). *Neurological Surgery, 37*(10), 973–981.
30. Lee, A., & Wu, H. Y. (2002). Diagnosis disclosure in cancer patients – when the family says "no!". *Singapore Medical Journal, 43*(10), 533–538.
31. Dégi, C. L. (2009). Non-disclosure of cancer diagnosis: An examination of personal, medical, and psychosocial factors. *Supportive Care in Cancer., 17*(8), 1101–1107.
32. Chittem, M., Norman, P., & Harris, P. R. (2013). Relationships between perceived diagnostic disclosure, patient characteristics, psychological distress and illness perceptions in Indian cancer patients. *Psychooncology, 22*(6), 1375–1180.
33. Chittem, M., & Butow, P. (2015). Responding to family requests for nondisclosure: The impact of oncologists' cultural background. *Journal of Cancer Research and Therapeutics, 11*(1), 174–180.

34. Mistakidu, K., Parpa, E., Tsilila, E., Katsouda, E., & Vlahos, L. (2004). Cancer information disclosure in different cultural contexts. *Supportive Care in Cancer, 12*, 147–154.
35. Ferraz Gonçalves, J., & Castro, S. (2001). Diagnosis disclosure in a Portuguese oncological centre. *Palliative Medicine, 15*(1), 35–41.
36. Shahidi, J. (2010). Not telling the truth: Circumstances leading to concealment of diagnosis and prognosis from cancer patients. *European Journal of Cancer Care, 19*, 589–593.
37. Parker, P. A., Ross, A. C., Polansky, M. N., Palmer, J. L., Rodriguez, M. A., & Baile, W. F. (2010). Communicating with cancer patients: What areas do physician assistants find most challenging? *Journal of Cancer Education, 25*(4), 524–529.
38. Rapoport, Y., Kreitler, S., Chaitchik, S., Algor, R., & Weissler, K. (1993). Psychosocial problems in head-and-neck cancer patients and their change with disease duration. *Annals of Oncology, 4*, 69–73.
39. Kreitler, S., Chaitchik, S., Kovner, F., & Kreitler, H. (1992). Information in breast cancer patients: The good and the bad news (Abstract). *Journal of Cancer Education, 7*(Suppl 1), 25.
40. Numico, G., Anfossi, M., Bertelli, G., Russi, E., Cento, G., Silvestris, N., Granetto, C., Di Costanzo, G., Occelli, M., Fea, E., Garrone, O., Gasco, M., Colantonio, I., & Merlano, M. (2009). The process of truth disclosure: An assessment of the results of information during the diagnostic phase in patients with cancer. *Annals of Oncology, 20*, 941–920.
41. Anguiano, L., Mayer, D. K., Piven, M. L., & Rosenstein, D. (2012). A literature review of suicide in cancer patients. *Cancer Nursing, 35*(4), E14–E26.
42. Crocetti, E., Arniani, S., Acciai, S., Barchielli, A., & Buiatti, E. (1998). High suicide mortality soon after diagnosis among cancer patients in central Italy. *British Journal of Cancer, 77*(7), 1194–1196.
43. Fang, F., Keating, N. L., Mucci, L. A., Adami, H. O., Stampfer, M. J., Valdimarsdóttir, U., & Fall, K. (2010). Immediate risk of suicide and cardiovascular death after a prostate cancer diagnosis: Cohort study in the United States. *[J] Journal of The National Cancer Institute, 102*(5), 307–314.
44. Yamauchi, T., Inagaki, M., Yonemoto, N., Iwasaki, M., Inoue, M., Akechi, T., Iso, H., Tsugane, S., & JPHC Study Group. (2014). Death by suicide and other externally caused injuries following a cancer diagnosis: The Japan Public Health Center-based Prospective Study. *Psychooncology, 23*(9), 1034–1041.
45. Walsh, M. C., Trentham-Dietz, A., Schroepfer, T. A., Reding, D. J., Campbell, B., Foote, M. L., Kaufman, S., Barrett, M., Remington, P. L., & Cleary, J. F. (2010). Cancer information sources used by patients to inform and influence treatment decisions. *Journal of Health Communication, 15*(4), 445–463.
46. Dey, A. (2004). Consumer health informatics: An overview of patient perspectives on health information needs. *Health Information Management Journal, 33*(4), 121–126.
47. de Bekker-Grob, E. W., Bliemer, M. C., Donkers, B., Essink-Bot, M. L., Korfage, I. J., Roobol, M. J., Bangma, C. H., & Steyerberg, E. W. (2013). Patients' and urologists' preferences for prostate cancer treatment: A discrete choice experiment. *British Journal of Cancer, 109*(3), 633–640.
48. Blinman, P., King, M., Norman, R., Viney, R., & Stockler, M. R. (2012). Preferences for cancer treatments: An overview of methods and applications in oncology. *Annals of Oncology, 23*(5), 1104–1110.
49. Begbie, S. D., Kerestes, Z. L., & Bell, D. R. (1996). Patterns of alternative medicine use by cancer patients. *The Medical Journal of Australia, 165*(10), 545–548.
50. Bar-Sela, G., Danos, S., Visel, B., & Mitnik, I. (2016). Understanding the attitudes of patients with cancer toward complementary and alternative therapies. *Journal of Palliative Medicine, 19*(5), 496–502.
51. Smith, P. J., Clavarino, A., Long, J., & Steadman, K. J. (2014). Why do some cancer patients receiving chemotherapy choose to take complementary and alternative medicines and what are the risks? *Asia-Pacific Journal of Clinical Oncology, 10*(1), 1–10.
52. Degner, L. F., & Sloan, J. A. (1992). Decision making during serious illness: What role do patients really want to play? *Journal of Clinical Epidemiology, 45*, 941–950.

53. Damm, K., Vogel, A., & Prenzler, A. (2014). Preferences of colorectal cancer patients for treatment and decision-making: A systematic literature review. *European Journal of Cancer Care, 23*(6), 762–772. Date of Electronic Publication: 20 May 2014.
54. Schmidt, K., Damm, K., Prenzler, Golpon, H., & Welte, T. (2016). Preferences of lung cancer patients for treatment and decision-making: A systematic literature review. *European Journal of Cancer Care, 25*(4), 580–591. Date of Electronic Publication: 17 Dec 2015.
55. Keating, N. L., Landrum, M. B., Arora, N. K., Malin, J. L., Ganz, P. A., van Ryn, M., & Weeks, J. C. (2010). Cancer patients' roles in treatment decisions: Do characteristics of the decision influence roles? *Journal of Clinical Oncology, 28*, 4364–4370.
56. Hodgson, K. D., Hutchinson, A. D., Wilson, C. J., & Nettlebeck, T. (2013). A meta-analysis of the effects of chemotherapy on cognition in patients with cancer. *Cancer Treatment Reviews, 39*, 297–304.
57. Tang, P. L., Wang, H. H., & Chou, F. H. (2015). A systematic review and metaanalysis of demoralization and depression in patients with cancer. *Psychosomatics, 50*(6), 634–643.
58. Wilbur, J. (2015). Surveillance of the adult cancer survivor. *American Family Physician, 91*, 29–36.
59. Garofalo, J. P., Choppala, S., Hamann, H. A., & Gjerde, J. (2009). Uncertainty during the transition from cancer patient to survivor. *Cancer Nursing, 32*(4), E8–E14.
60. Makubate, B., Donnan, P. T., Dewar, J. A., et al. (2013). Cohort study of adherence to adjuvant endocrine therapy, breast cancer recurrence and mortality. *British Journal of Cancer, 108*(7), 1515–1524. https://doi.org/10.1038/bjc.2013.116. Epub 21 Mar 2013.
61. Geller, B. M., Vacek, P. M., Flynn, B. S., Lord, K., & Cranmer, D. (2014). What are cancer survivors' needs and how well are they being met? *The Journal of Family Practice, 63*(10), E7–E16.
62. Etkind, S. N., Bristowe K., Bailey, K., Selman, L. E., & Murtagh, F. E. (2017). How does uncertainty shape patient experience in advanced illness? A secondary analysis of qualitative data. *Palliative Medicine, 31*(2), 171–180.
63. Koch, L., Jansen, L., Brenner, H., & Arndt, V. (2013). Fear of recurrence and disease progression in long-term (≥5 years) cancer survivors—a systematic review of quantitative studies. *Psychooncology, 22*, 1–11.
64. Kreitler, S. (2005). Fear of death. In P. L. Gower (Ed.), *New research on the psychology of fear*. New York: Nova Science Publishers.
65. Beresford, T. P., Alfers, J., Mangum, L., et al. (2006). Cancer survival probability as a function of ego defense (adaptive) mechanisms versus depressive symptoms. *Psychosomatics, 47*(3), 247–253.
66. Kreitler, S., & Barak, F. (2012). Nutrition and quality of life in cancer patients with advanced disease. *Supportive Care in Cancer, 20*(Suppl 1), S132–S133.
67. Barak, F., Livshits, S., Kaufer, H., Netanel, R., Siegelman-Danieli, N., Alkalay, Y., & Kreitler, S. (2015). Where to die? This is the question: A study of cancer patients in Israel. *Palliative and Supportive Care, 13*, 165–170.

Chapter 4
Determinants, Risk Factors, and Protective Factors for Cancer: Environmental, Physiological, and Demographic

General Interest in Determinants of Cancers

Two major tendencies may be detected in the attitude of the general public in diseases and their causes. One kind of attitude consists in denial. Many people just don't want to be worried, anxious, and scared by different potential diseases. They avoid hearing about diseases, doctors, hospitals, treatments, death, and all the affiliated associations. Their attitude is best expressed by claims such as "Anyway it won't help us to hear about all these illnesses," "We don't understand any of this stuff," and "It may just scare us and this harms our health." The other kind of attitude is just the opposite. It consists in looking actively for information about diseases and anything connected with them, especially causes and ways of prevention. The rationale is that the more they know about illnesses, the better they are equipped with means for avoiding them and prolonging their life. This attitude may lead to presumptuous declarations about medical issues that are based on misunderstandings that are to be expected in people who are not medical experts.

The trend described as interest in diseases is particularly strong and prevalent in regard to cancer. People of all ages and strata of society manifest interest in cancer, especially in its causes. Cancer is conceptualized as "the enemy from within" and is considered as one of the worst diseases. As such it evokes the desire to fight it so as to prevent it altogether or if it does occur – to overcome it. The tendency to learn about cancer is pitted against the fear of cancer. The fight against cancer that goes on in medicine and in science at large goes on privately and on a small scale within many individuals.

The causes for cancer are the theme that is most dominant in the public interest in cancer. Causes appear to be the crux of the whole issue. It is as if people assume that identifying the causes would bring about victory over the disease. However, there is a lot of misunderstanding hovering over the theme of causality of a disease in general and of cancer in particular.

S. Kreitler, *Psycho-Oncology for the Clinician*,
https://doi.org/10.1007/978-3-030-06126-5_4

Causes, Etiology, and Risk Factors

In order to be able to get and understand correctly the available information, it is necessary to clarify some of the involved concepts. Many individuals as well as sources of information about cancer use the major terms in an overlapping and sometimes misleading form. Causality has a long history in philosophy and is a major concept in the philosophy and practice of science. Admittedly causality is an unclearly defined concept. Sometimes *cause* stands for a totality that includes everything that results in the occurrence of cancer, whereby some undisclosed processes intervene between so-called causality and the outcome. Sometimes the term used is *causes* in the plural which may be confusing because it indicates there are multiple or different causes without specifying how they are interconnected or what is the principle or procedure determining the involvement of each in the process and the contribution each may have to the output. Moreover, there exists a whole set of "causes" in the arena, which is liable to add to the unclarity, for example, static and dynamic causes, instrumental and efficient (or agentive) causes, proximal and distal causes, necessary and sufficient causes, material and formal causes, and final or teleological causes – to mention just the major most commonly used ones. Causes may be replaced sometimes by the less committing terms antecedents or precursors, or they may be accompanied by the apparently affiliated term of correlation. In addition, there is the competing term *etiology* which is often used to denote a set of causes but also the manner of occurrence of cancer describing the processes through which the disease comes into being. Finally, there is the term *risk factors* that may replace the other constructs of causality or amplify them [1]. This brief introduction indicates that a practical, scientifically based approach to causality in medicine may be expected to be multifactorial rather than monocausal, relying on multiple convergent procedures of evidence [2].

The following clarification of the major mentioned terms is designed to help the practical understanding of these terms, without in any way delving into the rich and long epistemological history of causality in philosophy and science. Rather the clarification is based on a modern generally accepted approach in medicine and medical research, which takes account of the diverse determinants of a disease and allows for the integration of the physiological and environmental factors, leaving sufficient space for considering also the psychological influences.

Simply stated, the major tenet of this integrative approach is that in dealing with the cause for a disease like cancer, a distinction needs to be made between the pathogen and the risk factors. The distinction implies that in each case of a disease, some pathogen is assumed to be active or have been active, even if it has not been identified in general or has not been detected in the particular case of the patient. Pathogens are mostly viruses or bacteria. However, the mere act of contact between a pathogen and a living body does not result automatically in the occurrence of disease or, in the given case, of cancer. A pathogen is a necessary factor for the disease, but its potential activity and the result of the encounter between it and the human tissue or body depend on the existence of risk factors in the living body and sometimes its environment. It needs to be emphasized that both the pathogens and the risk factors are specific for the particular disease. Similarly since cancer is a family of diseases, it is to be expected that both the pathogens and the risk factors are specific for each of the particular cancer diseases.

At this point it needs to be emphasized that the integrative approach presented in this context differs completely from the biopsychosocial model [3] that has been promoted in recent years [4]. According to the biopsychosocial approach, the occurrence or the course of disease depend on the interaction between a variety of factors from the biological, psychological, and sociological domains. The major advantage of this model is that it broadens the scope of the biomedical classical approach by providing some kind of legitimacy to considering non-biological factors, namely, the psychological and social ones. But the major limitation of this approach is its holistic, unspecific nature and the absence of any specifications about the kind of variables that need to be considered, their interactions, and how they function together [5]. This limitation constitutes one difference between the biopsychosocial approach and the integrative approach. Another major difference is the emphasis on the involvement of the pathogen in the integrative approach, while in the biopsychosocial approach, this function is completely absent.

Pathogens for Cancer A survey of the literature shows that several classes of pathogens for cancer have already been identified. These include primarily members of the following four groups: viruses, microbes, parasites, and genes.

It is assumed that viruses are involved in about 12–20% of human cancers [6–8]. The often cited number of oncogenic viruses is seven, and these include hepatitis virus B (HBV) and hepatitis virus C (HCV), involved in liver cancer; human papilloma virus (HPV), involved in cervical cancer and perhaps also in thyroid cancer; as well as Epstein-Barr virus (EBV), human T-cell lymphoma virus 1 (HTLV-1), Merkel cell polyomavirus (MCPyV), and Kaposi's sarcoma virus also known as human herpes virus 8 (KSVH or HHV8). However, it is unlikely that the list is complete [9–11].

The list of oncogenic bacteria is longer and includes, for example, specimen of the following species or genera, *Helicobacter bilis*, *Helicobacter hepaticus*, *Chlamydia trachomatis*, and many others, targeting neoplasms in specific organs, often functioning through or together with an infection [12–14].

Parasites have also been identified as potential pathogens for some types of cancer [15]. They have been studied less probably because they are relatively rare in the Western world. Most often cited are *Opisthorchis viverrini* and *Clonorchis sinensis* which are a kind of flatworm potentially causing cancer in the bile ducts, and *Schistosoma haematobium* which is a parasite found in the water of some countries and has been linked to bladder cancer [16].

The largest amount of attention has been focused on oncogenes as likely pathogenic agents of cancer. At the risk of being outdated by the fast moving scientific discoveries in this domain, it may be mentioned that genes are involved in causing cancer most often when they have undergone mutations, which transform their functioning. Two kinds of mutations are distinguished: the first kind are germline mutations that are passed from parents to offspring and are assumed at present to include 70 genes, responsible for the so-called inherited cancers (which form about 5–10% of cancers). These mutations refer to genes that may activate processes, such as protein production, as well as inhibit processes, such as tumor suppressing genes. Often discussed examples include BRCA1 and BRCA2 that are involved in inherited breast cancer and ovarian cancer. The other kinds of mutations are acquired mutations, due to factors such as tobacco or ultraviolet radiation. They are more common (assumed at present to include 342 genes) and are involved in more cases of cancer occurrences. Often discussed examples include *HER2*, which is a specialized protein that controls cancer growth and the *ras* family of genes, which produce proteins involved in important cell functions such as communication, growth, and cell death [17].

A special subgroup of pathogens for cancer in the genetic domain goes under the heading of epigenetics. The domain of epigenetics refers to "heritable changes in gene expression that occur independent of changes in the primary DNA sequence" [18]. There is evidence about the involvement of epigenetic changes in the initiation of some cancers [19]. Changes of this kind seem to occur partly because of internal dynamics in the genes themselves and partly because of the action of external factors, such as compounds known as carcinogens, e.g., diethylstilbestrol, arsenite, hexachlorobenzene, and nickel compounds [20]. Epigenetics suggests the impact of external factors on gene functioning. Similarly important in the present context is the evidence that gene expression, for example, in regard to prostate cancer may be modulated by nutrition and lifestyle changes [21].

Risk Factors for Cancers

In medicine or epidemiology, a risk factor is defined as a variable or condition which increases the chances or likelihood that an individual will contract a certain disease. We would like to amend this definition by adding that the risk factor can be expected to enhance the chances of a disease only if there has been contact with a pathogen. There are many different kinds of risk factors, for cancer no less than for other diseases. Many of them are in a state of limbo, which means that there still is not enough evidence to support their status as risk factors or to describe the role they fulfill in regard to cancer. Moreover, risk factors differ in the manner in which they affect the occurrence of the disease. For example, some may contribute to the production of a pathogen (e.g., tobacco may contribute to producing a carcinogenic genetic mutation), others may affect the disease by activating a pathogen, or indirectly by weakening the immune system or by promoting infection. Furthermore, some risk factors may function singly, and some may function in groups or pairs.

Notably, not all risk factors are related to the outcome in the same manner. Some are more closely related, and others more distally. Sometimes a risk factor is merely a part of an environment or situation in which it is likely to encounter a pathogen or be exposed to it. A characteristic example is the association that has been detected between cervical cancer and starting intercourse early or the number of steady sexual partners [22]. Conditions such as these increase the chances for contracting the HPV virus in certain populations. The former conditions may be regarded as distal risk factors for cervical cancer. Furthermore, it is evident that risk factors for a disease may differ in the likelihood with which they contribute to a particular disease.

It is of special interest to note that risk factors may interact in different forms, whereby their joint impact may be greatly enhanced. For example, it was found that when intense alcohol consumption is combined with intense smoking, the risk for oral cavity cancer is increased by 64% and the risk for pharyngeal cancer is increased by 72% and for laryngeal it is increased by 89%, as compared to the percents in individuals who neither drink alcohol nor smoke cigarettes [23].

Risk factors are often detected by examining associations of a correlational kind between one or more characteristics or conditions and the outcome of interest. The frequencies of occurrence of the outcome in the presence and the absence of the tested conditions are compared. In case of a statistically significant result, it is concluded that the examined condition or conditions have at least potentially the status of a risk factor. This procedure is the way in which, for example, the effect of exposure to passive smoking on cancer has been detected [24]. In some cases research reveals that a whole set of variables that have been identified as likely risk factors for cancer are effective as risk factors through their association with a completely different factor. A case in point concerns breast cancer. It was found that nulliparity, late age at first birth, younger age, lower body mass index, hormone replacement therapy, alcohol consumption, low education, and smoking were all associated with increased percent density in the breast which could have been the crucial risk factors for breast cancer [25].

The present chapter is devoted to nonpersonal risk factors for cancer. These include environmental, physiological, and demographic factors. The more psychosocial and behavioral factors will be dealt with in Chap. 5.

Environmental Risk Factors

There is a lot of evidence that cancer varies in different geographical areas and in individuals of different occupations. Due to exposure to different environmental carcinogens, excess risks for cancer have been documented in several occupational groups, including miners and quarrymen, farmers, fishermen, masonry and concrete workers, machine operators, nurses, food industry workers, cooks, launderers, and dry cleaners. This evidence makes it likely that environmental factors play a role as risk factors for cancer [26]. According to the World Health Organization, 19% of all cancers in all countries are attributable to the environment, including work setting resulting in 1.3 million deaths each year [27].

Major among the environmental factors are tobacco, contact with certain toxins, and sun exposure.

Tobacco Concerning the effects of tobacco on cancer, there seems to be unclarity in many public and medical discussions. On the one hand, there are amply recorded correlations between the extent of smoking and cancer morbidity, particularly lung cancer. But on the other hand, there is ample information about people who have been lifelong smokers and did not get lung cancer or any other cancer and about people who never smoked but did get lung cancer. Even the Surgeon General's report about the harms of cancer [28] delved into the fine differences between, for example, causing cancer or being a significant cause of cancer. Over the years many doctors and other investigators raised their voice against the claim that smoking causes cancer and were blamed by others to the point of being suspected of having been bribed by the tobacco companies [29–31]. However, the different problems concerning the role of tobacco are resolved by viewing it simply as one risk factor for cancers in general and probably for lung cancer in particular.

There are three major forms through which tobacco affects the human body and hence the chances for cancer: smoking (cigarettes, cigars, pipes), chewing or snuffing, and exposure to tobacco smoke (i.e., passive smoking). Tobacco is being blamed for about 40% of cancer deaths in men and 20% of cancer deaths in women. Smoking cessation has been shown to be associated with decreased death and direct and indirect morbidity from cancer. Smoking contributes significantly not only to lung cancer but also to other kinds of cancer (oral, esophagus, larynx, bladder, stomach, pancreas, kidney, cervix, and leukemia) [32]. The cancer-promoting impact of cigarette smoking depends on the fact that the burning of a cigarette releases over 5000 different chemicals, many of which are poisonous and more than 70 may cause cancer, ranging from the poisonous arsenic to the radioactive polonium-210 [33]. Some of these chemicals are in general use, whereas others are found specifically in tobacco (tobacco specific nitrosamines). Some of the cancer-promoting chemicals are found in the tobacco plant itself, some are absorbed by the plant (from the ground, air, or fertilizers), some originate in the processing of the tobacco leaves or are added by the tobacco industry, and some form through the burning of the cigarette and are only present in the smoke.

The chemicals found in cigarettes contribute to cancer in different ways. For example, some chemicals make it harder for smokers to neutralize toxins and weaken their immune system in general; some cause directly DNA damage (e.g., benzene, nitrosamines), even to genes that inhibit cancer growth; others (e.g., chromium) render poisons like benzo(a)pyrene stick more strongly to DNA, thus increasing the chances for damage; some (e.g., arsenic, nickel) interfere with pathways for repairing damaged DNA. These different effects increase the chances that damaged cells will eventually turn malignant [34, 35].

Carcinogenic Materials Materials of different kinds that promote malignancy are found in the environment, all around us – in the soil, in the air we breathe, in the water we drink, in the food that we eat. As noted [27], it is evaluated that a fifth of cancers in all countries are attributable to environmental factors, to which one may be exposed in the environment, at home, and at work. Exposure at work is so salient that occupational cancers have come to be identified as a separate group [36].

Information about carcinogens is made regularly available by organizations, such as the National Toxicology Program (NTP), an interagency program of the US Department of Health and Human Services (HHS), and the International Agency for Research on Cancer (IARC), the cancer agency of the World Health Organization [36]. On the basis of research, different materials are identified as definite, likely, possible, and suspected carcinogens. The differences in the status of carcinogens reflect how high is the correlation between the substance and the occurrence of cancer, as well as the size of the sample on which it is based. Other likely contributors to the effect are not always considered in this type of studies. The number of carcinogens varies and is on the whole on the increase. The cited numbers at present are over 100 (107 mentioned by IARC). It is likely that the number will increase first because the means of investigation and the tools for exploration of carcinogens are improving and secondly because with the development of industry the number of carcinogenic agents and materials in the environment is bound to become larger. Carcinogens include chemicals, complex mixtures, and materials, such as all forms of asbestos, benzene, arsenic in the water, cadmium, ethylene oxide, benzo[a] pyrene, silica, as well as exposures to aluminum and coke production, iron and steel founding, or the rubber-manufacturing industry.

Further, some of the most potent and hazardous materials to which many of us are frequently exposed are: different kinds of pesticides found in the fruit, vegetables, and meat products we consume; dioxin found in commercial animal fats; chloroform found in the water; heavy metals found in aluminum cookware, certain types of fish, vaccines, dental amalgams, some toys, old lead pipes and lead-pigment paint; and mainly hundreds of artificial food additives and coloring in many of the foods we consume and materials (e.g., formaldehyde, parabens) used in cleansing, make-up, hygienic, and other body care products.

Air Pollution In the context of carcinogens, the IARC has identified air pollution as a cancer-causing agent in its own right [37]. This decision is based on the reasoning that outdoor air pollution is a major health hazard because of its ubiquity, the large number of people exposed to it all over the globe, and the continuous long duration of contact with air pollution. Indeed, it has long been known that outdoor air is carcinogenic because it includes carcinogens like diesel engine exhaust, solvents, metals, dust, and particulate matter which is a combination of tiny solid particles and liquid droplets in the air. However, the impact of air pollution is likely to increase because its major sources – transportation, industrial and agricultural emissions, energy generation, heating, and cooking – are likely to increase exponentially in the next decades. Recent studies unraveled some of the genetic pathways through which air pollution affects the occurrence of cancer [38]. According to the Global Burden of Disease Project air pollution was the fifth ranking mortality risk factor in 2015, responsible for 4.2 million deaths worldwide [39].

Radiation Ionizing radiation (i.e., radiation of specific wavelengths) has enough energy to damage DNA and is therefore considered as a risk factor for cancer. This kind of radiation includes radon (a radioactive gas emitted by rocks and soil in certain regions) and high-energy radiation, such as x-rays, gamma rays, alpha particles, beta particles, and neutrons [40, 41]. It is claimed that radiation from specific medical procedures, such as chest x-rays, computed tomography (CT) scans, positron-emission tomography (PET) scans, and radiation therapy for cancer may be also responsible for cell damage with carcinogenic potential. However, the risk is evaluated as minimal, especially when it is weighed against the benefits. Finally, lower-energy, non-ionizing forms of radiation, such as visible light and the energy from cell phones, microwave ovens, and electromagnetic fields are being investigated for carcinogenic effects with controversial findings so far. Other suspects include nighttime LED light and fluorescent lamps of all kinds.

Sunlight Exposure to UV radiation through sunlight, sunlamps, tanning booths, and other means was shown to be carcinogenic. It is particularly significant in regard to skin cancers, including melanoma, and possibly in regard to non-Hodgkin's lymphoma [e.g., 42]. The controversy about how certain we can be about the role of sun exposure in causing cancer [43] is misplaced in view of the fact that sunlight can be identified merely as one risk factor for skin cancers.

On the other hand, a certain modicum of sun exposure and certain levels of Vitamin D that may be produced by sun exposure have been shown to be protective factors for certain cancers, especially cancer of the colon, breast, prostate, ovary and leukemia [44].

Physiological Risk Factors

The physiologically based variables that have been identified as likely cancer-promoting factors include chronic inflammation, hormones, weakened immune system, and obesity.

Chronic Inflammation In contradistinction from regular inflammation involved in healing injured tissue, chronic inflammation may be caused by persisting infections or abnormal immune reactions to normal tissues. Over time, chronic inflammation can contribute to cancer by DNA damage, such as in the case of Crohn's disease [45, 46].

Weakened Immune System When the immune system is weak, it is less able to detect and destroy cancer cells or heal infections that may promote cancer. Any congenital or acquired immunodeficiency could in principle be a candidate to function as a risk factor for cancer. The immune system may be weakened by infection with HIV. Infection with HIV was shown to increase risk of lung cancer and mainly of cancers caused by infectious agents, including EBV; human herpesvirus 8 or Kaposi sarcoma-associated virus; HBV and HCV, which cause liver cancer; and human papillomavirus, which causes cervical, anal, oropharyngeal, and other cancers [47].

Another major reason for weakened immune system is immunosuppressive drugs given after organ transplants in order to prevent the rejection of the transplanted organ. Transplant recipients are particularly vulnerable to cancers caused by infectious agents, mainly non-Hodgkin's lymphoma (may be caused by Epstein-Barr virus) and liver cancer (may be caused by chronic infection with the hepatitis B (HBV) and hepatitis C (HCV) viruses, as well as lung and kidney cancers [48].

Over the years substantial evidence has accumulated about the effects of psychological stress on immune downregulation, acting through cellular and hormonal processes [49–51] (see Chap. 5).

Hormones Some hormones were shown to increase the chances for cancer. Best known are estrogen hormones, which may increase the chances for endometrial cancer, and estrogen together with progestin that increase the chances for breast cancer. Long exposure to high levels of these hormones, caused, for example, by starting menopause early, ending it late, or never having given birth, is considered as a risk factor for breast cancer. DES, a form of estrogen that had been used in the past in pregnancy treatment, was also shown to promote breast cancer. Similarly, IGF-1 and other factors related to sex hormones in women (specific oral contraceptives, hormonal replacement therapies, and hormonal treatments for increasing reproduction) seem to have carcinogenic potential for breast cancer or ovarian cancer [52, 53].

Previous Treatments, Diseases, or Cancer There is evidence showing that the occurrence of certain cancers may be followed after some time – short or long – by the occurrence of another kind of cancer, e.g., digestive and genitourinary primary neoplasms occurring often in adults who have survived pediatric cancers [54]. Other examples are the Lynch syndrome which may portend the occurrence of breast cancer [55] or Fanconi anemia that may portend the occurrence of prostate cancer [56]. The reasons could be reactions to treatments that have been undergone in the earlier cancer (e.g., radiotherapy), some common genetic source for the two kinds of cancer, or a weakened immune system due to the earlier neoplasm. Further, other possibilities are that there is a common source for the cancer and other diseases, as, for example, in the case of testicular cancer and hypoplasia and low fertility, whereby the latter may be regarded as a risk factor for the cancer [57]. In this context it may be appropriate to mention the possibility that some medications designed to cure specific disease may have side effects that enhance susceptibility to certain cancers. An example could be the diabetes medicine pioglitazone (Actos) which was announced by the FDA as possibly linked to an increased risk of bladder cancer if used over a year.

Obesity People who are obese may have an increased risk of several types of cancer [58], including cancers of the breast (in postmenopausal women), colon, rectum, endometrium (lining of the uterus), esophagus, kidney, pancreas, and gallbladder [59]. Possible mechanisms that could account for the documented increased risk for cancer are alteration in hormonal patterns, including insulin and insulin-like growth factors (IGFs), sex hormones, adipokines, and factors such as the distribution of body fat and changes in adiposity at different ages [60].

Food and Nutrition The impact of nutrition on cancer is a complicated issue, because nutrition includes a lot of different components, which might affect differently various cancers, and because it is mostly impossible to determine how much of the particular food is actually ingested by an individual. In any case, nutrition seems to be mainly a background factor that may impact cancer directly and indirectly, both as a risk factor and also as a protective factor [61].

There is a large body of data about the possible effects of specific nutrients on increasing or decreasing the risk for cancer, beyond the risk factors of additive chemicals, sweeteners, and food colorings mentioned above (materials and chemicals).

However, the evidence obtained in the laboratory studies has mostly not been supported sufficiently by epidemiological studies in large populations. Yet, there are some dietary materials for which there seems to be better scientific evidence. These include the following:

Heavy consumption of alcohol increases the risk of developing cancers of the oral cavity (excluding the lips), pharynx (throat), larynx (voice box), esophagus, liver, breast, colon, and rectum; higher intake of calcium appears to reduce the risk of colorectal cancer but probably not of other cancers and may even increase the risk for prostate cancer; cruciferous vegetables (cauliflower, broccoli) seem to reduce cancer risk; charred meat may be a risk factor for colorectal cancer [e.g. 62].

The guidelines of the American Cancer Society for the prevention of cancer include the following recommendations: focusing on vegetables, fruits, and whole grains and minimizing animal fat, salty products, and in general industrially prepared goods. The report emphasizes the absence of support for the contribution of vitamins A, C, and E [63].

Demographic Factors

Demographic background factors include variables that can be divided into two sets. The first includes age, gender, race/ethnicity, and marital status. The second includes variables, such as residential area, geographic region where one lives, education, income, and one's socioeconomic status. There is evidence that all the mentioned factors are related to cancer incidence or even mortality from cancer, but the kind of relation greatly differs for the variables of the first and the second sets. The variables of the first set affect cancer incidence more directly and may be considered as risk factors for cancer in some sense. The variables of the second set affect cancer incidence through the mediation of other factors, mainly availability of health services, possibility to undergo screening, and ease of access to medical diagnosis and treatment. Hence, the variables of the first set seem more directly related to cancer risk than the latter whose effect has a more distal character. The present section will therefore deal only with the variables of the first set.

Age Advancing age has been identified as one of the most important risk factors for cancer overall, as well as for many specific cancer types. The median age of cancer diagnosis in general is 66 and for specific common cancer types close to this age (e.g., prostate cancer 66, colorectal cancer 68, breast cancer 61) [64]. Statistics shows that the peak age range for cancer occurrence is 55–74 with a slow decline after 80 and low incidence up to 44. In older people the most common cancers are skin, lung, colorectal, breast (in women), and prostate (in men). Some cancers are more common in young adults, mainly leukemia and lymphoma. About 10% of leukemias are diagnosed in children and adolescents younger than 20, whereas cancer in general is on the whole less common in that age group.

It is generally assumed that the reason for the higher incidence of cancer in older adults is the accumulation of cellular damage with age. However, it needs to be emphasized that current statistics refer to the age of diagnosis and not to the age at which the cancer began, which is still mostly unidentified.

Gender In general cancer is less common in women than in men [65], except for specific cancers: breast cancer, the gynecological cancers and thyroid cancer. Overall, susceptibility is generally higher in males although some cancers are more common in women [66, 67]. Different studies uncovered genetic, molecular and hormonal factors that could account for the gender differences in cancer. One of the most intriguing hypotheses mentioned in order to account for the lower susceptibility of women to cancer is that women tend to mount higher innate and adaptive immune responses than males, which can result in faster destruction of pathogens. However, this same tendency can also contribute to enhanced susceptibility to inflammatory and autoimmune diseases in women than in men [66]. However, the likely impact of behavioral and lifestyle factors on gender disparity in cancer incidence cannot probably be ruled out [68].

Race/Ethnicity In the US the incidence of cancer is highest in African-Americans followed by Caucasians, Hispanics, Asian-Americans and American Natives [69]. Over 60% of new cancer cases world wide occur in Africa, Asia, and Central and South America [64]. These well known facts suggest strongly that race/ethnicity are a risk factor for cancer in general and undoubtedly also for specific cancers, e.g., black people are more prone to prostate cancer than white or Hispanic [70]. But the data does not yet allow at present to disentangle the network of genetic, environmental and socioeconomic factors responsible for these data.

Marital Status The results of large-scale studies about the relation of marital status to cancer risk are essentially unclear. While married individuals are a more homogenous group, the unmarried ones include widowed, divorced, separated, or never married individuals. This diversity of status could impact cancer risk differentially. On the whole the conclusion that is supported to some extent by diverse studies is that in itself marital status is not related negatively or positively to overall cancer risk but seems to be related to increased or decreased occurrence of specific cancers, for example, divorce was associated with increased risk for lung cancer and decreased risk for kidney or prostate cancer. Findings of this kind seem to be interpretable mainly as related to lifestyle habits such as smoking, physical activity, and diet, among others [71].

Afterthoughts About Protective Factors

A discussion of risk factors for cancer is incomplete without reference to protective factors. Protective factors constitute crucial elements in cancer prevention. Literature reviews show that there is less information about possible protective factors in regard to cancer than in regard to risk factors. Furthermore, there is little by way of theoretical or methodological clarification of the construct. In principle, protective factors could be defined as the obverse of risk factors, for example, if eating charred meat or being obese are considered as risk factors, it would be possible although not necessarily convincing to define low levels of these risk factors as protective factors. A better way would be to define protective factors in a positive manner in terms of variables that actively hinder the development of cancer. The latter could occur either by weakening directly or indirectly the agents or factors that promote cancer development or by strengthening those agents or factors that weaken or inhibit cancer development. Thus, in general terms in the context of the integrative model presented in this chapter, protective factors may be considered as factors contributing to lowering cancer risk either by weakening or moderating the effect of risk factors for cancer or by strengthening the action of factors that enhance the body's response to pathogens or risk factors for cancer.

Protective factors have been identified in different domains. At present most of the information concerns specific behaviors, medical procedures targeting specific cancers, and mainly nutrition [62] and physical exercise.

Specific Behaviors Specific behaviors are commonly known as having a protective value against cancer. These include avoiding active or passive smoking, using proper hygiene and protective measures in sexual behavior [21], and minimizing exposure to the sun and identified radioactive radiation sources.

Medical Procedures or Medications Targeting Specific Cancers Major examples concern various gynecological cancers. Examples of protective factors for ovarian cancer include breastfeeding, parity, and tubal ligation [72]; for endometrial cancer, the use of oral contraceptives [72]; for cervical cancer, vaccination against oncogenic HPV viruses [73]; for breast cancer, breastfeeding and possibly use of specific drugs [74]; and for prostate cancer, specific medications [75]. Preventive surgery has also been considered as a preventive measure mainly in regard to breast caster (mastectomy), ovarian cancer (oophorectomy or salpingo-oophorectomy), and endometrial cancer (hysterectomy).

Nutrition A large body of studies deals with identifying the major nutritional factors likely to contribute to reducing cancer occurrence or to act as protective factors in regard to particular cancers. The most often mentioned dietary components in this context are flax seed, especially its lignan fraction; fruits and vegetables, especially allium and cruciferous vegetables and broccoli sprouts being the densest source of sulforophane; antioxidants such as the carotenoids (alpha-carotene, beta-carotene, lycopene, lutein, cryptoxanthin); selenium; folic acid; vitamin B-12; vitamin D; chlorophyll; and possibly ascorbic acid, oral digestive enzymes, and probiotics [62]. In addition, there are nutritional recommendations for specific cancers, such as for prostate cancer, tomato lycopene, green tea epigallocatechin gallate, and soy phytoestrogens [76]; and for colorectal cancer, a diet rich in fruits and vegetables [77]. The evidence appears to be of a kind and at a level which seems to place the nutritional findings on the level of mere recommendations [63].

Physical Activity The information which links different kinds of physical activity with reduced risk for cancer is no less varied than the information concerning nutrition, in view of the need to consider amounts and kinds of physical activity for different kinds of individuals. Yet, on the whole the conclusions seem to be clearer. The findings support the recommendation of the American Cancer Society [63] and other national societies that a degree of physical activity which is continuous and at least moderate reduces the risk of different cancers in about 10% [78].

Summing Up and Some Conclusions

Our summary shows that on the whole, there is more information about risk factors than about the pathogens for cancer. Further, the number and variety of risk factors are really large. Yet, in most cases little is known about the duration of contact with the risk factor and the intensity of the risk factor that would actually impact the occurrence of cancer. A further complicating issue is that many of the risk factors tend to co-occur, sometimes due to an inherent factor as in the case of chlamydia that itself is not a risk factor for cervical cancer, but it tends to function with HPV in a way that promotes cancer growth [79]. Sometimes the co-occurrence of the risk factors may be more accidental, as in the case of a genetic propensity for cancer and the drinking of alcohol. It is likely that the impact of risk factors is cumulative, both horizontally and vertically in terms of time. The likelihood for the cofunctioning of several risk factors increases because of their sheer number and their ubiquitous nature. In other words, it is likely that a person may be a male, be exposed to several environmental carcinogenic materials, be overweight, and about 70 years old. Yet, in order to assess this person's potential risk for cancer, it would be necessary to know the kind, intensity, or severity of the environmental carcinogenic materials to which he has been exposed and for how long and of course also the extent and duration of his obesity. But even with this additional information, we would not be able to predict whether that person would get cancer. The bare minimum of missing information would be the extent of damaged DNA that that person would have, whether that person has been in contact with oncogenic pathogens, and the extent of protective factors that that person has. However, even improved information about the different risk and protective factors involved in cancer occurrence in general and in a specific case would merely serve as basis for the development and application of prediction models.

In sum, the complexity of the integrative approach to the occurrence of cancer carries essentially a positive message for all those interested in cancer prevention. The large number of involved risk and protective factors suggests that at least some are avoidable, and almost everyone can do something in order to safeguard oneself on the front of risk factors or protective factors.

Notably, the list of risk and protective factors in the present chapter will be extended by the psychosocial factors dealt with in Chap. 5.

References

1. Dowe, P. (2008). Causal processes. In E. N. Zalta (Ed.), *The Stanford encyclopedia of philosophy*. (Fall 2008 Edition). World Wide Web URL: https://plato.stanford.edu/. Stanford: The Metaphysics Research Lab Center for the Study of Language and Information, Stanford University.
2. Clarke, B. O. (2011). Causality in medicine with particular reference to the viral causation of cancers. A dissertation submitted in partial fulfillment of the requirements for the degree of Doctor of Philosophy of UCL Department of Science and Technology Studies UCL.
3. Engel, G. L. (1977). The need for a new medical model: A challenge for biomedicine. *Science, 196*, 129–136.
4. Frankel, R. M., Quill, T. E., & McDaniel, S. H. (Eds.). (2003). *The biopsychosocial approach: Past, present, future*. Rochester: University of Rochester Press.
5. Ghaemi, S. N. (2009). The rise and fall of the biopsychosocial model. *The British Journal of Psychiatry, 195*, 3–4.
6. Sarid, R., & Gao, S. J. (2011). Viruses and human cancer: From detection to causality. *Cancer Letters, 305*(2), 218–227.
7. Damania, B. (2007). DNA tumor viruses and human cancers: A long road of discovery of molecular paradigms. *Trends in Microbiology, 15*(1), 38–44.
8. Moore, P. S., & Chang, Y. (2014). Why do viruses cause cancer? Highlights of the first century of human tumor virology. *Clinical Microbiology Reviews, 27*(3), 463–481.
9. Zhang, X., Zhang, Z., Zheng, B., He, Z., Winberg, G., & Ernberg, I. (2013). An update on viral association of human cancers. *Archives of Virology, 158*(7), 1433–1443.
10. Mesri, E. A., Feitelson, M. A., & Munger, K. (2014). Human viral oncogenesis: A cancer hallmarks analysis. *Cell Host Microbe, 15*(3), 266–282.
11. Stamatiou, D. P., Derdas, S. P., Zoras, O. L., & Spandidos, D. A. (2016). Herpes and polyoma family viruses in thyroid cancer. *Oncology Letters, 11*(3), 1635–1644.
12. Cornwall, C. (2013). *Catching cancer: The quest for its viral and bacterial causes*. Lanham: Rowman & Littlefield Publishers.
13. Chang, A. H., & Parsonnet, J. (2010). Role of bacteria in oncogenesis. *Clinical Microbiology Reviews, 23*(4), 837–857.
14. Sinkovics, J. (2011). Molecular biology of oncogenic inflammatory processes. I. Non-oncogenic and oncogenic pathogens, intrinsic inflammatory reactions without pathogens, and microRNA/DNA interactions. *International Journal of Oncology, 40*, 305–349.

15. Khurana, S., Dubey, M. L., & Malla, N. (2005). Association of parasitic infections and cancers. *Indian Journal of Medical Microbiology, 23*, 74–79.
16. Mostafa, M. H., Sheweita, S. A., & O'Connor, P. J. (1999). Relationship between schistosomiasis and bladder cancer. *Clinical Microbiology Reviews, 12*(1), 97–111.
17. Matloff, E. (2013). *Cancer principles and practice of oncology: Handbook of clinical cancer genetics*. 1 Pap/Psc Edition. Philadelphia: Lippincott Williams & Wilkins, a Walters Kluver business.
18. Sharma, S., Kelly, T. K., & Jones, P. A. (2010). Epigenetics in cancer. *Carcinogenesis, 31*(1), 27–36. [see page 27].
19. Feinberg, A. P., Ohlsson, R., & Henikoff, S. (2006). The epigenetic progenitor origin of human cancer. *National Review of Genetics, 7*, 21–33.
20. Dumitrescu, R., & Verma, M. (2012). Cancer epigenetics: Methods and protocols. *Methods in Molecular Biology, 863*, 177–185.
21. Ornish, D., Magbanua, M. J., Weidner, G., Weinberg, V., Kemp, C., Green, C., Mattie, M. D., Marlin, R., Shimko, J., Shinohara, K., Hagg, C. M., & Carroll, R. R. (2008). Changes in prostate gene expression in men undergoing an intensive nutrition and lifestyle intervention. *Proceedings of the National Academy of Science, 105*(24), 8369–8374.
22. Herrero, R., Brinton, T. L. A., Reeves, W. C., Gaitan, E., Garcia, B. M., Rawls, W. E., Brenes, M. M., Tenorio, F., & De Britton, R. C. (1990). Sexual behavior, venereal diseases, hygiene practices, and invasive cervical cancer in a high-risk population. *Cancer, 65*, 380–386.
23. Hashibe, M., Brennan, P., Chuang, S. C., Boccia, S., Castellsague, X., Chen, C., et al. (2009). Interaction between tobacco and alcohol use and the risk of head and neck cancer: Pooled analysis in the international head and neck cancer epidemiology consortium. *Cancer Epidemiology Biomarkers Prevention, 18*(2), 541–550.
24. U.S. Department of Health and Human Services. (2006). *The health consequences of involuntary exposure to tobacco smoke: A report of the surgeon general*. Rockville: U.S. Department of Health and Human Services, Centers for Disease Control and Prevention, Coordinating Center for Health Promotion, National Center for Chronic Disease Prevention and Health Promotion, Office on Smoking and Health.
25. Vacho, C. M., Kuni, C. C., Anderson, K., & Sellers, T. (2000). Association of mammographically defined percent breast density with epidemiologic risk factors for breast cancer (United States). *Cancer Causes & Control, 11*(7), 653–662.
26. Siemiatycki, J., Richardson, L., Straif, K., Latreille, B., Lakhani, R., Campbell, S., Rousseau, M.-C., & Boffetta, P. (2004). Listing occupational carcinogens. *Environmental Health Perspectives, 112*(15), 1447–1459.
27. World Health Organization. (2011). *Environmental and occupational cancers: An overview of the evidence on environmental and occupational determinants of cancer*. Fact sheet N°350. Geneva: WHO.
28. Surgeon General's Report. (2012). *Smoking and tobacco use: Preventing tobacco use among youth and young adults*. Washington, DC: CDC: Centers for Disease Control and Prevention. Public Health Service.
29. Brennan, P., Crispo, A., Zaridze, D., Szeszenia-Dabrowska, N., Rudnai, P., Lissowska, J., Fabiánová, E., Mates, D., Bencko, V., Foretova, L., Janout, V., Fletcher, T., & Boffetta, P. (2006). High cumulative risk of lung cancer death among smokers and nonsmokers in central and eastern Europe. *American Journal of Epidemiology, 164*(12), 1233–1241.
30. Eysenck, H. J. (2000). *Smoking health and personality*. London: Transaction Press. (originally published 1965).
31. Siepman, J. P. (1999). Smoking does not cause lung cancer. *Journal of Theoretics. 1–4*. October/November Editorial. pp. 1–2.
32. Brandon, T. H., & Unrod, M. (2010). Tobacco use and cessation. In J. C. Holland, R. S. Breitbart, P. B. Jacobsen, S. Lederberg, M. J. Loscalzo, & R. McCorkle (Eds.), *Psycho-oncology* (2nd ed., pp. 15–21). New York: Oxford University Press. [especially p. 15].
33. World Health Organization, Agency for Research on Cancer. (2004). Tobacco smoke and involuntary smoking. IARC Monographs on the Evaluation of Carcinogenic Risks to Humans,

Vol 83, Working Group on the Evaluation of Carcinogenic Risks to Humans, which met in Lyon, 11–18 June 2002. Lyon.
34. Sobus, S. L., & Warren, G. W. (2014). Biologic effects of cigarette smoke on cancer cells. *Cancer, 120*(23), 3617–3626.
35. Xi, S., Xu, H., Shan, J., Tao, Y., Hong, J. A., Inchauste, S., Zhang, M., Kunst, T. F., Mercedes, L., & Schrump, D. S. (2013). Cigarette smoke mediates epigenetic repression of miR-487b during pulmonary carcinogenesis. *The Journal of Clinical Investigation, 123*(3), 1241–1261.
36. National Toxicology Program. (2014). *The report on carcinogens*. Washington, DC: National Institute of Environmental Health Sciences (NIEHS).
37. Straif, K., Cohen, A., & Samet, J. (Eds.). (2013). *Air pollution and cancer* (IARC Scientific Publications, No. 161). Lyon: International Agency for Research on Cancer. Distributed by WHO Press, World Health Organization, Geneva, Switzerland.
38. Viners, P. (2013). Biomarkers of air pollution: DNA and protein adducts. In K. Straif, A. Cohen, & J. Samet (Eds.), *Air pollution and cancer* (IARC Scientific Publications, No. 161) (pp. 149–164). Lyon: International Agency for Research on Cancer. Distributed by WHO Press, World Health Organization, Geneva, Switzerland.
39. Cohen, A. J., Brauer, M., Burnett, R., Anderson, H. R., Frostad, J., et al. (2017). Estimates and 25-year trends of the global burden of disease attributable to ambient air pollution: An analysis of data from the Global Burden of Diseases Study 2015. *The Lancer, 389*, 1907–1918.
40. IARC. (2000). *Ionizing radiation, part 1: X- and gamma-radiation, and neutrons, IARC monographs on the evaluation of carcinogenic risks to humans* (Vol. 75). Lyon: IARC.
41. IARC. (2001). *Ionizing radiation, part 2: Some internally deposited radionuclides* (IARC Monographs on the Evaluation of Carcinogenic Risks to Humans) (Vol. 78). Lyon: IARC.
42. Adami, J., Frish, M., Yuen, J., Glimelius, B., & Melbye, M. (1995). Evidence of an association between non-Hodgkin's lymphoma and skin cancer. *British Medical Journal, 310*, 1491–1495.
43. Lucas, R. M., McMichael, A., Armstrong, B., & Smith, W. (2008). Estimating the global disease burden due to ultraviolet radiation exposure. *International Journal of Epidemiology, 37*(3), 654–667.
44. Berwick, M., & Hay, J. (2010). Sun exposure and cancer risk. In J. C. Holland, R. S. Breitbart, P. B. Jacobsen, S. Lederberg, M. J. Loscalzo, & R. McCorkle (Eds.), *Psycho-oncology* (2nd ed., pp. 43–46). New York: Oxford University Press.
45. Khatami, M. (2016). Is cancer a severe delayed hypersensitivity reaction and histamine a blueprint? *Journal of Translational Medicine, 5*(1), 35.
46. Coussens, L. M., & Werb, Z. (2002). Inflammation and cancer. *Nature, 420*, 860–867.
47. Clifford, G. M., Polesel, J., Rickenbach, M., Maso, L. D., Keiser, O., Kofler, A., Rapiti, E., Levi, F., Jundt, G., & Fisch, T. (2005). Cancer risk in the Swiss HIV cohort study: Associations with immunodeficiency, smoking, and highly active antiretroviral therapy. *Journal of the National Cancer Institute, 97*(6), 425–432.
48. Dantal, J., & Soulillou, J.-P. (2005). Immunosuppressive drugs and the risk of cancer after organ transplantation. *New England Journal of Medicine, 352*(13), 1371–1373.
49. Kiecolt-Glaser, J. K., & Glaser, R. (1999). Psychoneuroimmunology and cancer: Fact or fiction? *European Journal of Cancer, 35*(11), 1603–1607.
50. McDonald, P. G., O'Connell, M., & Lutgendorf, S. K. (2013). Psychoneuroimmunology and cancer: A decade of discovery, paradigm shifts, and methodological innovations. *Brain, Behavior and Immunity, 30*(0), S1–S9.
51. Segerstrom, S. C., & Miller, G. E. (2004). Psychological stress and the human immune system: A meta-analytic study of 30 years of inquiry. *Psychological Bulletin, 130*(4), 601–630.
52. Lacey, J. V., Jr., Mink, P. J., Lubin, J. H., Sherman, M. E., Troisi, R., Hartge, P., Schatzkin, A., & Schairer, C. (2002). Menopausal hormone replacement therapy and risk of ovarian cancer. *JAMA, 288*(3), 334–341.
53. Chlebowski, R. T., Kuller, L. H., Prentice, R. L., et al. (2009). Breast cancer after use of estrogen plus progestin in postmenopausal women. *New England Journal of Medicine, 360*(6), 573–587.

54. Reulen, R. C., Frobisher, C., Winter, D. L., Kelly, J., Lancashire, E. R., Stiller, C. A., Pritchard-Jones, A., Jenkinson, H. C., Hawkins, M. M., & British Childhood Cancer Survivor Study Steering Group. (2011). Long- term risks of subsequent primary neoplasms among survivors of childhood cancer. *JAMA, 305*(22), 2311–2319.
55. Win, A. K., Lindor, N. M., & Jenkins, M. A. (2013). Risk of breast cancer in Lynch syndrome: A systematic review. *Breast Cancer Research, 15*(2), R27.
56. Chen, H., Zhang, S., & Wu, Z. (2014). Fanconi anemia pathway defects in inherited and sporadic cancers. *Translational Pediatrics, 3*(4), 300–304.
57. Schnack, T. H., Poulsen, G., Myrup, C., Wohlfahrt, J., & Melbye, M. (2010). Familial coaggregation of cryptorchidism, hypospadias, and testicular germ cell cancer: A nationwide cohort study. *Journal of the National Cancer Institute, 102*(3), 187–192.
58. Engguist, K. B., & Chang, M. (2011). Obesity and cancer risk: Recent review and evidence. *Current Oncological Reports, 13*(1), 71–76.
59. World Cancer Research Fund/American Institute for Cancer Research. (2007). *Food, nutrition, physical activity, and the prevention of cancer: A global perspective*. Washington, DC: AICR.
60. Nock, N. L., & Berger, N. A. (2010). Obesity and cancer: Overview of mechanisms. In N. A. Berger (Ed.), *Cancer and energy balance, epidemiology and overview* (pp. 129–179). New York: Springer.
61. Fitzgibbon, M. I., & Stolley, R. (2010). Diet and cancer. In J. C. Holland, R. S. Breitbart, P. B. Jacobsen, S. Lederberg, M. J. Loscalzo, & R. McCorkle (Eds.), *Psycho-oncology* (2nd ed., pp. 22–27). New York: Oxford University Press.
62. Donaldson, M. S. (2004). Nutrition and cancer: A review of the evidence for an anti-cancer diet. *Nutrition Journal, 3*(19), 1–21.
63. Kushi, L. H., Doyle, C., McCullough, M., Rock, C. L., Demark-Wahnefried, W., Bandera, E. V., Gapstur, Patel, A. P., Andrews, K., & Gansler, T. (2012). American Cancer Society guidelines on nutrition and physical activity for cancer prevention: Advisory Committee. Reducing the risk of cancer with healthy food choices and physical activity. Washington, DC.
64. Howlader, N., Noone, A. M., Krapcho, M., Miller, D., Bishop, K., Kosary, C. L., Yu, M., Ruhl, J., Tatalovich, Z., Mariotto, A., Lewis, D. R., Chen, H. S., Feuer, E. J., & Cronin, K. A. (Eds.). (April, 2018). *SEER cancer statistics review, 1975–2014, NCI's surveillance, epidemiology, and end results program*. Bethesda: National Cancer Institute.
65. Nguyen, S. P., Bent, S., Chen, Y. H., & Terdiman, J. P. (2009). Gender as a risk factor for advanced neoplasia and colorectal cancer: A systematic review and meta-analysis. *Clinical Gastroenterolgry and Hepatology, 7*(6), 676–681.
66. Dorak, M. T., & Karpuzoglu, E. (2012). Gender differences in cancer susceptibility: An inadequately addressed issue. *Frontiers in Genetics, 3*, 268.
67. Ferlay, J., Soerjomataram, I., Dikshit, R., Eser, E., Mathers, C., Rebelo, M., Parki, D. M., Forman, D., & Bray, F. (2015). Cancer incidence and mortality worldwide: Sources, methods and major patterns in GLOBOCAN. *International Journal of Cancer, 136*, E359–E386.
68. Demark-Wahnefried, W., Peterson, B., McBride, C., Lipkus, I., & Clipp, E. (2000). Current health behaviors and readiness to pursue life-style changes among men and women diagnosed with early stage prostate and breast carcinomas. *Cancer, 88*(3), 674–684.
69. American Cancer Society. (2011). *American Cancer Society. Global cancer facts and figures* (2nd ed.). Atlanta: American Cancer Society. 57 pp.
70. Farrell, J., Petrovics, G., McLeod, D. G., & Srivastava, S. (2013). Genetic and molecular differences in prostate carcinogenesis between African American and Caucasian American men. *International Journal of Molecular Sciences, 14*(1), 5510–5531.
71. Helgeson, V. S., & McUmber, A. I. (2010). Social environment and cancer. In J. C. Holland, R. S. Breitbart, P. B. Jacobsen, S. Lederberg, M. J. Loscalzo, & R. McCorkle (Eds.), *Psycho-oncology* (2nd ed., pp. 62–68). New York: Oxford University Press.
72. DeVita, V. T., Jr., Lawrence, T. S., Rosenberg, S. A., DePinho, R. A., & Weinberg, R. A. (2015). *Devita, Hellman, and Rosenberg's cancer: Principles and practice of oncology* (10th ed.). Philadelphia: Lippincott Williams & Wilkins.

73. Frazer, I. H. (2004). Prevention of cervical cancer through papillomavirus vaccination. *Nature Reviews Immunology, 4*, 46–55.
74. Moyer, F. A. (2013). Medications to decrease the risk for breast cancer in women: Recommendations from the U.S. Preventive Services Task Force recommendation statement. *Annals of Internal Medicine, 159*(10), 698–708.
75. Nordstrom, T., Clements, M., Karlsson, R., Adolfson, J., & Gronberg, H. (2015). The risk of prostate cancer for men on aspirin, statin or antidiabetic medications. *European Journal of Cancer, 51*(6), 725–733.
76. Adjakly, M., Ngolio, M., Dagdemir, A., Judes, G., Paion, A., Karsli-Ceppioglu, F., Boiteux, J. P., Bignon, Y., Guy, L., & Bernard-Gallon, D. (2015). Prostate cancer: The main risk and protective factors-epigenetic modifications. *Annals of Endocrinology, 76*(1), 25–41.
77. Slattery, M. L., Boucher, K. M., Caan, B. J., Potter, J. D., & Ma, K. N. (1998). Eating patterns and risk of colon cancer. *American Journal of Epidemiology, 148*(1), 4.
78. Pinto, B. M., & Hartman, S. J. (2010). Exercise and cancer. In J. C. Holland, R. S. Breitbart, P. B. Jacobsen, S. Lederberg, M. J. Loscalzo, & R. McCorkle (Eds.), *Psycho-oncology* (2nd ed., pp. 28–42). New York: Oxford University Press.
79. Josefson, D. (2001). Chlamydia increases risk of cervical cancer. *British Medical Journal, 322*(7278), 71.

Chapter 5
Psychosocial Risk Factors for Cancer

Psychosocial Risk Factors for Cancer: What Is the Problem?

Psychosocial variables seem to be in an inferior position insofar as their potential role as risk factors for cancer is considered. This is manifested in a pronounced skepticism about the role of psychological factors in regard to cancer that is expressed in a great number of reviews, chapters, studies, commentaries, etc. referring to this theme [1, 2]. This point of view is surprising especially since it is applied primarily in regard to psychological factors and not in regard to other possible risk factors like nutrition. While nutrition may not be acclaimed at least by some investigators as the source of important or convincing risk or protective factors, it is not laid low or even overlooked as psychological factors often are. The publicly presented rationale for this approach is in most cases methodological, e.g., the design of the studies dealing with psychological factors is inadequate, there is not enough control of other factors that could have affected the results, and there is no proof that the cancer was actually due to the psychological factors. These reasons are certainly convincing and applicable, but as already mentioned, they apply also in regard to other risk factors that have been adopted in this context, for example, sun exposure or physical activity. It is unlikely that factors such as weight, nutrition, genetic background, and comorbidities have been assessed in each study reporting some association between sun exposure and cancer, not to mention the fact that duration and frequency of exposure to the sun and radiation level have mostly not been checked. Despite these methodological shortcomings, sun exposure, for example, is considered seriously as a risk factor for cancer. Further, psychological studies are also criticized for lack of plausible mechanisms linking the psychological variables to cancer. Again, the same claim could be leveled against many of the commonly discussed risk factors. Moreover, when mechanisms are mentioned, they are mostly hypothetical.

In most reviews about psychosocial factors and cancer, several studies are presented with negative results. However, a computer search of Medline library resources conducted on February 18, 2017 brought up 139,796 research/study items

S. Kreitler, *Psycho-Oncology for the Clinician*,
https://doi.org/10.1007/978-3-030-06126-5_5

for the words “Personality or psychological risk factors for cancer.” It is unlikely that none of the presented studies fit the required methodological criteria. Even a rather superficial scan of this big file of studies readily reveals several high-quality studies. The theme of the controversial status of psychological factors in regard to cancer is dealt in the present context because of its importance for science in general, as well as for the status of psychology and for the role of psychology in regard to the study of cancer.

At the risk of being blamed for irrelevance, some possible reasons that might account for the somewhat odd attitude to psychosocial risk factors will be mentioned. One reason could be the problematic case of a whole set of studies about the association of personality with cancer by Hans J. Eysenck and Grossarth-Maticek published between 1981 and 1991 [3]. The reported findings were impressive. But unfortunately attempts at replication either failed or resulted in opposite findings [4, 5]. Furthermore, it turned out to be impossible to locate many of the subjects who have allegedly participated in these studies. There were many criticisms, countercriticisms, and a heated discussion focused on this body of research. Finally it was simply pushed aside and stayed in the scientific memory marked as possibly not quite veridical [3]. This impression was further enhanced by the suspicion that the authors may have had a personal interest in proving the effect of personality on cancer, possibly because among other things, they have been funded by the cigarette companies. Although these studies dealt more with psychological correlates of cancer and with their impact on mortality, they cast a shadow of distrust on the whole domain of personality and cancer. However, an even worse situation occurred when an outright accusation of fraud has been leveled against Cyril Burt’s work on intelligence. Yet, this has not resulted in a general distrust of work on intelligence.

To our mind, two aspects of the theme of personality and cancer deserve consideration. One aspect is of a methodological nature. Assigning legitimacy to the potential impact of personality on the risk of cancer may imply that psychological factors are involved also in the impact of other risk factors in regard to cancer, such as sun exposure, physical activity, nutrition, use of tobacco, and even contact with toxic materials. There are already studies suggesting that at least some of these risk factors depend on psychological tendencies. Thus, in order to understand the impact of a risk factor like sun exposure, it would be necessary to identify the antecedent psychological variables of this risk factor which may be involved in its activation and rendering the person vulnerable to the radiation effect [6]. Moreover, focusing on the relevant psychological factors may enhance the success of the different intervention procedures applied for reducing exposure to this or another risk factor.

And this is where the second consideration enters the scene. There is some kind of tendency to recoil from considering psychological factors as involved in the risk for cancer. The reason may be that many people tend to draw from this statement the implication that the situation is actually under their control and hence they are to blame for the cancer. People assume for some reason that psychological factors are not really serious variables and that they can be changed or manipulated at will so that if they get cancer, the responsibility for this resides in them. Moreover, since there is a general tendency to protect cancer patients from unnecessary suffering, even professionals do not necessarily gainsay the wrong conclusion that the involvement of psychological factors means that the person himself/herself is actually at least in some form responsible for the unfortunate outcome. It is as if they sacrifice psychology for the benefit of the patients.

In the following sections, the psychological factors including emotions and personality will be presented in the same form and following the same criteria as the other risk factors (Chap. 4).

Emotional Variables

Anti-emotionality

Different aspects of emotions have been studied as potential risk factors for cancer. Anti-emotionality figures as one of the most salient features whose potential role as a risk factor of cancer was explored. It goes under different labels, including suppression or repression of emotions, rationality, or emotional control, and sometimes it may be referred to as defensive style. It forms also part of the cancer-prone personality defined by Temoshok [7]. Earlier studies [8–11] often found evidence for the connection between anti-emotionality and the incidence of cancer, especially breast cancer. More modern studies mostly did not find evidence for this connection. For example, a methodologically exceptionally well-designed study published after a 6-year follow-up found that only anti-emotionality (i.e., no emotional behavior or lack of trust in one's feelings) had a weak relationship to the incidence of breast cancer [12], but a longer follow-up of 13 years did not confirm this finding or for that matter also not in regard to anxiety, anger, rationality, anti-emotionality, emotional expression-in, emotional expression-out, and emotional control [13]. Similarly a study of men showed no relation [14]. One study even showed a reverse relationship in that suppressed emotional expression was related to lower risk for breast cancer although rational anti-emotionality was related to a tendency for higher incidence of "other cancers" [15]. More indirect evidence for the positive correlation between cancer incidence and anti-emotionality comes from studies which showed that breast cancer risk was related to the use of defensive mechanisms, including denial, intellectualization, and rationalization [16], and to a tendency for reduced commitment to one's family and work [17] and higher scores in alexithymia [18], not always replicated [19]. Insight into the possible background of the tendency for anti-emotionality is provided by the following study which showed that defensiveness scores rose in the group of patients after they were diagnosed positively with breast cancer, whereas prior to the diagnosis, they did not differ in defensiveness or anxiety from those with benign breast disease or healthy controls [20, 21]. Hence it is likely that repression and anti-emotionality are not traits of cancer patients but coping mechanisms used for handling an anxiety bound with cancer.

A review of prospective longitudinal studies led to the intriguing conclusion that repression may have some kind of negative effect on cancer diagnosis, whereas denial and minimizing may have a positive effect [22]. Accordingly, in recent years the theme of anti-emotionality has been set aside, in the best case as irrelevant and in the worst case as wrong. One may well wonder how did this happen in regard to a psychological variable that originally seemed to have some psychological reality. The situation could resemble the development in regard to Type A in cardiology. It is likely that Type A referred originally to a real construct. However, when it became a theme for the media, individuals became reluctant to admit they had the Type A features so as not to be suspected of tendencies for cardiological diseases. Furthermore, at least some of those who learned about Type A may have undertaken changes in their behavior and attitudes so as to suppress or mitigate their Type A tendencies and thus overcome the risk of getting a heart attack. Hence, it is not unlikely that anti-emotionality was subjected to a similar fate by people scared of getting cancer.

Depression

Depression has been suspected for decades as a possible risk factor for cancer. This assumption has been enhanced by hypotheses about likely physiological pathways linking depression with cancer risk, for example, depression decreases the immune function, inhibits DNA repair mechanisms, and may underlie dysregulation of the stress hormone cortisol [23]. The results are mixed. Some studies show that depression in the years prior to the occurrence of cancer was predictive of breast cancer or other cancers (e.g., [24–26]), whereas other studies showed that there was no link between depression and onset of cancer [27–29]. One study even showed that depression had a protective role in regard to breast cancer [30]. Notably, in these studies, psychiatric diagnoses, self-reports, and different scales for assessing depression were used. In some studies, the follow-up period was over 15 years. However, two important considerations set serious doubt on the conclusions concerning the impact of depression on cancer risk. The first is that since cancer develops over a long period of time prior to the manifestation of external symptoms, the effects of depression need to be studied in correlation with the physiological development of cancer. Without this information, the occurrence of depression could be simply the reaction of the individuals to sensations of the developing cancer. Accordingly, a review of studies in this domain showed that studies with a longer follow-up had a better chance to indicate a relation between depression and the risk of cancer [31]. Secondly, since some antidepressants have been found to promote cancer, it is possible that the risk for cancer was promoted by the medication rather than by the depression which it was supposed to combat [32].

Anxiety and Anger

Anxiety and anger are two negative emotions whose potential role as cancer risk factors was studied. Anxiety seemed as a potential factor because of its ubiquity in cancer patients and strong component of stress that it includes. The status of anxiety in this context has been appreciably promoted by the finding that ATF3 which acts as the master gene for anxiety, activated when cells experience stressful conditions, may cause immune cells to malfunction and allow cancer cells to metastasize, promoting the development of cancer [33]. Some studies indicated that the overall cancer risk, including lung and prostate cancer, is elevated in patients diagnosed with generalized anxiety disorder [34] and that urological cancer risk is higher in patients suffering from anxiety disorders [35]. However, the role of anxiety as a risk factor for cancer was not confirmed in other studies [12, 13, 36]. There are even indications that cancer patients do not differ from control subjects prior to the diagnosis but score higher on anxiety only after getting the diagnosis [20].

Concerning anger, some studies showed that anger, mainly in the form of unexpressed or pent-up anger, may contribute to the risk of developing cancer [37, 38]. Other studies however showed that anger control or tendency to experience anger had no significant relation to cancer occurrence [13, 39, 40]. A more complicated set of findings indicates that anger control and negative affect are not associated with breast cancer, melanoma, or total cancer risk, although they may have a small role in risk of prostate, colorectal, and lung cancer [41].

Stress

Stress has been linked to cancer and other diseases in two major forms: as an explanatory construct for the occurrence of disease on the basis of physiological data and in terms of self-reported stress preceding the disease [42]. In the present context, stress is considered as an experienced emotion, as reported directly by the individuals. In some studies the intensity and frequency of reported stress were found to precede the diagnosis of cancer (e.g., [43, 44]). Notably, the interpretation of these findings may be difficult because experienced stress may result from multiple very different reasons. However, work-related stress of daily activities, for example, in large prospective cohorts of nurses over 6 years provided no evidence for a link between reported stress and the occurrence of cancer in women [45–48]. These findings indicate that probably only specific kinds of stress contribute to cancer occurrence (for the effects of chronic stress, see below complicated grief).

Life Events and Traumas

Reported stress is often closely linked with reported stressful life events. Stressful life events are the oldest suspected psychological risk factor for cancer. Two kinds of life events are often distinguished. One type refers to relatively recent life events. Several studies showed that stressful life events in the years preceding the occurrence of cancer increased the chances for cancer [8, 49, 50]. Stressful life events often refer to loss of a spouse or another family member by death sometimes accompanied by prolonged bereavement known as "traumatic grief" including despair, loss, anger, frustration, and hopelessness. The evidence that the presence of traumatic grief symptoms about 6 months after the death of the spouse predicted cancer 13–25 months follow-up (15.4% in the group with traumatized grief vs 0% in the other) suggests that the risk consists not in the stress bereavement as such but in the mental health complications to which it gives rise [51]. Thus, a study performed with the Finnish twin cohort who responded to the standard life events questionnaire showed that both the total number of life events in the 5 preceding years and especially events as divorce/separation, death of a husband, and death of a close relative or friend were associated significantly with increased risk of breast cancer [45]. Another study of particular interest compared the incidence of cancer over a period of over 20 years in 6284 Jewish Israelis who lost an adult son in the Yom Kippur War or in an accident between 1970 and 1977 and in non-bereaved members of the population. The results showed an increased incidence of lymphatic and hematopoietic malignancies and melanomas among parents of accident victims and among war-bereaved parents, as well as more lung cancer cases in accident-bereaved parents [52]. There is further evidence that exposure to war conditions increases the risk for cancer. Thus, individuals who lived through the Leningrad famine or other serious famines had an increased risk for cancer in later years [53]. The same phenomenon was found in regard to holocaust survivors [54]. A study which compared cancer rates in Jewish people who immigrated to Israel after 1945 (so that they had been exposed to the holocaust) or before found 17% increase in risk for all types of cancer in the former group. The effect was particularly pronounced in the case of children and toddlers. Survivors born between 1940 and 1945 had a higher overall risk of cancer than those not exposed to the holocaust (3.5 times higher in males and 2.3 higher in females) [55].

Another type of life events refers to early traumata, conforming to what has been defined as adverse childhood experiences (ACE), such as physical torture, beatings, starvation, physical neglect, or sexual molestation [56]. Several studies showed that individuals who have been exposed to ACE in their childhood had a higher chance of getting cancer in adulthood. Compared to persons without ACEs, the risk of lung cancer for those with at least six ACEs was increased about threefold. With control over smoking, the effect turned insignificant but still those with over six ACES were about 13 years younger when the cancer appeared than the others [57]. Again, a study based on the 1958 cohort in Britain showed that the chances of women getting cancer before the age of 50 was twofold higher for those who had over two ACEs versus those with none [58]. Cancer in adulthood was found to be associated especially with sexual abuse variables of ACE [59]. A review of the literature showed that especially physical and psychological abuse victimization in early childhood was associated with risk of any cancer and that sexual abuse was associated more with the risk for cervical cancer [60]. Only in some studies, there was a relation between specific kinds of abuse and specific cancers rather than any cancer.

Personality

Personality Traits

As early as AD 200, Galen noted the personality traits of women with breast cancer whom he considered to be higher in melancholy and lower in sanguine tendencies. The personality traits investigated in modern times focus mainly on a rather limited set. A preliminary study by Kissen and Eysenck [61] claimed that lung cancer patients scored high on extraversion and low on neuroticism. The results of further studies that focused on these tendencies using mostly the Eysenck Personality Test were controversial. Some found evidence for an association of extraversion or neuroticism with some kinds of cancer [62, 63], but other studies in large samples, different cultures, long periods of follow-up, and control over several relevant variables found no evidence for any relation between neuroticism and extraversion with any type of cancer [13, 39, 40, 45, 64–66].

Beliefs, Attitudes, and Meanings

The studied traits were shown to be unrelated to cancer risk. However, there are additional individual tendencies that can be examined for the role they may play in regard to cancer [67]. The approach based on the cognitive orientation theory assumes that beliefs of specific kinds representing meanings relevant for specific disorders could be identified and their function as potential risk factors for cancer may be explored. This assumption has been tested in regard to different disorders, such as cardiological disorders, diabetes Type 2, or high blood pressure [68]. The two major theoretical components of cognitive orientation are the motivational disposition and operational program. The motivational disposition defines the direction of the involved processes, for example, health, recovery, or disease. The operational program defines the manner in which it is carried out, focusing on the processes involved in implementing the motivational disposition, including the overall program, the strategy, and the different operational steps. The motivational disposition answers as it were the implicit question "where to," whereas the operational program answers the implicit question "how, in which manner." Both are essential for the performance or occurrence of a disorder. Although beliefs and meanings contribute to the motivational disposition, it is not based on a conscious decision; it does not reflect some consideration of pros and cons and is not under voluntary control. It can however become conscious if one gets adequate guidance. This is being done in the framework of the cognitive orientation intervention for patients.

The Cognitive Orientation Approach: The Motivational Disposition

The motivational disposition is a vector that is grounded in four types of beliefs which represent specific themes. The four types of beliefs are (a) *beliefs about oneself*, which express information about oneself, such as one's habits, actions, or feelings (e.g., "I often get angry," "I was born in a big city"); (b) *general beliefs*, which express information concerning others, situations, and the environment (e.g., "The world is a dangerous place," "Small lies may solve big problems"); (c) *beliefs about rules and norms*, which express ethical, esthetic, social, and other rules and standards (e.g., "One should not be aggressive," "In order to succeed one should work hard"); and (d) *beliefs about goals*, which express actions or states desired or undesired by the individual (e.g., "I want to be respected by others"). The beliefs must not necessarily be logical or veridical, although they may be both.

Formally, the beliefs differ in two respects. Firstly, they differ in the subject of the belief – in beliefs about self and goals, the subject is the self, and in general beliefs and norms, it is nonself; and secondly, they differ in the relation between the subject and the predicate: in beliefs about self and general beliefs, the relation is factual, in norms the relation is the desirable, and in goals the relation is the desired [69–71].

All four belief types should be involved in the motivational disposition for any state of health. Exceptions may occur in cases, for example, when one or more belief types are simply missing (e.g., for lack of relevant beliefs in one or more belief types) or when two belief types coalesce (e.g., beliefs about goals represent what one thinks one should do, or general beliefs represent not how things actually are but how one thinks they should be).

Thus, the motivational disposition in regard to each state of health consists formally of the four belief types, but in each case, the contents of the beliefs differ, representing themes that are relevant specifically for the particular state of health. Relevance is defined in this context in terms of relations of meaning. The role of meaning is clarified by the procedure used for identifying the themes. The procedure consists of two major stages. *The first stage* is devoted to identifying potential themes by a systematic stepwise interviewing of a small number of individuals with the particular diagnosis and without it. The interviewing consists in a stepwise exploration of meaning which starts with the general interpersonally shared meaning of the studied state of health and proceeds to questions about the personal-subjective meaning of the answer provided previously. This procedure is applied sequentially three times, each time reaching deeper levels of meaning. The interviewing stops at the third level, which was found to contain the themes likely to be most relevant for identifying underlying motivations for disorders. In contrast, themes identified on a deeper level are too general, and those on a more superficial level prove to be too close to the explicit meanings of the disorder itself. After interviewing a sample of pretest individuals with the disorder and a sample of pretest individuals without the disorder, the themes identified in at least 50% of the former sample and in less than 50% of the latter sample are pulled together. The interviewing continues until at least 8–12 themes corresponding to the mentioned criteria can be identified. Usually the required sample size is about 10–20 subjects of both groups together. The first stage ends when the expected number of themes has been identified in the preliminary interviews. The identified themes at the end of the first stage are merely hypothetical themes that need to be confirmed empirically.

The second stage consists in examining empirically the extent to which the identified themes differentiate between a group with the disorder and control subjects. For this purpose, the themes are phrased in the form of beliefs of the four types. For example, a theme such as "striving for perfection" will be phrased in the form of the four types of beliefs as follows: "In whatever I do I strive for perfection" (belief about self); "Striving for perfection usually leads to frustration" (general belief, opposite direction); "One should always strive for perfection even if the chances for its attainment are meager" (belief about norms); and "I would like to stop striving for perfection" (belief about goal, opposite direction). The beliefs of each type are grouped together and are presented in the form of a questionnaire of four parts, in random order, referring to the four belief types. Each part is preceded by instructions explaining the specific type of belief. The beliefs themselves are presented as separate statements each followed by four response alternatives: very true, true, not true, and not at all true. The subjects are requested to check for each belief their degree of acceptance. The beliefs do not refer in any way to the cancer type or disorder that is being examined but only to the themes that have been identified as potentially underlying the disorder. A questionnaire of this kind is called "a cognitive orientation questionnaire" of the particular disorder studied. The scores reflect the basic direction of the questionnaire supporting some state of health or disease (see examples of themes and specific beliefs in Tables 5.1, 5.2, and 5.3).

Table 5.1 Themes and Conflicts Characterizing Breast Cancer Patients

A. Themes characteristic for breast cancer patients:
1. Perfect external behavior. Includes perfect social behavior and no anger manifestations, adjusting to frameworks and regulations.
2. Giving up oneself and one's needs.
3. One's task in life is to take care of others.
4. Obsessive compulsive tendencies: cleanliness, order, perfect external appearance, and obedience; concern about certainty, need for knowing what exactly to expect in every situation.
5. Giving to others without any limitations (despite no intimate close relations with others); giving for the purpose of control.
6. Emotional control and inhibition; tendency not to share with others one's inner world; tendency not to disclose to others what oppresses or bothers oneself.
7. Striving for success (mainly in order to contribute to society rather than to advance oneself); fear of failure.
8. Feeling that one is controlled from outside, accepting the judgments of others about oneself.
9. Dissociation from oneself (in order to get positive evaluation from others).
10. Unclarity about one's identity, e.g., as mother, woman, wife, career person, and professional person (related to the ability to feel what others feel, ability to identify with others).
11. Keeping one's freedom of decision (failure and disease limit this freedom).
12. Achievement motivation.
13. Pleasing others.
14. Striving to be accepted/approved/loved fully by others, for what one is rather than for what one does or achieves.
15. Getting along, managing (flexible, adapting, no need for help).
16. Striving for perfect honesty, fighting injustice, and doing things for the common welfare.
17. Others and their needs are always more important than one's own needs.
B. Major clusters of themes:
1. Giving to others and giving up one's own needs (Themes 2, 3, 5, 17)
2. Self-effacement (Themes 1, 2, 8, 9, 10, 15)
3. Concern with success (Themes 7, 12)
4. Pleasing others (Themes 1, 5, 13, 14)
C. Characteristic conflicts:
1. Striving to be accepted/approved/loved fully by others, for what one is rather than what one does or achieves (Theme 14) vs achievement motivation (Theme 12)/striving for success (Theme 7)

(continued)

Table 5.1 (continued)

2. Self-effacement (perfect external behavior, Theme 1; giving up oneself, Theme 2; controlled from the outside, Theme 8; dissociation from oneself, Theme 9; unclarity about one's identity, Theme 10; getting along, Theme 15) vs striving to be accepted/approved/loved fully by others, for what one is rather than what one does or achieves
3.Controlling others (Theme 5) vs pleasing others (perfect external behavior, Theme 1; giving to others, Theme 5; pleasing others, Theme 13; striving to be accepted, Theme 14)
4. Feeling that one is controlled from outside (Theme 8) vs keeping one's freedom of decision (Theme 11)
5. Getting along and managing (Theme 15) vs perfect external behavior (Theme 1)

Table 5.2 Themes and Conflicts Characterizing Prostate Cancer Patients

A. Themes characteristic for prostate cancer patients:
1. Striving for perfection in everything one does
2. Striving to be always involved in action
3. Perfect punctuality
4. Keeping one's promises regardless of prevailing conditions
5. Striving for a peaceful life without any problems or tensions
6. Insisting on doing things only in one's own way
7. Striving for good and perfectly harmonious relations in the family
8. Avoiding help from others
9. Concern with maintaining one's own freedom of action without accepting any limitations or compromises
10. Accepting reality and considering one's own limitations
11. Behaving strictly according to the rules
12. Taking responsibility even if not directly involved, in order to maintain adherence to regulations and justice
13. Planning actions down to the last detail prior to starting any action
14. Not sharing with others one's inner world
15. Expressing anger openly
16. Not to violate the freedom of others and not to intervene in the life of others
B. Major clusters of themes:
1. Complete freedom (Themes 6, 8, 9)
2. Strict adherence to regulations (tendencies for compulsiveness) (Themes 1, 3, 4, 11, 12)
3. Realistic approach (Themes 10, 11)
4. Expressing anger openly vs striving for harmonious relations in the family (Themes 10, 11)
5. Keeping distance from others (Themes 6, 8, 14,15)
6. Striving for perfection and control (Themes 11, 1, 3, 13)
C. Potential conflicts:
1. Expressing anger openly (Theme 15) vs striving for good and perfectly harmonious relations in the family (Theme 7)/striving for a peaceful life (Theme 5)
2. Insisting on doing things only in one's own way (Theme 6) vs striving for good and perfectly harmonious relations in the family (Theme 7)/striving for a peaceful life (Theme 5)
3. Concern with maintaining one's own freedom of action without accepting any limitations or compromises (Theme 9) vs accepting reality and considering one's own limitations (Theme 10)/behaving strictly according to the rules (Theme 11)

Table 5.2 (continued)

4. Not to violate the freedom or others (Theme 16) vs striving for a peaceful life (Theme 5)
5. Striving for good and perfectly harmonious relations in the family (Theme 5) vs expressing anger openly (Theme 15)
6. Striving for perfection in everything one does (Theme 1) vs accepting reality and considering one's own limitations (Theme 10)

Table 5.3 Themes Characterizing Colorectal Cancer Patients

A. Themes and examples of beliefs of the cognitive orientation questionnaire of colorectal cancer	
Themes	Examples of beliefs from the cognitive orientation questionnaire of colorectal cancer
Promoting peace and quiet in one's environment	I would like to behave so that there would be no tension and fights among the people close to me (Go)
Cleanliness	It is impossible to live in an environment that is not perfectly clean (GB)
Orderliness	It disturbs me a lot if there is around me any kind of disorder (BS)
Heavy load of responsibility	I undertake many commitments and take carc of many things which actually I do not have to do (BS)
Keeping promises and commitments	Keeping promises means doing what is required and on time without considering circumstances and obstacles (GB)
Work as the most important thing in life	One should consider one's work as the most important thing in life (N)
Giving all to others	I want to give to others all I can without any limitations or considerations (Go)
Doing for oneself only the bare minimum	I do very little for myself (BS)
Need for signs of love and affection from others	One should not depend on signs of affection from others (N-)
No demands for oneself	I would like not to have any demands from life (Go)
Refraining from getting help from others	I want never and under no circumstances to ask others for help (Go)
Avoid getting orders from others	A person ought to be able to get orders from others (N-)
Complying with routines, rules, and regulations	I keep strictly all the socially accepted rules concerning proper conduct among friends, at work, etc. (BS)
Avoiding anger	One should avoid anger at all costs (N)
Avoiding the expression of anger	I want to hide my anger deep inside me (Go)
Not sharing any negative emotions and weaknesses	I want to share with others everything I experience (Go-)
Insisting on getting one's due and rights	It irritates me if I do not get precisely what I deserve (BS)
Getting everything exposed out in the open	It is important to me that everything should always be open and clear, without any secrets or things done behind one's back (BS)
Telling others one's opinion of them even if they don't like it	I want to state my views even if it will not please others (Go)

(continued)

Table 5.3 (continued)

Having to prove oneself (as in an exam)	I feel as if I were constantly standing up for an exam, trying to prove myself (BS)
Ignoring problems and avoiding solving them	Unpleasant things should simply be overlooked (N)
Trying to correct injustice	I am upset by each instance of injustice (BS)
Setting duty prior to pleasure	Entertainment should not be an option for anyone who has not completed all one's duties (N)
Not letting oneself make any mistakes	It is forbidden to make any mistakes in any domain of one's life (N)
Striving for perfection	I expect from myself to perform up to perfection in every domain (BS)

BS beliefs about self, *GB* general beliefs (about others and reality), *N* beliefs about standards and norms, *Go* beliefs about goals; a minus sign denotes that the item supports the direction opposed to colorectal cancer

B. Theme clusters	
Cluster	Themes
1. Compulsiveness	Cleanliness; orderliness; punctuality; avoid spending money
2. Control, especially over ones' emotions and anger	Avoid fighting with others; control over others; controlling events; control of emotional expression and experiencing; control over one's body; avoiding the experience and expression of anger (despite feeling a lot of anger within oneself); not sharing any negative emotions and weaknesses
3. Self-effacement	Setting others before oneself; doing for oneself only the bare minimum; no demands for oneself; giving up success for other things in life; ignoring one's problems and avoiding solving them
4. Pleasing others	Promoting peace and quiet in one's environment; giving all to others; need for signs of love and affection from others; pleasing others; being nice and accommodating
5. Asserting oneself	Insistence on getting one's due and rights; getting everything exposed and discussed out in the open; telling others one's opinion of them even if they don't like it; having to prove oneself (as in an exam)
6. Distancing oneself from others	Refraining from getting help from others; avoid getting orders from others
7. Keeping regulations	Need to specify demands and expectations; complying with routines, rules, and regulations; trying to correct injustice
8. Performing commitments to perfection	Heavy load of responsibility; keeping promises and commitments; work as the most important thing in life; pressuring oneself for maximum performance; setting duty prior to pleasure; not letting oneself make any mistakes; striving for perfection

C. Potential conflicts characterizing patients with colorectal cancer
1. Self-effacement (cluster 3) vs asserting oneself (cluster 5)
2. Promoting peace and quiet in one's environment (theme in cluster 4) vs getting everything exposed and discussed out in the open (theme in cluster 5)
3. Pleasing others, being nice, and accommodating (themes in cluster 4) vs telling others one's opinion of them even if they don't like it (theme in cluster 5)

The cognitive orientation questionnaire of the particular cancer is administered to a sample of individuals with the disease, and one or more control groups that may include in addition to healthy individuals also other groups that differ according to the cancer types. Thus, in regard to breast cancer, control groups may include individuals with benign breast tumors; in regard to thyroid cancer, control groups may include not only healthy individuals and those with benign tumors but also those with functional thyroid disorders. Items or themes that do not differentiate significantly between the groups are dropped from the final questionnaire which is then administered to other samples of groups with and without the disorder [72].

The scores provided by the cognitive orientation questionnaire range per item from 1 to 4, in line with the direction of the questionnaire. The questionnaire provides two kinds of scores: four scores representing the sums or means for each of the four belief types across all themes and scores for each of the themes across all four belief types. The latter are usually factor analyzed so that the factors (often 1–4) represent clusters of themes. The scores of the four belief types are used for identifying or predicting membership in the group characterized by the state of health (e.g., sick or healthy), while the scores for the themes are used for getting insight into the psychological dynamics of the particular state of health.

Up to now the cognitive orientation approach has been applied in regard to over ten different kinds of cancer, for example, breast cancer [73, 74], prostate cancer [75], colorectal cancer [76], cervical cancer [77, 78], and ovarian cancer [79]. Tables 5.1, 5.2, and 5.3 present the themes for a selected group of cancers illustrating the findings and the themes characteristic for different cancers. In the former paragraphs, we have described in detail the rationale and procedure that have yielded the results about the correlates of the different cancers. The reason is that it is highly likely that the rationale and procedure are responsible for the findings we present about personality correlates of cancer types where other procedures such as the use of standard personality questionnaires have been much less successful in this regard.

Themes of the Cognitive Orientation of Breast, Prostate, and Colorectal Cancers

The approach adopted by cognitive orientation consists in focusing on each cancer type separately without assuming a priori any similarities or differences with other types of cancer. Table 5.1 presents the themes for breast cancer. The major tendencies reflected in the list of 17 characteristic themes are giving to others everything they may need and which one can give, self-effacement, pleasing others, and striving for achievement and success. The detailed presentation of the themes reveals specific potentially unexpected features, such as the possible relation of the tendency of giving to others with controlling others (Theme 5) or the relation between the achievement motivation with the desire to promote the social well-being and welfare (Theme 7). Notably, some of the themes indicate potential sources of stress and tension, for example, unclarity about one's identity (Theme 10) or feeling that one is controlled from the outside (Theme 8). Although on the whole the set of themes describes a fairly homogenous approach, some of the themes contradict others, so that they constitute foci of potential conflicts. Five sets of this kind are mentioned in Table 5.1. The most characteristic one is probably the contradiction between striving to be accepted and loved for who one is and achievement motivation. Evidently, if one satisfied one's achievement motivation, one can never be sure whether the love of others is due to one's achievements or to one's being as such. Possibly, the tendency to direct one's achievements toward the common welfare rather than for promoting oneself is some kind of an attempt to resolve the conflict. In addition, also the four kinds of beliefs define domains of potential contradictions. In breast cancer patients, there are mainly the inconsistencies between different kinds of goals (e.g., success and being accepted for oneself) as well as between beliefs about oneself and beliefs about norms which may generate, for example, the guilt feeling that one does not give to others as much as one should [73, 74].

Table 5.2 presents the themes for prostate cancer. The major tendencies reflected in the list of 16 themes are the striving for complete freedom and independence from others, strict adherence to regulations, realistic approach, and keeping distance from others. The themes that appear to be potentially foci of tension are mainly those involved in the strict adherence to rules and regulations and the striving for perfection and control. Despite the overall impression of a fairly homogenous set of tendencies describing a realistic and pedantic individual, intent on keeping to oneself, doing things one's own way, and maintaining both freedom and control, there are evidently contradicting themes that may generate conflicts. For example, expressing anger openly and insisting on doing things one's own way may render the striving for a peaceful life and perfectly harmonious relations in the family rather difficult to maintain. In addition, prostate cancer patients may suffer from tension generated by beliefs of the four types, for example, between the beliefs about one's goals in regard to attaining perfection and the general beliefs concerning the actual attainments that may fall short of the desired ideal [75].

Table 5.3 presents the themes for colorectal cancer. The eight major clusters of themes refer to compulsiveness, control mainly over oneself, self-effacement, pleasing others, asserting oneself, distancing oneself from others, keeping regulations, and performing commitments to perfections. The three major foci of these tendencies are perfect duty performance and two contradictory pairs: self-effacement versus self-assertion and closeness to others versus distancing from others. A closer analysis revealed that the main factor is the striving to maintain peace and quiet around oneself. This desired state is promoted, on the one hand, by doing specific things, such as taking care of orderliness, focusing on work, and controlling one's body and emotional expressions, and on the other hand, by refraining from doing certain things, such as avoiding fights and renouncing all demands that concern oneself. The focus of this factor is self-restraint, exercised in regard to fulfilling one's own needs, spending money, striving for success, and emotional expression. It is further promoted by the tendencies represented by the second factors, namely, striving to fulfill perfectly all one's duties and commitments in regard to cleanliness and punctuality, fulfilling the expectations of others in regard to oneself, keeping one's promises, and complying with rules and regulations. The themes represented by the two major factors of maintaining peace and quiet around oneself and attaining self-restraint are likely to function as sources of tension, both singly and in combinations, for example, pleasing others and expressing openly one's views. The tension may derive both from the difficulty of conforming to the themes themselves and behaving accordingly, e.g., suppressing anger or doing things to perfection. In addition, there are tension-generating inconsistencies between beliefs of the four types, for example, between norm beliefs and self-beliefs concerning the control over anger [76].

General Conclusions About the Cognitive Orientation of Cancer Diseases

Tables 5.1, 5.2, and 5.3 present the relevant themes for each of the three cancers – breast cancer, prostate cancer, and colorectal cancer. Each list includes 10–20 themes. It is evident that the themes do not represent any psychiatric categories but refer rather to quite common individual tendencies that do not represent any systematic approach to personality, emotions, attitude, cognitions, or behaviors. The detailed presentation of the themes enables to get very precise insight into the underlying meanings, which sometimes deviate from the expected. For example, in the framework of breast cancer, doing things for others is related more to the tendency to control others than to the tendency to please others. Or, in the framework of colorectal cancer restraining one's anger is a means for controlling situations and events.

Although some of the themes identified by the cognitive orientation approach resemble tendencies discussed by other investigators, for example, under the heading of anti-emotionality (see this chapter, above), there are several advantages to the approach represented by cognitive orientation. The first is that the themes for each cancer diagnosis represent a complete set in terms of the applied theory and methodology rather than one or more themes selected on the basis of different theoretical or empirical approaches. The second related advantage is that the themes are embedded in a firm theoretical framework that provides a good basis for further empirical and interventional studies and allows for embedding cancer diseases in a broader psychological theory of personality and motivation. The third advantage is that the matrices of themes and beliefs represented in cognitive orientation questionnaires enable identifying precancerous tendencies in medically unclear disorders or disorders that have a malignancy potential (e.g., Crohn's disease), as well as in healthy individuals for purposes of scanning (e.g., for breast cancer). The fourth advantage of the cognitive orientation approach is that the identified themes and beliefs serve as basis for interventions designed to enable control the diseases and their manifestations (see Chap. 8).

Beyond the differences between the lists in the themes and their significance, as noted, here are two major features characterizing the lists. The first is that each contains one or more themes that in themselves could serve as a source of stress. For example, the list of themes for prostate cancer contains the themes of doing things only in one's own way or of striving for perfection. The list for colorectal cancer contains the theme of feeling constantly that one is standing up for an examination. The second feature is that each list contains several potential conflicts that may also serve as sources of stress. Thus, in regard to breast cancer, there is the mentioned conflict between the striving for perfect unconditional love and the striving for achievement and excellence. In regard to colorectal cancer, there is the conflict between striving for perfect harmony and peaceful relations in the family and the tendency to control the behavior of others and to maintain perfect disclosure about all issues.

It is suggested to call this kind of conflicts "chronic conflicts" because they tend to recur since they cannot be resolved once and for all by some specific act. They differ from so-called action-oriented conflicts that can in principle be resolved since they refer to some specific action, such as eating a piece of cake, divorcing, purchasing something, opening or closing a business, disclosing some information, and so on. Conflicts of the latter kind are in principle soluble and disposable. Indeed, sometimes people delay a decision in regard to conflicts of this kind, but then it is rather because they cannot make up their mind due to the issue in question or personal difficulties, for example, in regard to assuming responsibility. However, the conflicts we have detected in the context of cancer are in principle insoluble and undisposable because even if a decision has been met in one instance, it does not prevent the reappearance of the same conflict in another instance. Conflicts of this kind require for their solution a different procedure and psychological elaboration than the action-oriented conflicts.

The lists of themes corresponding to the cancer types may be considered as cognitive orientation sets. They consist of contents that are specific to the type of cancer for which they have been identified. Unlike personality traits that can be applied to different diseases, they are not adequate for characterizing other types of cancer. The cognitive orientation questionnaire of colorectal cancer did not differentiate significantly between breast cancer patients and healthy controls or between prostate patients and healthy controls [80]. These findings support the conclusion that the cognitive orientation clusters are unique for each cancer. One may add that they are unique in their contents and in their dynamics.

Further, the cognitive orientation clusters are sets of themes. As such, it is not necessary that all the themes are functional or accepted by every patient with the particular cancer diagnosis. Empirical studies showed that in order to qualify as diagnostic, it is necessary that the person adopts the beliefs of at least one half of the themes of the relevant set, provided that they represent at least three of the four belief types. There are three important implications to this finding. The first is that in order to be identified as a member of a specific diagnostic group, two different individuals may be characterized by different themes that may not even be overlapping. Hence, the psychological correlates of the disease leave space for individual differences. A second implication is that there may be different degrees of identification with the diagnostic group, reflecting different degrees of adopting the relevant beliefs by the individuals. Hence, it is possible that individuals would manifest tendencies for a specific cancer that are below the threshold, namely, below the mean score characterizing members of the group. This enables identifying individuals with subthreshold tendencies for that cancer. Support for this implication was obtained by showing that patients with DCIS had lower scores on the cognitive orientation of breast cancer than patients with breast cancer but higher scores than healthy controls [73, 74]. Another example concerns individuals with Crohn's disease, which is a nonmalignant gastrointestinal disease with malignant potential for colorectal cancer, especially if left untreated. On the cognitive orientation questionnaire of colorectal cancer, Crohn's patients score lower than patients with colorectal cancer but higher than healthy controls [76]. Finally, the third implication is based on the finding that when a person adopts a lower number of the themes in the cognitive orientation set relevant for a certain cancer, the strength of the psychosocial support for the cancer is lower. Hence it is likely that reducing support for at least some of the themes in the set by psychosocial means (see Chap. 8) might weaken the strength of the tendency for that cancer on the psychological level. This goal may be attained also by mitigating the stress-generating foci of specific themes and particularly of the conflicts in the framework of the particular cognitive orientation set.

Is There a Cancer-Prone Personality?

The findings of the different discussed approaches to the issue of personality and cancer do not support the conclusion that there is a cancer-prone personality. One reason for this conclusion is that it is not justified to refer to cancer as one disease, on the medical or psychosocial levels. Although little concern has been paid to the differential character of the cancer diseases in studies on personality traits or traumas, the cognitive orientation approach has started from the assumption that there is a separate cognitive orientation cluster corresponding to each cancer disease. The findings up to now concerning several cancer diseases show that the different cognitive orientation sets actually differ appreciably and may be considered to be cancer specific. Studies designed to examine the issue of how specific are the cognitive orientation sets supported this conclusion. For example, the cognitive orientation questionnaire of colorectal cancer was administered to two groups of subjects: male subjects of the following three groups – colorectal cancer patients, prostate cancer patients, and healthy controls – and female subjects of the following three groups, colorectal cancer patients, breast cancer patients, and healthy controls. The results showed that in each set, the cognitive orientation questionnaire of colorectal cancer differentiated between the colorectal cancer patients and the other two groups but did not differentiate between the other two groups. Hence the cognitive orientation questionnaire of colorectal cancer was not adequate for identifying prostate cancer patients in males or breast cancer patients in women [80].

Indeed, there are some themes that appear in different sets, for example, the themes of striving for perfection or self-effacement. But it needs to be considered that the recurrent themes are few in number, do not define a whole cognitive set for any type of cancer, and are shared by two or three sets at the utmost. The sharing of several themes by the cognitive orientation set of two or more cancer diseases has inspired the attempt to identify the cognitive orientation cluster corresponding to a family of cancer diseases that relate, for example, to similar or close organs or share the same pathogenesis. Two studies of this kind are being carried out at present in our laboratory – one referring to the gynecological cancers and the other to cancers of the gastrointestinal tract.

However, the issue of the cancer-prone personality refers to "personality." Yet most of the studies and the findings concerning psychological risk factors for cancer do not actually address the issue of personality at large. Even if one or more personality traits are found to characterize one or more cancer types, in the best case the conclusion would refer to those personality traits, each of which has a limited range of impact or of manifestations rather than to personality at large. Similarly, even though the cognitive orientation approach refers to specific cancer types, a cognitive orientation set in no way defines a personality type. The most adequate interpretation of a cognitive orientation type is that it represents a set of tendencies out of which several may turn into focal with more or less salient manifestations. The focal position of some of the tendencies may be temporary and be replaced by other tendencies of the same set or by none at all. The application of a cognitive orientation set is fluid. Finally, even if a certain cognitive orientation set turns into a stable set of tendencies, it would represent only a certain part of psychosocial risk factors for that particular kind of cancer.

The major implications of the stated conclusions are scientific in nature. They should or could be further explored in a scientific framework so as to determine whether the findings in regard to psychological variables qualify at all to be considered as potential risk factors. The road seems to be still quite long since the relations of the described psychological variables with major other risk factors of cancer would have to be first examined in regard to different kinds of cancer and in different stages of cancer manifestations.

What does this approach imply for the individual patient? At present the individual patient may learn about the kind of psychological factors that are being examined, their nature, and their possible role and that changing them or some of them requires real expertise and guidance with the help of an experienced psychooncologist (see Chap. 8).

References

1. Bergelt, C. (2016). Psychosoziale Risikofaktoren bei der Entsehung einer Krebserkrankung. In A. Mehnert & U. Koch (Eds.), *Handbuch Psychoonkologie* (pp. 113–120). Goettingen: Hogrefe.
2. Johansen, C. (2010). Psychosicial factors. In J. C. Holland, W. S. Breitbart, P. B. Jacobsen, M. S. Lederberg, M. J. Loscalzo, & R. McCokle (Eds.), *Psycho-oncology* (2nd ed., pp. 57–61). New York: Oxford University Press.

3. Kreitler, S. (2016). Hans Eysenck as a health psychologist. *Personality and Individual Differences, 103*, 153–156.
4. Amelang, M. (1997). Using personality variables to predict cancer and heart disease. *European Journal of Personality, 11*, 319–342.
5. Pelosi, A. J., & Appleby, L. (1993). Personality and fatal diseases. *BMJ, 306*, 1666–1667.
6. Keesling, B., & Friedman, H. S. (1987). Psychosocial factors in sunbathing and sunscreen use. *Health Psychology, 6*(5), 477–493.
7. Themoshok, L. (1990). *Type C and cancer*. New York: Random House.
8. Forsen, A. (1990). Psychosocial aspects of breast cancer. *Psychiatria Fennica, 21*, 189–200.
9. Eysenck, H. J. (1994). Cancer, personality and stress: Prediction and prevention. *Advances in Behavioral Research Therapy, 16*, 167–215.
10. Gross, J. (1989). Emotional suppression in cancer onset and progression. *Social Science Medicine, 12*, 1239–1248.
11. Persky, V. W., Kempthorne-Rawson, J., & Shekelle, R. B. (1987). Personality and risk of cancer: 20-year follow-up of the Western Electric Study. *Psychosomatic Medicine, 49*, 435–449.
12. Bleiker, E. M. A., Henk, M., van der Ploeg, H. M., Hendriks, H. C. L., & Adir, A. J. (1996). Personality factors and breast cancer development: A prospective longitudinal study. *Journal of the National Cancer Institute, 88*(20), 1478–1482.
13. Bleiker, E. M. A., Hendriks, J. H. C. L., Otten, I. D. M., Verbrek, A. L. M., & van der Ploeg, H. M. (2009). Personality factors and breast cancer risk: A 13 year follow up. *Journal of National Cancer Institute, 100*, 213–218.
14. Tijhuis, M. A. R., Elshout, I. R. A. F., & Feskens, E. J. M. (2000). Prospective investigation of emotional control and cancer risk in men (the Zutphen Elderly Study) (The Netherlands). *Cancer Causes and Control, 11*(7), 589–595.
15. Lemogne, C., Consoli, S. M., Geoffroy-Perez, B., Coeuret-Pellicer, M., Nabi, H., Melchior, M., Limosin, F., Zins, M. L., Ducimetière, P., Goldberg, M., & Cordier, S. (2013). Personality and the risk of cancer: A 16-year follow-up study of the GAZEL cohort. *Psychosomatic Medicine, 75*(3), 262–271.
16. Ollonen, P., Lehtonen, J., & Eskelinen, M. (2005). Coping and defending as risk factors for breast cancer in patients with breast disease; a prospective case-control study in Kuopio, Finland. *Anticancer Research, 25*, 4623–4630.
17. Eskelinen, M., & Ollonen, P. (2011). Assessment of 'cancer-prone personality' characteristics in healthy study subjects and in patients with breast disease and breast cancer using the commitment questionnaire: A prospective case-control study in Finland. *Anticancer Research, 31*(11), 4013–4017.
18. Eskelinen, M., & Ollonen, P. (2011). Sifneos alexithymia questionnaire in assessment of general alexithymia in patients with breast disease and breast cancer: A prospective case-control study in Finland. *Anticancer Research, 31*(9), 3101–3106.
19. De Vries, A. M. M., Forni, V., Voellinger, R., & Stiefel, F. (2012). Alexithymia in cancer patients: Review of the literature. *Psychotherapy & Psychosomatics, 81*, 79–86.
20. Kreitler, S., & Kreitler, H. (1990). Repression and the anxiety-defensiveness factor: Psychological correlates and manifestations. *Personality & Individiodual Differences, 11*, 559–570.
21. Kreitler, S., & Kreitler, H. (1991). Cognitive orientation and physical disease or health. *European Journal of Personality, 5*, 109–129.
22. Garssen, B. (2004). Psychological factors and cancer development: Evidence after 30 years of rese. *Clinical Psychology Review, 24*, 315–338.
23. Spiegler, D. (2003). Depression and cancer: Mechanisms and disease progression. *Biological Psychiatry, 54*(3), 269–282.
24. Goldacre, M. J., Wotton, C. J., Yeates, D., Seagroatt, V., & Flint, J. (2007). Cancer in people with depression and anxiety: Record-linkage study. *Social Psychiatry and Psychiatric Epidemiology, 42*, 683–689.

25. Chen, Y.-H., & Lin, H.-C. (2011). Increased risk of cancer subsequent to severe depression-A nationwide population-based study. *Journal of Affective Disorders, 131*, 200–206.
26. Liang, J.-A., Sun, L.-M., Muo, C.-H., et al. (2011). The analysis of depression and subsequent cancer risk in Taiwan. *Cancer Epidemiology, Biomarkers & Prevention, 20*, 473–475.
27. Kroenke, C. H., Bennett, G. G., Fuchs, C., Giovanucch, E., Kawachi, I., Scherenhammer, E., Holmes, M. D., & Kubzansky, L. D. (2005). Depressive symptoms and prospective incidence of colorectal cancer in women. *American Journal of Epidemiology, 162*, 839–848
28. Dalton, S. O., Mellemkjær, L., Olsen, J. H., Mortensen, P. B., & Johansen, C. (2002). Depression and cancer risk: A register-based study of patients hospitalized with affective disorders, Denmark, 1969–1993. *American Journal of Epidemiology, 155*(12), 1088–1095.
29. Zonderman, A. B., Costa, P. T., & McCraae, R. R. (1989). Depression as a risk for cancer morbidity and mortality in a nationally representative sample. *JAMA, 262*(9), 1191–1195.
30. Nyklicek, I., Louwman, W. J., Van Nierop, P. W., et al. (2003). Depression and the lower risk for breast cancer development in middle-aged women: A prospective study. *Psycological Medicine, 33*, 111–1117.
31. Pössel, P., Adams, E., & Valentine, J. C. (2012). Depression as a risk factor for breast cancer: Investigating methodological limitations in the literature. *Cancer Causes Control, 23*(8), 1223–1229.
32. Cosgrove, L., Shi, L., Creasey, D. E., Anaya-McKivergan, M., Myers, J. A., & Huybrechts, K. F. (2011). Antidepressants and breast and ovarian cancer risk: A review of the literature and researchers' financial associations with industry. *PLoS One, 6*(4), e18210.
33. Chris, C., Wolford, S. J., McConoughey, S. P., Jalgaonkar, M. L., Anand, S. M., Johnna, L. D., Xin, Y., Yiseok, C., Zmuda, E. J., O'Toole, S. A., Millar, E. K. A., Roller, S. L., Shapiro, C. L., Ostrowski, M. C., Sutherland, R. L., & Hai, T. (2013). Transcription factor ATF3 links host adaptive response to breast cancer metastasis. *Journal of Clinical Investigation, 123*(7), 2893.
34. Shen, C. C., Hu, Y. W., Hu, L. Y., Hung, M. H., Su, T. P., Huang, M. W., Tsai, C. F., Ou, S. M., Yen, S. H., Tzeng, C. H., Chiou, T. J., Chen, T. J., & Liu, C. J. (2013). The risk of cancer in patients with generalized anxiety disorder: A nationwide population-based study. *PLoS One, 8*(2), e57399.
35. Chen, Y. C., Kao, L. T., Lin, H. C., Lee, H. C., Huang, C. C., & Chung, S. D. (2016). Increased risk for urological cancer associated with anxiety disorder: A retrospective cohort study. *BMC Urology, 16*(1), 67.
36. Aro, A. R., De Koning, H. J., Schreck, M., Henriksson, M., Anttila, A., & Pukkala, E. (2005). Psychological risk factors of incidence of breast cancer: A prospective cohort study in Finland. *Psychological Medicine, 35*(10), 1515–1521.
37. Faller, H., Lang, H., & Schilling, S. (1996). [Causal "cancer personality" attribution–an expression of maladaptive coping with illness?]. Kausalattribution "Krebspersönlichkeit" – ein Ausdruck maladaptiver Krankheitsverarbeitung? (German). *Zeitschrift Fur Klinische Psychologie, Psychiatrie Und Psychotherapie, 44*, 1431–8172.
38. Bruno, A., Pandolfo, G., Scimeca, G., Leonardi, V., Cedro, C., Racchiusa, S., Zoccali, R. A., & Muscatello, M. R. (2014). Anger in health, benign breast disease and breast cancer: A prospective case-control study. *In Vivo (Athens, Greece), 28*(5), 973–977.
39. Stürmer, T., Hasselbach, P., & Amelang, M. (2006). Personality, lifestyle, and risk of cardiovascular disease and cancer: Follow-up of population based cohort. *BMJ (Clinical Research Education), 332*(7554), 1359.
40. Wakai, K., Kojima, M., Nishio, K., Suzuki, S., Niwa, Y., Lin, Y., Kondo, T., Yatsuya, H., Tamakoshi, K., Yamamoto, A., Tokudome, S., Toyoshima, H., Tamakoshi, A., & JACC Study Group. (2007). Psychological attitudes and risk of breast cancer in Japan: A prospective study. *Cancer Causes Control, 18*(3), 259–267.
41. White, V. M., English, D. R., Coates, H., Lagerlund, M., Borland, R., & Giles, G. G. (2007). Is cancer risk associated with anger control and negative affect? Findings from a prospective cohort study. *Psychosomatic Medicine, 69*(7), 667–674.
42. Cohen, S., Janicki-Deverts, D., & Miller, G. E. (2007). Psychological stress and disease. *JAMA, 298*(14), 1685–1687.

43. Segerstrom, S. C., & Miller, G. E. (2004). Psychological stress and the human immune system: A meta-analytic study of 30 years of inquiry. *Psychological Bulletin., 130*(4), 601–630.
44. Nielsen, N. R., Zhang, Z.-F., Kristensen, T. S., Netterstrøm, B., Schnohr, P., & Grønbæk, M. (2005). Self-reported stress and risk of breast cancer: Prospective cohort study. *BMJ, 331*(7516), 548.
45. Lillberg, K., Verkasalo, P. K., Kaprio, J., Teppo, L., Helenius, H., & Koskenvuo, M. (2003). Stressful life events and risk of breast cancer in 10,808 women: A cohort study. *American Journal of Epidemiology, 157*(5), 415–423.
46. Kroenke, C. H., Hankinson, S. E., Schernhammer, E. S., Colditz, G. A., Kawachi, I., & Holmes, M. D. (2004). Caregiving stress, endogenous sex steroid hormone levels, and breast cancer incidence. *American Journal of Epidemiology, 150*(11), 1019–1027.
47. Scherenhammer, E. S., Hankinson, S. E., Rosner, B., et al. (2004). Job stress and breast cancer risk. The nurses health study. *American Journal of Epidemiology, 160*, 1079–1086.
48. Nielsen, N. R., Stahlberg, C., Strandberg-Larsen, K., et al. (2008). Are work-related stressors associated with diagnosis of more advanced stages of incident cases of breast cancer? *Cancer Causes Control, 19*, 297–303.
49. Kruk, J., & Aboul-Enein, H. Y. (2004). Psychological stress and the risk of breast cancer: A case-control study. *Cancer Detection & Prevention, 28*(6), 399–408.
50. Kruk, J. (2012). Self-reported psychological stress and the risk of breast cancer: A case-control study. *Stress, 15*(2), 162–171.
51. Prigerson, H. G., Bierhals, A. J., Kasl, S. V., Reynolds, C. V., III, Shear, M. C., Day, N., Beery, L. C., Newsom, J. T., & Jacobs, S. (1997). Traumatic grief as a risk factor for mental and physical morbidity. *American Journal of Psychiatry, 154*, 616–623.
52. Levav, I., Kohn, R., Iscovich, J., Abramson, J. H., Tsai, W. Y., & Vigdorovich, D. (2000). Cancer incidence and survival following bereavement. *American Journal of Public Health, 90*(10), 1601–1607.
53. Koupil, I., Plavinskaja, S., Parfenova, N., Shestov, D. B., Danziger, P. D., & Vågerö, D. (2009). Cancer mortality in women and men who survived the siege of Leningrad (1941–1944). *International Journal of Cancer, 124*(6), 1416–1421.
54. Kenan-Boker, L., Vin-Raviv, N., Liphshitz, I., Linn, S., & Barchana, M. (2009). Cancer incidence in Israeli Jewish survivors of world war II. *JNCI: Journal of the National Cancer Institute, 101*(21), 1489–1500.
55. Vin-Raviv, N., Liphshitz, I., Linn, S., Keinan-Boker, L., & Barchana, M. (2006). Incidence and survival characteristics of diseases among holocaust survivors that have immigrated to Israel (abstract). *Early Human Development, 82*, 532.
56. Felitti, V. J., Anda, R. F., Nordenberg, D., Williamson, D. F., Spitz, A. M., et al. (1998). Relationship of childhood abuse and household dysfunction to many of the leading causes of death in adults. The Adverse Childhood Experiences (ACE) Study. *American Journal of Preventive Medicine, 14*, 245–258. [PubMed].
57. Holman, D. M., Ports, K. A., Buchanan, N. D., Hawkins, N. A., Merrick, M. T., Metzler, M., & Trivers, K. F. (2016). The association between adverse childhood experiences and risk of cancer in adulthood: A systematic review of the literature. *Pediatrics, 138*(Suppl 1), S81–S91.
58. Brown, D. W., Anda, R. F., Felitti, V. J., Edwards, V. J., Malarcher, A. M., et al. (2010). Adverse childhood experiences are associated with the risk of lung cancer: A prospective cohort study. *BMC Public Health, 10*, 20.
59. Kelly-Irving, M., Lepage, B., Dedieu, D., Lacey, R., Cable, N., Bartley, M., Blane, D., Grosclaude, P., Lang, T., & Delpierrre, C. (2013). Childhood adversity as a risk for cancer: Findings from the 1958 British birth cohort study. *BMC Public Health, 13*, 767.
60. Brown, M. J., Thacker, L. R., & Cohen, S. A. (2013). Association between adverse childhood experiences and diagnosis of cancer. *PLoS One, 8*(6), e65524.
61. Kissen, D. M., & Eysenck, H. J. (1962). Personality in male lung cancer patients. *Journal of Psychosomatic Research, 6*, 123–127.
62. Coppen, A., & Metcalfe, M. (1963). Cancer and extroversion. *BMJ, 2*, 18–19.

63. Morris, T., Greer, S., Pettingale, K. W., & Watson, M. (1981). Patterns of expressing anger and their psychological correlates in women with breast cancer. *Journal of Psychosomatic Research, 25*, 111–117.
64. Nakaya, N., Tsubono, Y., Hosokawa, T., Nishino, Y., Ohkubo, T., Hozawa, A., Shibuya, D., Fukudo, S., FukaoIchiro, A., & Shigeru, T. (2003). Personality and the risk of cancer. *Journal of the National Cancer Institute, 95*(11), 799–805.
65. Hansen, P. E., Floderus, B., Frederiksen, K., & Johansen, C. (2010). Personality traits, health behavior, and risk for cancer: A prospective study of Swedish twin court. *Cancer, 103*, 1082–1091.
66. Nakaya, N., Bidstrup, P. E., Saito-Nakaya, K., Frederiksen, K., Koskenvuo, M., Pukkala, E., Kaprio, J., Floderus, B., Uchitomi, Y., & Johansen, C. (2010). Personality traits and cancer risk and survival based on Finnish and Swedish registry data. *American Journal of Epidemiology, 172*(4), 377–385.
67. Kreitler, S., & Chaitchik, S. (1994). The psychological profile of the breast-screened woman. *International Journal of Oncology, 5*(Suppl), 384.
68. Kreitler, S. (1999). The cognitive orientation for health: A tool fot assessing health-pronrness. In R. Schwarzer (Ed.), *Advances in health psychology research [CD-ROM]*. Berlin: Freie Universitaet Berlin. Institut fuer Arbeits-Organizations- und Gesundheitspsychologie. [ISBN 3-00-002776-9].
69. Kreitler, S. (2004). The cognitive guidance of behavior. In J. T. Jost, M. R. Banaji, & D. A. Prentice (Eds.), *Perspectivism in social psychology: The yin and yang of scientific progress* (pp. 113–126). Washington, DC: American Psychological Association.
70. Kreitler, S., & Kreitler, H. (1891). Cognitive orientation and physical disease or health. *European Journal of Personality, 5*, 109–129.
71. Kreitler, S., Weissler, K., Kreitler, M. M., & Barak, F. (2013). Physical health and cognition. In S. Kreitler (Ed.), *Cognition and motivation: Forging an interdisciplinary perspective* (pp. 238–269). New York: Cambridge University Press.
72. Kreitler, S., & Kreitler, H. (1998). Cognitive orientation and disease in cancer patients. *Psycho-Oncology, 7*(Suppl 174).
73. Kreitler, S., Kreitler, H., Chaitchik, S., Shaked, S., & Shaked, T. (1997). Psychological and medical predictors of disease course in breast cancer: A prospective study. *European Journal of Personality, 11*, 383–400.
74. Kreitler, S., Kreitler, M. M., Yaal-Hahoshen, N. & Inbar, M. (2006, July 22–26). *Personality correlates of breast cancer*. 13th European conference on personality, Athens, Greece.
75. Kreitler, S., Ariely, J., Gai, M., & Muriel, E. (2006, September 29–October 3). *The psychological correlates of prostate cancer*. 31st ESMO Congress, Istambul, Turkey.
76. Kreitler, S., Kreitler, M. M., Len, A., Alkalay, Y., & Barak, F. (2008). Psychological risk factors for colorectal cancer? *Psycho-Oncologie, 2*, 131–145.
77. Kreitler, S., Kreitler, M. M., & Inbar, M. (2006, October 18–21). *The cognitive orientation of cervical cancer*. In Symposium "Cancer in women: Personality correlates and coping", 8th world congress of psycho-oncology, (organized by IPOS: International Psychooncology Society). Venice, Italy.
78. Kreitler, S., Levavi, H., & Bornstein, G. (1996). Personality factors and cervical premalignancy. *Personality and Individual Differences, 21*, 883–890.
79. Kreitler, S., Kreitler, M. M., Weissler, K., & Safra, T. (2006, October 18–21). *The cognitive orientation of cancer of the ovaries*. In Symposium "Cancer in women: Personality correlates and coping", 8th world congress of psycho-oncology, (organized by IPOS: International Psychooncology Society). Venice, Italy.
80. Kreitler, S., Kreitler, M. M., & Barak, F. (2013). Psychosocial risk factors of cancer diseases: How specific are they? *Open Journal of Social Sciences, 1*(6), 81–86.

Chapter 6
The Impact of Cancer

Every chronic disease impacts the patient's life in many respects. However cancer does so to a more prominent degree, or at least it has the reputation and image for doing so. Getting cancer is a major event in the life of any person, at any age. The reasons are the broad range of effects, the severity of the effects, the treatments, and all through the inescapable association with death, which is highly prominent at least in the Western world. In this chapter major impacts of cancer in the different domains of life are described. The chapter refers to several domains, the major ones in which changes occur, and in each domain several major changes are described. Evidently, not every cancer patient undergoes all of the described changes, but at least a few of the different domains would be familiar to most patients and clinicians. The description is necessarily sequential, focusing on each domain separately. However, psychologically this style of presentation involves a distortion because the importance of each domain and the interrelations between the domains differ for different individuals. For some individuals, changes in body image may be of crucial importance, manifested in depression and even aggression, while for others difficulties at work may be the cause for depression.

Emotional Impact of Cancer

The impact of cancer on emotions is manifested most clearly in regard to *emotional control*. This tendency is conceptualized in terms of a dimension which runs from emotional suppression, through emotional regulation to the other pole of emotional lack of control. In cancer patients there is evidence for both extreme tendencies. Suppression becomes evident mainly in the initial phases [1–3], whereas outbursts of lack of control occur all along, slightly more in later phases [4].

There is almost no emotion which is not impacted by cancer. The most frequently discussed emotions are anxiety and depression. *Anxiety* has been identified in about 10–30% of cancer patients, which is similar to the 12% assessed in patients with

S. Kreitler, *Psycho-Oncology for the Clinician*,
https://doi.org/10.1007/978-3-030-06126-5_6

chronic medical diseases [5–9] but tends to be higher than the about 10% rate in the population at large [10–11]. The relatively wide range in results of assessment is due to differences in assessment tools, some of which include more physical symptoms that maybe reflect rather effects of treatment of the disease [12]. In cancer patients, it tends to be high in the first phase following diagnosis but is reported to decline after the beginning of treatment [13]. It is then often identified as adjustment disorder with anxiety [14]. However, many patients continue to suffer from at least low-grade anxiety for prolonged periods of time, often evoked by specific triggers, such as disease recurrence or the passing away of another patient with whom one shared some treatment phase, undergoing of medical tests, some change in treatment, or the occurrence of a new symptom. Cancer patients sometimes report specific fears which at least to some extent may be shared also by other chronic patients, such as fear of loss of dignity, loss of independence, and loss of motivation to live. Essentially anxiety consists in the feeling of insecurity and threat. In contrast to fear which is assumed to refer to external situations, it is defined as focused on internal thoughts and concerns. The difference is however hardly sustainable, especially in the case of cancer where the internal and external aspects intermingle indistinguishably. It has been noted that anxiety in cancer patients may appear together with other trauma-related disorders and different forms of anxiety mixed with somatic preoccupation, panic reactions, or depression. The anxiety may also develop into a generalized anxiety disorder, in which case psychiatric intervention may be recommended [13].

Depression is possibly even more common in cancer patients than anxiety and like anxiety suffers from unclarity in assessment. Thus its range runs from 0% to 38% for major depression and 0–58% for depression spectrum syndromes, as compared with 6.6–16.6% in the general population [15, 16]. It is estimated that 22% of cancer patients suffer from at least subthreshold depressive disorders [17]. The relatively high scores of depression that cancer patients get in different assessment scales are due at least partly to the fact that they include several of the physical symptoms caused by most anticancer treatments (e.g., fatigue, lack of energy) [12]. Further, depression is associated with particular medications (e.g., corticosteroids, vincristine) and tends to be higher in specific cancer types (e.g., pancreatic, oropharyngeal, and lung) [18, 19]. Depression affects negatively the patients' quality of life and may weaken their motivation to adhere to the treatment and continue it and to go on coping with the different difficulties of the disease [20]. It may also enhance suicidal thoughts and desire for death [21]. When depression is severe or prolonged, in some clinics, antidepressants are offered in a standard regular manner to all oncology patients from the very beginning of treatment.

In addition to depression per se, cancer patients often suffer from different emotions reflecting negative mood. Since they are characteristic of cancer patients, they will be mentioned separately rather than under the common descriptive heading of depression. This cluster of emotions includes *demoralization, mental pain, despair, distress, hopelessness, suffering, existential distress, meaninglessness of life (or loss of meaningfulness of life), and even grieving over oneself.* Notably, these emotions are characteristically not from the domain of psychiatry but rather from the sphere of daily life and suffering, although they may acquire psychiatric overtones as in the case of demoralization. The mentioned constructs are sometimes used as explanatory terms for the patient's state which may be described, for example, as due to his/her "hopelessness" or "existential despair" or as constructs describing the patient's actual emotional experience which may be, for example, "demoralization" or "distress." However, most of these terms are used to denote a set of negative descriptors focusing on hopelessness, despair, and kind of stoic surrender to the situation.

Some of the terms have more characterizing features. Thus, demoralization is defined as a state that includes despair, hopelessness, and loss of purpose in life but differs from depression mainly in the low emphasis on anhedonia and strong emphasis on the fear of loss of dignity and of dependence on others, impotence, and loss of desire to live. It is often manifested also as loss of interest in activities, people, or social events and as a kind of lethargy and lack of initiative or motivation to engage in activities of any kind [22]. Loss of meaningfulness of life is an increasingly frequent complaint of patients which expresses mainly their feeling of disorientation, in both internal and external realities, compounded by loss of direction and comprehension of what goes on (see later section, this chapter). Grieving over oneself is an emotion of a different order. It is a kind of self-centered bereavement reaction evoked by treating one's losses – bodily, psychological, and behavioral – as stages in the process of gradual dying. Some patients express thoughts such as "what a pity that this beautiful body of mine will not be loved any more" or "I will never again plan a vacation on a beach." Another aspect is emphasized by mental pain, which has been identified in cancer patients and survivors [23]. It denotes an emotion that is distinct from physical pain but is its correlative on the psychological level. It represents the experience of irreversibility, loss of control, narcissistic wounds, emotional flooding, freezing, estrangement, confusion, social distancing, and emptiness. Distress is a more general term that has come to be used increasingly in order to refer to the often unidentified psychological unmet needs of about 30–50% of cancer patients [24]. These emotions affect negatively the patients' quality of life and possibly also their chances for survival [25]. Some of the mentioned emotions develop mainly in the course of the disease. Psychosocial treatment is indicated for helping the patient maintain a tolerable level of quality of life and of coping with the disease (see Chap. 8).

The negative emotions that are frequent in cancer patients include also *tension and stress*. These are definitely unpleasant emotions, of varying intensity, marked especially by being relatively nonspecific. They are often manifested as restlessness, nervousness, impulsivity in reactions, or claims about loss of patience. Since their triggers are unidentified by the person, they are difficult to reduce and are often treated by tension-reducing drugs which provide at least temporary relief.

A different set of emotions impacted by cancer is focused on *anger, frustration, dissatisfaction, annoyance, passive aggression, hostility, and irritability*. Emotions of this kind appear in various forms in the different stages of cancer and often even at the very beginning after disclosure of the diagnosis. Since anger is a frequent reaction to the appearance of some obstacle to the attainment of one's goals or a hindrance in one's way of acting, it is to be expected in cancer patients for whom the disease is an immense block or barrier, unexpected, undeserved, and unjustified. Additionally, the anger may also be a deflection from another emotion bound with the patient's misery [26]. Be it as it may, anger is a difficult emotion for the patients to handle since it is so hard to express it in a controlled and acceptable manner. It is no less difficult for the caretakers including the health professionals to handle it when it is expressed by the patients because they are quite helpless in regard to it and may feel blame or guilt for no evil done on their part. Sometimes the anger evoked by the disease and the attendant limitations and difficulties absorb pent-up anger that the patient may carry inside, so that it explodes in an uncontrolled manner, not infrequently against the inadequate object. Sometimes the anger manifests itself in uncontrolled screaming or crying, which may be embarrassing for everyone involved. More problematic are different forms of destructiveness expressive of the anger. These may lead to breaking up of relations, distancing oneself from friends and acquaintances, and destroying different projects in which one is involved. Anger may be directed even against oneself and be manifested as self-destructiveness, psychologically or physically. Under certain circumstances, it may lead to suicidal behavior [21].

A separate heading should be reserved for other forms of *emotional misery*, which include feeling worthless, dependent, incompetent, and weak, in sum a human being without any role or dignity. Emotions of this kind are not unique to cancer patients and actually not very frequent in the regular course of events, but they may be expected and identified especially in the palliative stage.

Characteristic components of emotional misery are *socially grounded emotions* of loneliness, seclusion, withdrawal, feeling rejected, unwanted, feeling estrangement, being different from other people whose right to live has not been so to say abrogated, and "no one understands me" [27, 28]. Sometimes patients complain of experiencing jealousy of healthy friends or relatives but resent this feeling which they have rarely felt before being sick. They often consider it as an improper emotion reflecting their sense of inferiority. There are further emotions of a different order that are often reported by cancer patients and considered by them as enhanced by the disease. These include compassion for the suffering of others and need for forgiveness. The former may be grounded in one's own suffering, and the latter may possibly reflect the desire to overcome one's sense of guilt and self-blame.

There are also characteristic changes in cancer of *positive emotions*. Most prominent among these is hope, which is often enhanced and promoted not in the least because it is believed to be of benefit in coping with the disease [29]. Hope is sometimes presented as optimism, especially in the context of the often promoted so-called positive thinking. By now it is evident that positive thinking as such is of controversial status for cancer patients because it emphasizes the importance of experiencing only positive emotions while subduing or overlooking the negative emotions. This advice is barely possible to implement because the negative emotions are there and are difficult to overlook. Further, implementing "positive thinking" may be harmful both because curtailing emotional experiences of any kind may impair also the ability to experience positive emotions and because experiencing in general is advocated for cancer patients (see Chap. 8).

The Cognitive Impact

There are two major kinds of cognitive impact of cancer: one relates to different kinds of cancer and the anticancer treatments, whereas the other refers to central nervous system tumors. The present section is devoted only to the first kind of impairments (for the second, see Chap. 14). The effect of cancer and/or anticancer treatments on cognitive functioning has been suspected for several decades, particularly due to the complaints of cancer patients. Consequently many studies have been conducted in order to clarify the issue. The results indicate that the major effects are manifested in disruptions in thinking, concentration, attention, speed of acquiring and processing information, memory, multitasking, and different cognitive abilities (e.g., verbal, mathematical, spatial) [30, 31]. There is also evidence for impulsive decision-making due to limited consideration of the different options and too fast dismissal of options. Its main causes are different treatments, chemotherapy (causing, e.g., direct neurotoxic effects, oxidative stress, and DNA damage); biologic, hormonal, and supportive medication; brain surgery; and brain radiation, as well as associated conditions (poor nutrition, sleep disorders, fatigue, pain, inactivity, anemia, anxiety, and depression). However, there is evidence that already at diagnosis, there are signs of cognitive impairment, for example, in 33% of breast cancer patients [32] and in 17–41% of AML/MDS patients [33, 34]. In some cases the specific cognitive impairments were found to be correlated with specific medical indices, for example, higher IL-6 levels were associated with poorer executive function [34]. There is evidence from animal studies about changes in the brain due to penetration of chemotherapeutic materials [35]. An additional essentially psychological factor that could affect impairment in cognitive performance is preoccupation with the disease, manifested sometimes in continuous attention to one's physical state or fear about possible reactions. Manifestations of this kind may require resources that could lower the level of cognitive performance [31]. Another possibility is that anxiety of cognitive deterioration may prompt special efforts on the part of patients to compensate for the cognitive impairments they have noted. However, the impact of factors such as the patient's age, hormonal status, surgery, and comorbidity on the cognitive impairment should not be overlooked [31].

The reported incidence of cognitive impairment in cancer patients varies from 15% to 50% and is reported to last for even 10–20 years [36]. In regard to breast cancer, it was found that in 61%, the impairment persisted for 3 weeks after termination of chemotherapy, in 45% it persisted for 1 year, and in 45% there was improvement [32]. In some cases (30–35% of patients), the impairment becomes evident only posttreatment [37].

Various impairments in cognitive functioning have been reported also for pediatric cancer patients, especially those who have undergone radiotherapy [38]. Cranial radiotherapy (CRT) is used for brain tumors but also for leukemia and lymphoma in pediatric patients. The major cognitive effects of CRT are declines in general intelligence and specific deficits in nonverbal and verbal cognitive functions, mainly memory and attention, that increase with time since radiotherapy and are especially notable in children who have received it at a younger age. The amount and severity of cognitive impairment depend also on the dose and location of radiotherapy.

In adult patients it appears that many of the cognitive impairments are reversible but probably not all and not soon after treatment termination. An attempt to summarize the results shows that effects on cognitive functioning undoubtedly exist, but their extent, severity, and persistence depend in the very least on the diagnosis (so far, more often in breast cancer, lymphoma, and brain), the age of the patient (e.g., more when older), the kind of treatment (e.g., more after cranial radiotherapy) and the additional medications administered, and the kind of cognitive functions tested (more memory and concentration than reasoning) [39–41].

The cognitive impact of cancer and its treatments affect negatively the quality of life of cancer patients in the course of treatment and afterward and even their decisions concerning undergoing treatment at all or going back to work.

There is however evidence that cognitive treatment rehabilitation could have positive effects on reducing the extent of the cognitive deficits and improving cognitive functioning in general in both adults and children [42].

Impact on Beliefs and Worldview

It is not surprising that cancer may exert an impact on the patients' beliefs in different domains and even their worldview in general. One of the initial reactions to the diagnosis of cancer that many patients have is "why me," "I don't deserve this at all." Getting sick is viewed as a kind of punishment, an unjust consequence for the proper and moral behavior that the individual attributes to oneself. Getting cancer is considered as a violation of the "just-world" hypothesis when or if the person considers himself as one whose behavior does not justify this kind of suffering [43]. The *just-world hypothesis* assumes that the world is a stable, balanced, well organized, and rule-determined complex. Upholding this view presumably contributes to one's peace of mind and overall well-being. According to the hypothesis of a just-world, people get what they deserve, so that if something bad happens to a person, that person has most probably done something to deserve it. This kind of thinking may get the individual into a dilemma. In order to uphold the just-world hypothesis, one is expected to regard oneself as having done something to deserve the disease. Identifying in oneself the cause for the disease contributes to enhancing one's sense of guilt, and if that cause cannot be changed or reversed, it may contribute to one's sense of hopelessness-helplessness in regard to the disease. However, if one does not identify in oneself the cause for the disease, then this enhances one's confusion and unclarity concerning oneself. Evidently, if one does not tend to blame oneself for the disease, then it is difficult to maintain the belief in the just world. Considering oneself as responsible for the disease upholds the just-world hypothesis but breeds guilt feelings and an inferior view of oneself; considering oneself as free of guilt undermines the just-world hypothesis which is important for one's overall sense of security and well-being.

Doubts are likely to be evoked in cancer patients also concerning other views and beliefs they may have had prior to the disease. One such issue is *religion, spirituality*, and belief in God. Atheistic reflections may be nurtured in religious people because – like the biblical figure of Job – they find it difficult to believe that God could allow so much suffering and pain for a devout human being. On the other hand, other patients may be induced by the situation to feel closer to God precisely because they assume that only God can be expected to be able to help them to overcome the difficulties they face. Thus, cancer may turn some believers into non-believers and some non-believers into believers [44, 45].

Some patients feel induced to change also their conceptions about *friendship and friends*. It is not unusual that people who have been considered as friends for many years may withdraw from the cancer patient when the diagnosis becomes known. Even if they stay around, the patient may find out that they are unwilling or unable to provide the help or understanding he or she may need. Experiences of this kind may undermine one's conceptions about friendship in general (viz., "a friend in need is a friend indeed"), especially since it is often the case that people whom one hardly knew before the disease do provide needed support and help [46].

Other attitudes that may change following cancer concern the overall scale of one's *life preferences* with implications for one's life narrative. The scale of life preferences or life plan includes in some order the set of goals, duties, wishes, and habitual actions that one has adopted or constructed over the years, for example, career, family, or acquisition of possessions. This scale is being set up for reevaluation due to cancer. This may sometimes occur already after the diagnosis, because of the time schedule of treatments that may occupy time and require some changes in one's daily life. But more often it occurs later in time close to the termination of treatments; because of a prolonged pause due to treatments or because at the verge of the termination of treatments, it is necessary to make up one's mind about how to proceed. It is then that cancer patients may start thinking about their life, its goals, and management. Usually the goals uppermost in the scale are reconsidered seriously, and their location in the scale may be altered. It is quite common for cancer patients to concentrate on their personal needs and wishes and decide to devote more interest and motivation to taking care of oneself and one's pleasure and well-being, doing things one has wanted to do for a long time but had no time or opportunity to do them, and doing something creative, something that expresses one's inner being. The mentioned goals often enjoy an upgrading in one's scale of goals, whereas performing one's duties and obligations may be downgraded if one's financial and familial situation allows it.

Another important change may take place in regard to *time*. Originally preceding the disease, most patients in the Western world live as if time is an endless resource and as if living forever is the normal situation. After the diagnosis of cancer, these assumptions are likely to change. Patients feel that their time is measured and limited, and at any case, it is not limitless [47]. Of the three aspects of time – past, present, and future – the one that suffers the most is the future. Its state may be so bad that patients sometimes do not dare to make a plan or to accept a commitment for the next days since it often happens that they need to change their decisions and commitments. In cases such as these, it may be necessary to apply a procedure for reconstructing the future. The training consists in establishment of small steps of future events in the very close future over which the patient feels he or she has a modicum of control, before extending the planning of events to further time points in the future.

Loss of the future dimension contributes to the overall sense of insecurity that may characterize the general experience of cancer patients in their life span. This sense of uncertainty is nourished by what they experience in regard to the major components in their life space, viz., body, disease, self, beliefs, faith, and friendship.

Changes in one's life preferences constitute part of possible changes in one's *meaningfulness of life*. Meaningfulness of life consists of a set of items representing potential areas that are evaluated positively or desired by an individual, such as relations with others, possessions, being active, undergoing adventures, etc. [48]. These areas form part of the overall domain of meaning. Most people base their meaningfulness of life on four to eight areas, and the number of areas is correlated positively with the overall rating of one's meaningfulness of life. In cancer patients both the number of areas constituting one's meaningfulness of life and the rating of one's meaningfulness of life are lower than in healthy controls. Another difference consists in the overall background of thinking tendencies characterizing individuals with high meaningfulness of life. Healthy controls with high meaningfulness of life are focused on reality, on interpersonally shared meanings, and actional-dynamic aspects complemented by emphases on experiential-cognitive and sensory aspects. Further, their thinking is goal-oriented, focused, complex, yet orderly and systematic. However, cancer patents are focused rather on experiential-cognitive and sensory aspects of reality; on personal-subjective meanings; on associative and metaphoric constructs supporting creativity tendencies, relying also on images and other nonverbal forms of expression [49]. These findings indicate that cancer patients suffer from loss of various domains constituting their meaningfulness of life and are involved in reconstruction of their meaningfulness of life. It may involve merely maintenance of the remaining areas which have neither been lost nor destroyed. But if it involves reconstruction and production of new areas for inclusion in one's meaningfulness of life, the above-described focus on personal-subjective and metaphoric meanings may be helpful [47, 50]. Changes in the meaningfulness of life may involve temporary insecurity and even anxiety but may also eventually end up with a rewarding reconstruction of one's meaningfulness of life attended by improvement in quality of life.

Sense of Self

The sense of self includes a variety of aspects relating, for example, to one's feelings, memories, qualities, functions, plans, interpersonal relations, goals, and evaluations. All of these and other similar aspects make up one's sense of self, which is sometimes called self-concept, self-image, and self-identity. The sense of self is one of the most important components that contribute to one's sense of security and stability in life [51]. When changes take place in regard to several of the characterizing items, for example, one's state of health, bodily appearance, attractiveness, or self-control, one's sense of self may undergo changes with implications in regard to one's role in life, one's identity, and the evaluation of one's competence. Cancer patients may often be heard saying "I don't know any more who I am," or "I am unsure about what I should do in life." Expressions of this kind reflect the loss of self-confidence and self-control that often accompanies the changes that may take place in one's view of oneself [52]. As long as this state lasts, the person feels anxiety and sometimes even panic. When it passes, not in the least because of the tendency to overcome the unpleasantness of anxiety, the patient may emerge with a new view of oneself which may be even broader and more stable and rewarding than the previous one (see Chap. 9 on Coping with Cancer).

The Social Impact

Cancer may impact significantly the social life and behavior of the patients. As is well documented, cancer often evokes compassion, pity, and a desire to help and provide support on the part of family members, friends, acquaintances, and even strangers. Thus, at least in the beginning of the disease, a cancer patient may get a lot of warm companionship, social interest, and support from others. Cancer patients are often pleasantly surprised by this overflow of warm friendship which they tend to attribute to their special skills and personality. However, with time other aspects of social contacts become apparent. While the support fades somewhat, patients may discover that it involves dependence on others which results in a sense of weakness and temptation to rely on others in regard to things one could do oneself. This may induce fear of loss of independence and limitations in regard to one's privacy.

Other problems that may influence the social life of cancer patients may arise because patients may feel that there is a big gap between the things that concern them and the interests of other people. In meeting other people, cancer patients often desire to talk about issues that have nothing to do with cancer and their treatments. But the other people whom they meet may feel compelled to talk about issues related to cancer because they are convinced that the patients would like to do so or in the very least expect others to show interest in their disease. Healthy people may feel somewhat insecure in their relations with cancer patients. They are not sure what is expected of them in general and by the patients in particular. They would like to do what is required and helpful but are not sure what these things are. Sometimes they would like to withdraw from the relations with cancer patients because they assume they would have to provide more help and support than they are ready or willing to. Maybe some of them would like to have as little as possible to do with the issues of cancer. This situation may result in the withdrawal of close friends from contact with cancer patients. Needless to mention that the effect on the patients is detrimental. It is not infrequent that loss of friends comes with the cancer (see also conceptions about friends and friendship, earlier this chapter) [53, 54].

Be it as it may, patients sometimes feel increasingly alienated from daily interests of healthy people [55]. They may even feel jealous of the health of other people and resentful that they do not share it. On the other hand, when cancer patients meet primarily with other cancer patients, there is a smaller gap of interests and greater sharing of relevant information concerning the disease, but the negative outcome may be that the patients feel increasingly estranged from the normal community. This feeling may be further enhanced by awareness of the stigma against cancer that is still quite frequent and strong as well as by the tendency to withdraw from regular social contacts due to external physical symptoms such as loss of hair and skin anomalies [56, 57].

Thus, cancer patients may feel different from others, and the others may feel uneasy in their company. This situation may engender social difficulties for the patients, which were shown to impact negatively their quality of life and sense of dignity [56]. Improving the situation may require some psychological work focused on clarifying the involved fears and various misunderstandings.

Impact on Behavior

The noted potential changes in the life of cancer patients may have implications also for the patients' behavior. One most important change in behavior is probably the change that may take place in the patients' work behavior. Many surveys and studies have documented the fact that unemployment, shifting to part-time work or early retirement, is frequent in cancer patients and cancer survivors, more than in healthy controls comparable in age, gender, education, ethnicity, and previous work history (e.g., [58, 59]). Some of the reasons why many cancer survivors do not return to work after treatment termination may be the fatigue that plagues many of them [60], loss of routine to work following long periods of sickness leave, or loss of working place due to long absence during the treatments [61] as well as changes in one's scale of preferences and in one's meaningfulness of life [61]. Some patients claim they would like to have more time for themselves, some would like to use the remaining time of life for enjoying things and doing things they may have missed in the past, such as traveling, doing something creative (especially if they consider their work as not creative), or leaving some kind of legacy for future generations. Considerations of this kind may underlie other changes – for example, in regard to spending money, living quarters, lifestyle, and social contacts.

Different behavioral changes have been observed in cancer patients in treatment and afterward. Some adopt a much freer lifestyle than they have led before and minimize commitments, load of obligations, and performance of duties toward others. There is evidence for increased sexual behavior and health behaviors in general in adolescents who are survivors of pediatric cancer, especially when they are healthy [62, 63]. Yet, also more sexual dysfunctions have been found in this group [64]. Others focus on doing things they would like to finish, such as a piece of art or a scientific publication or a record of their biography. Still others concentrate on enjoyment, creating social relations, or simply leading a quiet existence. Individual differences in this domain are dominant.

Physiological Impact

The physiological impact of cancer is the clearest and most salient of all kinds of impact. It is manifested in the disease itself which involves a disorder in the form of a tumor or other malignant manifestations and characteristic symptoms in different systems and parts of the body. The kind, location, and severity of the symptoms vary with the disease. Some depend directly on the tumor or its metastases, for example, pain caused by pressure of the tumor on an organ like the kidneys, jaundice caused by blocked bile ducts through pancreatic cancer, or weakness and dizziness caused by elevated blood calcium levels through hormone-like substances released by some lung cancers. Common effects of the disease may include pain, persistent cough, difficulty in swallowing, fever, weakness, unusual bleeding, disturbances in eating, sleeping and bowel movement, weight loss, confusion, and forgetfulness. This list demonstrates that the range of symptoms caused by cancer is very large and that the symptoms vary in kind and in the sites of the body which they affect. Some are more specific, like a localized pain, and some are more general, like fatigue [65–67].

The physiological effects of the cancer may be enhanced or alleviated by the common therapeutic measure of surgery. Sometimes surgery results in the loss of an organ (e.g., the breast, ovary, uterus, limb), distorted limb or part of the face, damaged skin, scars, different forms of disfigurement, or functional difficulties (e.g., walking, swallowing).

The symptoms caused by chemotherapy are no less varied or limited in their number. Their kind and severity depend on the substances used in the treatment protocol. Some chemotherapeutic agents are highly toxic and affect a wide range of cells, regardless of whether they are healthy or not. The common toxicities affect the heart, kidneys, liver, skin, digestive tract, blood, lungs, and the nervous system [68]. Certain kinds of chemotherapy are attended by sensory symptoms, such as prickly sensations or change in tastes and smelling. Some symptoms are not only unpleasant but actually dangerous such as myelosuppression with possible anemia. The most troubling symptoms for the patient include alopecia, nausea and vomiting, mouth ulcers, infertility, and impaired wound healing [68].

Further therapeutic agents include immunotherapy and other biological or targeted therapies. These therapies may also have side effects. Pain, swelling, soreness, redness, itchiness, and rash at the site of infusion are common as well as flu-like symptoms, including fever, chills, tiredness, dizziness, nausea or vomiting, muscle or joint aches, fatigue, headache, breathing difficulties, lowered or heightened blood pressure, and allergic reactions [69].

Other common treatments also have troubling side effects. Hormone therapy used mainly for breast cancer and prostate cancer may cause tiredness, headaches, loss of bone density, decreased muscle mass, hair loss, digestive problems, weight gain, blood clots, memory problems, mood swings, and increased risk for diabetes and cardiological problems (e.g., [70]).

Finally radiotherapy has common side effects in the skin (e.g., dryness, itching, peeling, or blistering) and further symptoms dependent on the site of the radiation. For example, the head and neck (difficulty swallowing, dry mouth, nausea, mouth and gum sores, jaw stiffness, and tooth decay), chest (breath shortness, difficulty swallowing, breast soreness, and shoulder stiffness), stomach and abdomen (vomiting, nausea, or diarrhea), or pelvis (rectal bleeding, incontinence, sexual and urination problems) [e.g., [71]).

Sometimes the side effects themselves need to be treated by drugs, as in the case of severe allergies or decline in different blood counts. Treatment of the side effects may also have side effects of their own, such as Neupogen for anemia or corticosteroids for allergy.

The side effects of the different treatments affect the whole body, including internal processes and external manifestations, and are often intense and of long duration, extending sometimes beyond the termination of the treatment itself. Many patients are concerned also about prolonged harm to their bones, muscles, and nerves that may be caused by the treatments. Moreover, patients are often afraid of possible later or delayed developments, including effects on fertility, reduced chances for pregnancy, and even the occurrence of other cancers, such as endometrial or leukemia following specific treatments [72].

Fatigue is a special symptom on which a lot of attention has been focused. It is a symptom that occurs with high frequency, in many different kinds of patients, following different diagnoses and treatments, and may often continue after termination of the treatments. It is often severe, does not appear as a result of activity or effort, and does not diminish appreciably after sleep or resting. It affects seriously the patients' quality of life because it reduces their ability or motivation to work, socialize, or plan their future.

The Impact on Body Image

Patients often do not differentiate between the physiological effects of the disease and of the treatments. For them it is mostly one big and protracted load. The symptoms are so extensive and intense that they may change the whole experience of one's body. Patients often report that they feel as if they have a "changed body," that the whole experience of their body is different, that they are in sense strangers who have slipped inadvertently into a body that does not quite belong to them, or that they do not belong to it. One result may be that patients feel a kind of estrangement from themselves, enhanced through the changes in the body experience. Another frequent result is that their sense of confidence in themselves and in their ability to act is hurt and may be seriously diminished. Patients may feel more vulnerable physically, worried that they may not be able to complete some action or that they may break some part of their body or that something physically unexpected may happen. For example, they may feel insecure in engaging in physical activities or even mild sport actions. Experiences of this kind often enhance the sense of insecurity and incompetence in social settings that patients may feel as well as the anxiety that they would be rejected by others [73, 74].

One frequent manifestation of changes in the body image following cancer may be presented as a change in the implicit contract an individual has with one's body. According to this contract, the body is a trustworthy partner on whose services and unquestionable cooperation one can rely. However, many patients repeat the claim that "the body has betrayed me." This claim expresses the feeling that the body has not fulfilled its expected role which was supposedly to stay healthy, to fight successfully all threats to one's health, to react as necessary to all medical treatments, and if all fails so in the very least to announce the problem so that adequate measure can be applied in time. However, as the patient sees the situation, the body has not behaved in line with any of these expectations, so that the individual feels that the body cannot be trusted anymore. This is especially unsettling since the individual considers the behavior of the body as unjustified and not attributable to anything the individual has done to it. A further aspect of the so-called assumed perfidy of the body is the change in the mutual relations of the individual and the body. The situation in which the body is in the role of serving the individual and maintaining one's well-being is replaced by the situation in which the individual is expected henceforth to serve the body, for example, by providing the body the right kind of medical treatments, drugs, and attention.

A special issue concerns weight. The impacts of cancer and cancer treatments on weight may vary greatly from loss of weight to gaining weight. So do the reactions of the patients. Gaining weight as a result of treatments or medications is an unpleasant result for many patients who may consider it as a disfigurement. On the other hand, losing weight is interpreted by many patients as an indication of disease progression, possibly even as nearness to death. Hence, the weight issue may become the focus of conflicts and anxiety [75].

Patients who have undergone gynecological surgery or breast surgery often feel that they have lost an important part of their femininity and experience serious difficulties in dating and in reinstating sexual behavior. So do men undergoing hormonal therapy for prostate cancer who may experience decline in their sexual behavior [76].

A Final Note About the Gap Between the View from Inside and Outside

In discussing the issue of the impact of cancer, it is important to note that there may be a gap between the way the patients feel about themselves and the impression that others get of them. In many cases the patients may feel that they have barely changed, while others may get the impression that the patient is not himself/herself anymore. In other cases, the situation may be reversed: the patients may feel that they have completely changed, while others may barely notice the difference between their current and previous state. Some of the reasons for this gap reside in the motivation for feeling changes in oneself. It may be that patients do not feel the change in themselves because they have invested a lot of effort to keep their image and life unchanged or because they are afraid of change or because they rely on others who insist – for reasons of their own – on convincing them that they have barely changed. On the other hand, patients may feel that they have changed a lot for reasons, such as the beliefs that an event like a cancer diagnosis is bound to produce changes in the person or that changes in the person are a kind of requirement for a positive turn in their state of health. Be it as it may, the gap between the way one feels about oneself and the way others see one is a theme that requires attention on the part of cancer patients and their therapists.

References

1. Kreitler, S., Kreitler, H., & Chaitchi, S. (1993). Repressiveness: Cause or result of cancer? *Psycho-Oncology, 2*, 43–54.
2. Iwamitsu, Y., Shimoda, K., Abe, H., Tani, T., Okawa, M., & Buck, R. (2005). Anxiety, emotional suppression, and psychological distress before and after breast cancer diagnosis. *Psychosomatics, 46*, 19–24.
3. Brandão, T., Tavares, R., Schulz, M. S., & Matos, P. M. (2016). Measuring emotion regulation and emotional expression in breast cancer patients: A systematic review. *Clinical Psychology Review, 43*, 114–127.
4. Warren, M. (2010). Uncertainty, lack of control and emotional functioning in women with metastatic breast cancer: A review and secondary analysis of the literature using the critical appraisal technique. *European Journal of Cancer Care, 19*(5), 564–574.
5. Roy-Byrne, P. P., Davidson, K. W., Kessler, R. C., Asmundson, G. J., Goodwin, R. D., Kubzansky, L., Lydiard, R. B., Massie, M. J., Katon, W., Laden, S. K., & Stein, M. B. (2008). Anxiety disorders and comorbid medical illness. *General Hospital Psychiatry, 30*(3), 208–225.
6. Roth, A., Nelson, C. J., Rosenfeld, B., Warshowski, A., O'Shea, N., Scher, H., Holland, J. C., Slovin, S., Curley-Smart, T., Reynolds, T., & Breitbart, W. (2006). Assessing anxiety in men with prostate cancer: Further data on the reliability and validity of the Memorial Anxiety Scale for Prostate Cancer (MAX-PC). *Psuchosomatics, 47*(4), 340–347.
7. Wittchen, H. U. (2002). Generalized anxiety disorder: Prevalence, burden, and cost to society. *Depression Anxiety, 16*(4), 162–171.
8. Wells, K. B., Goldin, J. M., & Burnam, M. A. (1989). Chronic medical conditions in a sample of the general population with anxiety, affective, and substance use disorders. *American Journal of Psychiatry, 146*(11), 1440–1446.
9. Harter, M. C., Conway, K. P., & Merikongas, K. R. (2003). Associations between anxiety disorders and physical illness. *European Archives of Psychiatry & Neuroscience, 253*, 313–320.
10. Australian Bureau of Statistics. (2008). *National survey of mental health and wellbeing: Summary of results*, 2007. Cat. no. (4326.0). Canberra: ABS.
11. Baxter, A. J., Vos, T., Scott, K. M., Ferrari, A. J., & Whiteford, H. A. (2014). The global burden of anxiety disorders in 2010. *Psychological Medicine, 44*(11), 2363–2374.
12. Kroenke, K., Spitzer, R. L., Williams, J. B. W., & Löwe, B. (2010). The patient health questionnaire somatic, anxiety, and depressive symptom scales: A systematic review. *Journal of Hospital Psychiatry, 32*, 345–359.
13. Korfage, I. J., Essink-Bot, M.-I., Janssens, A. C. J. W., Schröder, F. H., & de Koning, H. J. (2006). Anxiety and depression after prostate cancer diagnosis and treatment: 5-year follow-up. *British Journal of Cancer, 94*(8), 1093–1098.

14. Li, M., Hales, S., & Rodin, G. (2015). Adjustment disorders. In C. Holland, W. S. Breitbart, P. N. Butow, P. B. Jacobsen, M. J. Loscalzo, & R. McCorkle (Eds.), *Psycho-oncology* (3rd ed., pp. 274–279). New York: Oxford University Press.
15. Kessler, R. C., Chiu, W. T., Demler, O., & Walters, E. E. (2005). Prevalence, severity, and comorbidity of twelve-month DSM=IV disorders in the national comorbidity survey replication (NCS-R). *Archives of General Psychiatry, 62*(6), 617–627.
16. Massie, M. J. (2004). Prevalence of depression in patients with cancer. *Journal of the National Cancer Institute Monographs, 32*, 57–71.
17. Mitchell, A. J., Chan, M., Bhatti, H., Halton, M., Grassi, L., Johansen, C., & Meader, N. (2011). Prevalence of depression, anxiety, and adjustment disorder in oncological, haematological, and palliative-care settings: A meta-analysis of 94 interview-based studies. *Lancet Oncology, 12*(2), 160–174.
18. Brintzenhofe-Szoc, K. M., Levin, T. T., Li, Y., Kissane, D. W., & Zabora, J. R. (2009). Mixed anxiety/depression symptoms in a large cancer cohort: Prevalence by cancer type. *Psychosomatics, 50*(4), 383–391.
19. Lo, C., Zimmermann, C., Rydall, A., Walsh, A., Jones, J. M., Moore, M. J., Shepherd, F. A., Gagliese, L., & Rodin, G. (2010). Longitudinal study of depressive symptoms in patients with metastatic gastrointestinal and lung cancer. *Journal of Clinical Oncology, 28*(18), 3084–3089.
20. DiMatteo, M. R., & Haskard-Zolnierek, K. B. (2011). Impact of depression on treatment adherence and survival from cancer. In D. W. Kissane, M. Maj, & N. Sartorius (Eds.), *Depression and cancer* (pp. 101–124). Chichester: Wiley & Blackwell.
21. Breitbart, W., Pessin, H., & Kova, E. (2011). Suicide and desire for hastened death in people with cancer. In D. W. Kissane, M. Maj, & N. Sartorius (Eds.), *Depression and cancer* (pp. 125–150). Chichester: Wiley & Blackwell.
22. Robinson, S., Kissane, D. W., Brooker, J., & Burney, S. (2016). A review of the construct of demoralization: History, definitions, and future directions for palliative care. *American Journal of Hospice and Palliative Care, 33*(1), 93–101.
23. Orbach, J., Mikulincer, M., Sirota, P., & Gilbora-Schechtman, E. (2003). Mental pain: A multidimensional operationalization and definition. *Suicide and Life-Threatening Behavior, 33*(3), 219–230.
24. Bultz, B. D., & Johansen, C. (2011). Special issue: Screening for distress, the 8th vital sign. *Psycho-Oncology, 20*, 569–674.
25. Kim, G. M., Kim, J. S., Song, S. K., Kim, H. R., Kang, B. D., Noh, S. H., Chung, H. C., Kim, K. R., & Rha, S. Y. (2017). Prevalence and prognostic implications of psychological distress in patients with gastric cancer. *BMC Cancer, 17*, 283.
26. Taylor, E. J., Baird, S. B., Malone, D., & McCorkle, R. (1993). Factors associated with anger in cancer patients and their caregivers. *Cancer Practice, 1*(2), 101–109.
27. Adams, R. N., Mosher, C. E., Abonour, R., Robertson, M. J., Champion, V. L., & Kroenke, K. (2016). Cognitive and situational precipitants of cancer patients' loneliness: A qualitative analysis. *Oncology Nursing Forum, 43*(2), 156–163.
28. Deckx, L., van den Akker, M., & Buntinx, F. (2014). Risk factors for loneliness in patients with cancer: A systematic literature review and meta-analysis. *European Journal of Oncology Nursing, 18*(5), 466–477.
29. Clarke, D. (2003). Faith and hope. *Australasian Psychiatry, 11*, 164–168.
30. Tannock, V. J. (2007). Cognitive function after chemotherapy in adults with solid tumours. *Critical Reviews in Oncology/Hematology, 63*(3), 183–202.
31. Moore, H. C. (2014). An overview of chemotherapy-related cognitive dysfunction, or 'chemobrain'. *Oncology, 28*(9), 787–804.
32. Wefel, J. S., Lenzi, R., Theriault, R., Buzdar, A. U., Cruickshank, S., & Meyers, C. A. (2004). Chemobrain' in breast carcinoma? A prologue. *Cancer, 101*, 466–475.
33. McDonald, B. C., Conroy, S. K., Ahles, T. A., et al. (2012). Alterations in brain activation during working memory processing associated with breast cancer and treatment: A prospective functional MRI study. *Journal of Clinical Oncology, 30*, 2500–2508.

34. Meyers, C. A., Albitar, M., & Estey, E. (2005). Cognitive impairment, fatigue, and cytokine levels in patients with acute myelogenous leukemia or myelodysplastic syndrome. *Cancer, 104*, 788–793.
35. Seigers, R., & Fardell, J. E. (2011). Neurobiological basis of chemotherapy-induced cognitive impairment: A review of rodent research. *Neuroscience and Biobehavioral Reviews, 35*(3), 729–741.
36. Koppelmans, V., Breteler, M. M., Boogerd, W., Seynaeve, C., Gundy, C., & Schagen, S. B. (2012). Neuropsychological performance in survivors of breast cancer more than 20 years after adjuvant chemotherapy. *Journal of Clinical Oncology, 30*(10), 1080–1086.
37. Ahles, T. A., Root, J. C., & Ryan, E. L. (2012). Cancer- and cancer treatment-associated cognitive change: An update on the state of the science. *Journal of Clinical Oncology, 30*(30), 3675–3686.
38. Kreitler, S., Weyl Ben Arush, M., Krivoy, E., Golan, H., Yalon, M., & Toren, A. (2016). Psychosocial aspects of radiotherapy for the child and family with cancer (Chapter 26). In L. S. Constine, N. J. Tarbell, & E. C. Halperin (Eds.), *Pediatric radiation oncology* (7th ed., pp. 1–12). Alphen aan den Rijn: Wolters Kluwen Health.
39. Mandelblatt, J. S., Hurria, A., McDonald, B. C., Saykin, A. J., Stern, R. A., VanMet, J. W., McGuckin, M., Traina, T., Denduluri, N., Turner, S., Howard, D., Jacobsen, P. B., & Ahles, T. (2013). Cognitive effects of cancer and its treatments at the intersection of aging: What do we know; what do we need to know? Thinking and Living With Cancer Study. *Seminars in Oncology, 40*(5), 709–725.
40. Lee, P. E., Tierney, M. C., Wu, W., Pritchard, K. I., & Rochon, P. A. (2016). Endocrine treatment-associated cognitive impairment in breast cancer survivors: Evidence from published studies. *Breast Cancer Research and Treatment, 158*(3), 407–420.
41. Simó, M., Vaquero, L., Ripollés, P., Jové, J., Fuentes, R., Cardenal, F., Rodríguez-Fornells, A., & Bruna, J. (2016). Brain damage following prophylactic cranial irradiation in lung cancer survivors. *Brain Imaging and Behavior, 10*(1), 283–295.
42. Kreitler, S. (submitted). Cognitive rehabilitation effects of cognitive treatment for pediatric cancer patients with CNS malignancies. *Journal of Palliative Care* (under review).
43. Lerner, M. J., & Montada, L. (1998). An overview: Advances in belief in a just world theory and methods. In L. Montada & M. J. Lerner (Eds.), *Responses to victimizations and belief in a just world* (pp. 1–7). New York: Plenum Press.
44. Puchalski, C. M. (2012). Spirituality in the cancer trajectory. *Annals of Oncology, 23*(Issue Suppl 3), 49–55.
45. Penson, R. T., Yusuf, R. Z., Chabner, B. A., Lafranceska, J. P., MCelhinny, M., Axelrad, A., & Lynch, T. J., Jr. (2001). Losing God. *The Oncologist, 6*, 286–297.
46. Kenen, R., Ardern-Jones, A., & Eeles, R. (2006). "Social separation" among women under 40 years of age diagnosed with breast and carrying a BRCA1 or BRCA2 mutation. *Journal of Genetic Counseling, 15*(3), 149–162.
47. Martino, M. L., & Freda, M. F. (2016). Meaning-making process related to temporality during breast cancer traumatic experience: The clinical use of narrative to promote a new continuity of life. *Europe's Journal of Psychology, 12*(4), 622–634.
48. Kreitler, S. (2014, July 5–8). Meaning-based assessment of the meaningfulness of life. *European conference on psychological assessment ECPA 14*. Lisbon.
49. Kreitler, S. (2016). Meanings of meaningfulness of life. In A. Batthyany (Ed.), *Logotherapy and existential analysis* (Vol. 1, pp. 95–106). Vienna: Springer.
50. Kreitler, S. (2016). Meaningfulness of life and its impact on quality of life. In C. Pracana & M. Wang (Eds.), *International psychological applications and trends (InPact)* (pp. 392–394). Lisbon: W.I. R.
51. Kreitler, S., & Kreitler, H. (1987). Psychosemantic aspects of the self. In T. M. Honess & K. M. Yardley (Eds.), *Self and identity: Individual change and development* (pp. 338–358). London: Routledge and Kegan Paul.

52. Kreitler, S. (2017). Who am i? A meaning-based approach to assessing the self image. In C. Pracana & M. Wang (Eds.), *International psychological applications and trends (InPact)* (pp. 429–433). Lisbon: W.I. R. S.
53. Podmore, E. J., Bingham, A. C., Roberts, K. M., Selby, P. J., & Velikova, P. W. G. (2009). Routine assessment of social difficulties in cancer patients: Are we opening Pandora's box? *Supportive Care in Cancer, 17*, 1425–1432.
54. Kreitler, S. (2014). Special aspects of social issues in cancer (Chapter 9). In H. van Halteren (Ed.), ESMO *handbook on rehabilitation issues during cancer treatment and follow-up*. European Society for Medical Oncology (ESMO), *Annals of Oncology*.
55. Figueiredo, M. I., Fries, E., & Ingram, K. M. (2004). The role of disclosure patterns and unsupportive social interactions in the well-being of breast cancer patients. *Psycho-Oncology, 13*(2), 96–105.
56. Philipp, R., Mehnert, A., Lehmann, C., Oechsle, K., Bokemeyer, C., Krüll, A., & Vehling, S. (2016). Detrimental social interactions predict loss of dignity among patients with cancer. *Supportive Care in Cancer, 24*(6), 2751–2758.
57. Trusson, D., & Pilnick, A. (2016). Between stigma and pink positivity: Women's perceptions of social interactions during and after breast cancer treatment. *Sociology of Health & Illness, 39*(3), 458–473.
58. De Boer, A. G., Taskila, T., Ojajärvi, A., Van Dijk, F. J., & Verbeek, J. H. (2009). Cancer survivors and unemployment: A meta-analysis and meta-regression. *The Journal of the American Medical Association, 301*(7), 753–762.
59. Ratzon, N., Uziely, B., De Boer, A. G., & Rottenberg, Y. (2016). Unemployment risk and decreased income 2 and 4 years after thyroid cancer diagnosis: A population based study. *Thyroid, 26*(9), 1251–1258.
60. Spelten, E. R., Verbeek, J. H., Uitterhoeve, A. L., Ansink, A. C., van der Lelie, J., de Reijke, T. M., Kammeijer, M., de Haes, J. C., & Sprangers, M. A. (2003). Cancer, fatigue and the return of patients to work-a prospective cohort study. *European Journal of Cancer, 39*(11), 1562–1567.
61. Mehnert, A. (2011). Employment and work-related issues in cancer survivors. *Critical Reviews in Oncology/Hematology, 77*, 109–130.
62. Klosky, J. L., Foster, R. H., Peasant, C., Howell, C. R., Mertens, A. C., Robinson, L. L., & Ness, K. K. (2014). Risky sexual behavior in adolescent survivors of childhood cancer: A report from the Childhood Cancer Survivor Study. *Health Psychology, 33*(8), 868–877.
63. Lown, E. A., Hijiya, N., Zhang, N., Srivastava, D. K., Leisenring, W. M., Nathan, P. C., Castellino, S. M., Devine, K. A., Dilley, K., Krull, K. R., Oeffinger, K. C., Hudson, M. M., Armstrong, G. T., Robison, L. L., & Ness, K. K. (2016). Patterns and predictors of clustered risky health behaviors among adult survivors of childhood cancer: A report from the Childhood Cancer Survivor Study. *Cancer, 122*(17), 2747–2756.
64. Bober, S. L., Zhou, E. S., Chen, B., Manley, P. E., Kenney, L. B., & Recklitis, C. J. (2013). Sexual function in childhood cancer survivors: A report from Project REACH. *Journal of Sexual Medicine, 10*(8), 2084–2093.
65. Kirkova, J., Davis, M. P., Walsh, D., Tiernan, E., O'Leary, N., LeGrand, S. B., Lagman, R. L., & Russell, K. M. (2016). Cancer symptom assessment instruments: A systematic review. *Journal of Clinical Oncology, 24*, 1459–1473.
66. Dupuis, L. L., Ethier, M.-C., Tomlinson, D., Hesser, T., & Sung, L. (2012). A systematic review of symptom assessment scales in children with cancer. *BMC Cancer, 12*, 430.
67. Reilly, C., Bruner, D. W., Mitchell, S. A., Minasian, L. M., Basch, E., Dueck, A. C., Cella, D., & Reeve, B. B. (2013). A literature synthesis of symptom prevalence and severity in persons receiving active cancer treatment. *Supportive Care in Cancer, 21*(6), 1525–1550.
68. Tipton, T. M. (2015). Side-effects of chemotherapy. In S. M. Khleif, O. Rixe, & R. T. Skeel (Eds.), *Skeel's handbook of cancer therapy* (9th ed., pp. 632–656). Riverwoods: Wolters Kluver Health.

69. Janik, J. E. (2015). Side-effects of immunotherapy. In S. M. Khleif, O. Rixe, & R. T. Skeel (Eds.), *Skeel's handbook of cancer therapy* (9th ed., pp. 857–666). Riverwoods: Wolters Kluver Health.
70. Lin, J. J., Chao, J., Bickell, N. A., & Visniwetsky, J. P. (2017). Patient-provider communication and hormonal therapy side effects in breast cancer survivors. *Women & Health, 57*(8), 976–989.
71. Janssen, S., Käsmann, L., Fahlbusch, F. B., Rades, D., & Vordermark, D. (2018). Side effects of radiotherapy in breast cancer patients: The internet as an information source. *Strahlentherapie Und Onkologie*. *194*(2), 136–142.
72. Oh, H. S., & Seo, W. S. (2011). Systematic review and meta-analysis of the correlates of cancer-related fatigue. *Worldviews on Evidence-Based Nursing, 8*(4), 181–201.
73. Miaja, M., Platas, A., & Martinez-Cannon, B. A. (2017). Psychological impact of alterations in sexuality, fertility, and body image in young breast cancer patients and their partners. *Revista De Investigacion Clinica, 69*(4), 204–209.
74. Lehmann, V., Hagedoorn, M., & Tuinman, M. A. (2015). Body image in cancer survivors: A systematic review of case-control studies. *Journal of Cancer Survivorship: Research and Practice, 9*(2), 339–348.
75. Stamataki, Z., Burden, S., & Molassiotis, A. (2011). Weight changes in oncology patients during the first year after diagnosis: A qualitative investigation of the patients' experiences. *Cancer Nursing, 34*(5), 401–409.
76. Oberguggenberger, A., Martini, C., Huber, N., Fallowfield, L., Hubalek, M., Daniaux, M., Sperner-Unterweger, B., Holzner, B., Sztankay, M., Gamper, E., & Meraner, V. (2017). Self-reported sexual health: Breast cancer survivors compared to women from the general population – An observational study. *BMC Cancer, 17*, 599.

Chapter 7
Major Decision in the Life of Cancer Patients

Involvement of Patients in Decisions

One may expect that getting a cancer diagnosis implies assuming henceforth a passive role in life and adopting decisions of others concerning one's health and treatments. Actually most patients learn soon enough that nothing is less true. Becoming a cancer patient implies that an increasing number of issues become open for decision-making. Those who are scared that others will take the lead regarding their life and will control them may wonder at some point whether it would not have been better to give up some of the control which they had to assume.

There are a great number of issues in regard to which the patient expects others to take the lead, and there are many issues that the patient expects oneself to be capable of assuming the decision-maker role. The former relates to medical decisions, the latter more to personal life decisions. In reality mostly it does not turn out to be the case. The patient is often engaged or even pressured to participate in decision-making in regard to medical issues, and others are often mobilized to participate in decisions regarding the patient's private or personal life.

Decisions Regarding Medical Issues

The Problem of Patient Participation

It is unlikely that there is any other domain in medicine in which patients are called upon to participate in the crucial decisions about their health and treatments to the same extent as in cancer. This may seem surprising in view of the fact that cancer diagnosis and treatment require a lot of highly professional medical information and experience. The information is complicated; it is based on expertise in a variety of domains including genetics, physiology, pharmaceutics, surgery, etc.; it refers to

S. Kreitler, *Psycho-Oncology for the Clinician*,
https://doi.org/10.1007/978-3-030-06126-5_7

different systems and organs in the body and is constantly updated in view of research and FDA decisions. Moreover, even in the domain of medicine, no one doctor can be proficient in aspects, organs, and all kinds of treatment of cancer. In addition to a lot of precise information, the medical decisions in regard to cancer benefit from prolonged experience of the doctor and the other involved health professionals.

The involvement of patients in the processes of medical decisions has been prompted initially mainly by the pressure of the patients themselves. The original reasons may have been lack of trust of the patients in the doctors because they did not always get all the information about the disease. This reason is not valid anymore because the imparting of information to patients is complete or highly advanced in many countries. Nevertheless, patients still tend to consider the issue of participation in decisions as part of the information provision requirement [1]. This attitude is supported by the logical need for information in order to express any kind of attitude in regard to a medical treatment or other therapeutic issue.

However, now that the habit of enabling patients to participate in the decisions has been established, patients feel almost compelled to get involved in the decisional procedures as if their recovery or survival depended on it, at least to some extent. Doctors on their side also started viewing decisions about cancer treatments as "personal decisions" by the patients and got used to involving patients in these decisions. Some of them at least confess that they prefer in a way to share the responsibility with the patients [2].

Getting involved in medical decisions may be difficult for some patients, because they may feel incompetent and maybe also because they would not like to hurt their doctor by expressing in this way their possible lack of trust in him or her. Moreover, not a few patients would like to rely on the authoritative decision of the expert health professionals instead of taking a stand in these matters. But they find it hard to insist because of the pressure of family and friends who tend to consider such behavior as evasive, prompted by denial and fear, and running against the current trend of empowerment by the patient. Consequently, many patients suffer from a kind of implicit conflict between accepting the doctor's decision and making their own decision, solving this dilemma by stating that they got convinced by the choices and arguments of their doctor [3].

Decisions About Medical Issues in Which Patients May Be Called upon to Participate

The major decisions concern the kinds of treatment, their sequence, the time at which they will be started or ended, the location (hospital or clinic) where they will be administered, and the doctor who will be in charge.

Concerning *treatment options*, it is necessary to consider that their kind and number depend on the specific disease. In regard to prostate cancer, there are initially more options than in the case of some other cancer diseases, for example, active surveillance, hormonal treatment, or surgery. Patients may be faced with the decision whether to opt for hormonal therapy or surgery. Patients with prostate cancer may reject surgery because they may be unwilling to endanger their urinary control or erection. In regard to ductal carcinoma in situ (DCIS) diagnoses in breast cancer, the decision addresses the issue whether to undergo surgery or continue with recurrent biopsies. Another kind of decision concerns bilateral mastectomy after the occurrence of cancer in one breast or even as precaution prior to diagnosis [4], or undergoing radiation therapy instead of surgery in the case of thyroid cancer [5]. In some cases, patients are faced with the option of two kinds of surgery, differing in how radical, extensive, damaging, or protective against disease recurrence they are, as in breast surgery, prostate cancer, laryngectomy, and thyroid cancer. Concerning breast cancer treatment, patients may be advised by the doctor to undergo excision of the ovaries, which they may decide to do right away together with the breast surgery or later at some point in time or not at all. Sometimes patients are faced with the decision to opt between two different chemotherapy protocols differing in the severity of side effects. At other times, breast cancer patients, for example, may be faced with the situation of choosing between different maintenance drugs, such as Femara, Arimidex, or tamoxifen.

In many medical centers, it is habitual to offer patients in-treatment psychiatric medication, primarily antianxiolytic and antidepressants. Patients may accept these drugs or not, on the basis of personal considerations. Similar attitudes may be evoked in patients concerning different adjuvant drugs designed to take care of different functions, such as blood counts, nausea, weight in the course of treatments, pain control and more recently to the offers to use cannabis. In regard to all these medications, sometimes the patients resist, sometimes they consent, and sometimes they consent but do not fully adhere to ingesting these drugs for the required periods (see *Decisional Conflicts*).

Some treatments are required after termination of the major phases and depend on the patients' adherence to the regulations for prolonged periods of time (see above Femara and tamoxifen) [6].

There are two kinds of treatments about which it is usually the patient who decides. These are complementary or alternative treatments and the psychosocial treatments. Although in some medical institutions complementary treatments are encouraged or even offered to the patient in the course of medical treatments, it is still up to the patient to decide whether he or she would like to undergo them. In an increasing number of cases, patients choose to accept the offer and try these treatments. In regard to psychosocial treatments, patients may have more reservations because of the potential connotations of personal weakness, incompetency, and failing mental health (see Chaps. 6 and 8).

Concerning the *sequence of treatments*, patients sometimes participate in deciding for example whether to undergo chemotherapy prior to surgery (in breast cancer or colorectal cancer) or following it, or which sequence of treatments to apply in the case of renal cancer [7]. Other similar decisions are whether to start chemotherapy prior to biological treatments, in case the choice is at all given [8]. A question about sequence may arise also in regard to alternative or complementary treatments. Patients may be aware or may be advised that some alternative treatments may collide with the standard medical treatments, for example, by reducing their impact.

Hence, it may be necessary or advisable to decide about some kind of sequence in regard to the standard and alternative treatments.

Concerning *the time of starting treatment*, in cases of dormant lymphoma or leukemia which have been only followed up for some time, when it seems advisable to start active treatment, patients often have their say about when to start it, within the range of days or a few weeks. Similarly, patients often participate in determining the time of surgery as well as the days of the week on which they undergo chemotherapy, for example. The freedom of choice that patients may have regarding the starting of treatment or when to undergo it makes it possible for many of them to maintain their routine way of life or go on working despite the treatments.

The *termination or stopping of treatments* is a more controversial issue. Patients may decide to discontinue a treatment they have already begun, because it is too difficult for them. This decision is particularly controversial when the doctor is opposed to it and considers a good chance for a beneficial effect of the treatment. In some cases, patients opt not even to start the treatment, usually of chemotherapy, often because they consider that it has toxic dangerous effects. If patients tend or consider resisting treatment, then it is most often chemotherapy that they decide not to undergo. Surgery is less often resisted. Patients more often undergo surgery which they consider an aggressive one-time single-coup radical treatment that may solve their medical problem [9].

There may be additional reasons for the decision to stop or *discontinue specific kinds of treatment*. Thus, in regard to medication prescribed for maintenance for longer periods of time (e.g., tamoxifen for breast cancer or medication like Gleevec for leukemia), patients may stop taking it after a certain period of time. Their decision may be prompted by the desire to feel "healthy" since they tend to believe that people who take medication regularly cannot be considered healthy. Another reason may be the desire to avoid some of the side effects of the treatments, such as gaining weight (sometimes in the case of tamoxifen), fatigue, or mood effects.

The situation is different for patients with advanced disease who have already undergone more than one cycle of treatment. Decisions concerning the discontinuation of treatment at this point are more complicated because the patients are already weaker and their expectations about the benefits of treatments are lower than initially. They have already experienced the difficult and scary phase of disease recurrence and do not trust treatments as much as originally. In general it is evident to all involved that the expected benefits of improvement are not as great in view of the patient's state but that the cost in terms of decline in quality of life may be appreciable. At this stage also, the doctors are less convinced of the necessity or utility of the treatments, and their arguments for continuation of the treatment may be less forceful. However, even if patients tend to terminate treatments at this stage, they may still surrender to the explicit or implicit pressure or expectations of family members who would like to continue treatments at any cost, sometimes for no other reason than in order to make sure that everything possible has been done for the patient.

In some cases the decision to discontinue treatment in an advanced stage of the disease does not mean complete cessation of all treatment but only discontinuation of active curative treatment and its replacement by palliative treatment. The point in time when this decision is implemented is suggested by the doctor, but the actual decision is made by the patient [10].

An issue that need not be overlooked in the present context is the decision of some patients *not to undergo any treatment at all.* The reasons may be lack of trust in the utility of medical treatments, fear of the damage the treatments may cause, reliance on one's physical constitution and internal health-supporting forces, reliance on higher powers like God, reliance on psychological therapies or procedures like guided imagery or shamanic practices, etc., or trust in the support of spiritual communities. Finally, the reasons for avoidance of treatment may include also desire to die, desire to avoid the pain of treatments and the involved suffering, or desire to get punished for something one has done and which one considers as a crime deserving death.

Another issue that patients may be able to decide concerns *the location of undergoing the treatment*, for example, whether it will be in a hospital or a clinic, close to their home or in another city. Whether decisions of this kind are at all possible depends on the country, the area, and sometimes the socioeconomic state of the individuals or their families. Different locations may provide different services or amenities, even better forms of treatment, and better care. Sometimes decisions about location involve also decisions about the doctor who will be in charge (see Chap. 11).

Location for treatment may refer also to the last phases of a patient's life. After a patient passes from the curative to the palliative stage of treatment, the decision which the patient faces is where to stay. The options include one's home (which is actually – in the community), a nursing home, or a hospice. Not all options are always available or available for everyone. Some people cannot stay at home because they may need more help than is available at home or they cannot afford paying for it. In some locations, no hospice is available. Hence, some patients may need to stay in the hospital [11].

Further Decisional Issues of Medical Relevance

There are further important medical decisions which patients make or in which they participate. One frequent case is *getting a second opinion.* Getting the opinion of another doctor or medical center concerning one's diagnosis or recommended treatment is a first-rate medical decision. It has implications in regard to trusting one's doctor and in regard to personal empowerment, even if the trust in one's doctor is unswerving. In the domain of cancer, getting a second opinion is a highly common practice, so much so that even the doctors themselves sometimes encourage the patients to engage in it and may even participate in the process by suggesting second-opinion consultants. Sometimes the decision to address a second opinion source is made under the pressure of one's family and friends. However it may be, one's doctor is often consulted by the patient for the final decision, especially in cases where the two opinions do not match. Yet, it is also not rare that the patient decides to switch doctors and engage the second-opinion doctor as the main one [12].

Sometimes patients participate in deciding *whether to undergo different medical tests* in the course of their treatment. For example, tests of this kind may help in determining the extent to which a chemotherapy protocol is likely to benefit the patient (or rather, whether it belongs to treatments that do not benefit the patient), or making tests at the termination of treatment to establish the extent to which the treatment has benefitted the patient. Surprisingly, some patients do the former tests even though they have to pay for them personally. The reasons may be to get an assurance that the choice of treatment was right or in order to test the doctor or just in order to establish one's participation in the decision process. In contrast, some patients do not do the latter tests even though they constitute part of the protocol for which they do not need to carry the costs. The reasons may be to avoid confronting the unpleasant option of finding out that the change in the disease is less than has been expected or in order to feel that they have not ended their relationship with the hospital or the treatment and continue in a way to be protected medically.

Breast reconstruction is another theme about which patients often decide by themselves or share the decision with an expert. The decision involves not only whether to perform the reconstruction but also the time for the surgery – in the course of the primary surgery for extraction of the tumor or separately and later. Considerations supporting a positive decision are, for example, the patient's desire to preserve her bodily appearance and sense of femininity, whereas a negative decision is often based on fear that the reconstructed breast may endanger early detection of potential recurrence of the disease [13].

Testing for genetic tendencies is another controversial decisional issue for cancer patients. The tests concern usually BRCA1 and BRCA2 concerning primarily breast cancer and ovarian cancer and HNPCC (or Lynch syndrome) concerning uterine and colon cancer. Many aspects can be involved in the decision for genetic testing. Apart from the possible implications of the genetic findings for the medical treatment, a great number of psychosocial aspects may be involved in genetic testing. The major ones concern cancer risk for oneself and others. For example, the finding that one carries a genetic propensity implies the possibility that one will get cancer or an additional cancer, and that one's children may get cancer. Information of this kind affects relations to others in the family from whom one may have inherited the genetic tendency, as well as to one's children and other blood relatives who may be directly or indirectly influenced by the findings. It may affect one's plans for having children at all or when (e.g., as early as possible prior to excision of ovaries), one's life narrative and one's financial decisions [14, 15].

Fertility concerns constitute one of the most basic and disturbing themes for cancer patients. Cancer as a disease and the different treatments devised for it may affect fertility in various ways, in both men and women, and even in cases of pediatric cancer. Different procedures for the preservation of fertility have been devised for cancer patients. The major ones include pharmacological protective means against damage by chemotherapy (GnRH analogues), IVF and cryopreservation of embryos, oocyte or sperm cryopreservation, ovarian transposition, or transplantation of ovarian tissue. In view of the multiplicity of options and the urgency of action, many patients undergo a serious decisional crisis. They need to study the options: the chances of success, the difficulties, the risks, the benefits, and the need of possibly delaying cancer treatment in regard to some options. The decision is harder in the case of single women who have not yet had children or childless men [16, 17].

Participating in clinical trials may constitute another decisional issue for patients. The option of participating in clinical trials is often proposed to patients, especially in more advanced stages of the disease when it may appear that the standard treatments are not sufficiently efficient. Clinical trials are a necessary requirement for developing and testing new drugs for cancer treatment. They are conducted in four major phases with human subjects. However, it is well known that recruitment is slow and that patients do not always readily volunteer to participate [18]. The decision to participate in clinical trials is one of the most difficult issues for patients. Considerations that support a positive decision on the part of patients include the desire to exploit any flicker of hope that could contribute to their health or at least to delaying death; the financial benefit which is sometimes offered; the tendency to please their doctor who suggested participation; readiness to contribute to the welfare of others in general or to science specifically; wish to perform a good deed in general or as a response to the good treatment they have previously got in the hospital; and interest in the study itself [19–21]. On the other hand, there are considerations that may function as barriers to consent to participate. These include the feeling that one is exploited without being given sufficient retribution, misgivings about possible harm that may be caused by a drug that has not been sufficiently studied, fear of being included in a placebo arm of the study, and fear of missing out on the regular treatment that could have perhaps benefitted the patient [22–24].

The Effects of Shared Decisions

Studies show that the majority of patients would like to get a lot of information about the disease and the available treatments [25]. Yet, most patients feel there is a gap, varying in size, between the degree to which they would like to get information and be involved in the decisions and the degree to which these objectives are actually implemented. The extent to which the patients desire participation in decisions varies in the different diagnoses. It is highest (around 90%) in healthy individuals or newly diagnosed prostate cancer patients but lower (about 64%) in breast cancer patients [26–28]. Additionally, the higher the degree of patients' participation in decisions, the higher is their satisfaction, as well as the degree to which they feel self-efficacy [29], and the rating they assign to the quality of treatment [30]. Also, patients who have participated in the decision are less likely to stop treatment prior to its termination. Patients who participated as they desired felt less depression, anxiety, and fatigue after the consultation and were less depressed also later [31]. The findings reported in this section have contributed largely to shaping the generally accepted conception about the positive effects of patients' participation in the decision process.

Decisional Conflicts

There are many reports of the conflicts that cancer patients experience in regard to the decisions that need to be undertaken. Conflicts of patients concerning decisions can vary in severity. Sometimes they may be described as mere doubts, while at other times they may be so severe and even prolonged that they act like paralyzing forces. The decisional conflict scale [32] assesses three kinds of states concerning decisions: uncertainty in selecting options; factors contributing to uncertainty such as feeling uninformed, unclarity about personal values involved in the decision, and lack of support in decision-making; and effective decision-making reflecting the feeling that the decision is based on adequate information, conforms to one's values, includes the intent to implement it, and is accompanied by a sense of satisfaction with the whole process [33]. These various possibilities are assessed by the decisional conflict scale.

There is evidence that decisional conflict in patients is related to getting more information from the health professionals [34]. It is possible that patients who present a decisional conflict start a discussion that results in actually getting more information. This is supported by studies showing that having sufficient information results in low levels of decisional conflict [35].

Studies show that patients who have been exposed to inconsistent information experience more decisional conflict [36]. In a complementary manner, those who got more information feel more self-efficacy and experience less decisional conflict [37]. Personal uncertainty, also called "decisional conflict," is more prevalent when patients are uninformed, have unclear values, and do not feel adequately supported [31]. In general, patients who have had decisional conflict feel more satisfied with their decision and feel less regret up to 6 months after treatment [34]. A decisional conflict must not necessarily result in a satisfactory decision. When this is not the case, the decision is attended by regret and feelings of having been deceived or misled or not having obtained enough help or support from the health professionals. In such cases the patient may manifest only partial adherence to the treatment regulations or requirements.

Most decisional conflicts arise in regard to the medical issues themselves. However, some may concern the very problem of participating as a patient in the decision-making process, with which the patients are not completely in accord, namely, they may not feel comfortable with participating in the decision process (see next section).

Factors Which Affect the Patient's Decisions

There are various kinds of factors likely to impact the patients' decisions. The reason for the variety is that the decisions are of different kinds and the contexts vary with the patients' personalities, needs, and background as well as with the doctors, diagnoses, and disease stage. The present section will focus on some of the most salient and common factors. The doctors' recommendations carry a lot of weight. One set of general factors are the characteristics of the doctor. Patients tend to accept the recommendations of a doctor who is assertive and clear in the options he/she proposes to the patient and exudes confidence accompanied by empathy and readiness to listen to the patient [38, 39]. Even mere clarity in the outlined options may function as a factor affecting decisions [40]. Further, patients are likely to respond favorably to doctors who are known as experts in their field, behave in an authoritative manner, and easily provide the relevant information [41, 42].

Studies showed that exposure to psychoeducational materials and different tools that improve the patients' understanding of the involved medical issues plays an important role as a factor affecting the patients' decisions. The major influence is to render the patients more receptive to logical and relevant arguments [38, 43] which may even spare them post-decisional regret [44].

Patient-related factors that could impact the patients' decisions are the perceptions of patients about the attitudes of family members and acquaintances in regard to the considered issues. Thus, at least some patients tend to adhere to views expressed by family members, friends, and acquaintances in general. A possible reason may be the wish to ascertain support of family and friends in implementing the selected option. A special weight may be assigned also to the views of other patients encountered in the hospital and clinics because they are assumed to be relatively experienced and impartial in regard to the selected option. In recent years social networks have become an increasingly important factor impacting health decisions. Despite the widespread awareness of the unreliability of this source of information, there seems to be something enticing in the reports of individuals worldwide who share their opinions and experiences often without disclosing their identities or bases of evidence [45, 46]. In this context a particularly interesting important factor, whose impact is however transitory, is the media and internet presentation of the behavior or selected options by celebrities. It is as if the patient assumes implicitly that "if this option has been selected by or for the celebrity it must also be good enough for me."

Factors related to the patients' personality may also impact decisions. Thus, some patients feel more comfortable when they assume a passive role in regard to decisions while others prefer an active role [47, 48]. Some patients try to minimize their involvement so as to reduce their responsibility for the decision and regret concerning the outcome. Involving patients of this kind in active decision-making may increase their anxiety [49, 50].

The Difficulties of Shared Decisions: For Patient and for Doctor

The prevalence of decisional conflicts and the variety of reactions following decisions and shared decisions, ranging from satisfaction to regret, indicate that the situation of decision-making may be fraught with difficulties. For doctors the situation in which they are expected to discuss medical issues with patients and their relatives may be experienced as an extra load, a requirement in which they may not be at their best. It is likely that at least some doctors are not used to discussing or explaining medical issues in popular terms and may even consider this task as useless or superfluous. This is not surprising because patients cannot be expected to have the necessary information for discussions of this kind, and even if they have acquired this information they do not master the habitual medical jargon used for discussing the medical issues in question. Studies show that there are big differences in understanding and communication between experts and non-experts in regard to themes they may be discussing, regardless of their educational and informational background [51, 52]. Further, the need to explain the medical issues to patients may not be a pleasant task for some doctors who may even believe that it is of only limited benefit for the patients [53].

Patients too may feel uneasy in the situation in which they are expected – by themselves and their family members – to share in decision-making regarding medical issues. Some patients may have low self-esteem in general and especially in the unfamiliar situation in which they are required to undertake decisions in regard to medical questions. The low self-esteem may inhibit them in posing the relevant questions to their doctors or expressing their opinions at all.

Further, many patients are not used at all to making decisions on their own, or at least not in regard to issues in which they understand very little. Many individuals did not have the chance to acquire decision-making habits in general and especially not decision-sharing habits in the contexts of their families and schools where they have learned rather to follow the decisions made by others, mostly people in authority. Accordingly, many patients may have little experience and practice in making decisions or sharing decision-making.

Additionally, in many cases, patients are attended in the decision situation contexts by their spouses, relatives, and friends, who come on their own or are invited by the patient in order to provide help and support [26, 29]. It is often difficult for the patient to adopt a decision that is contrary to that upheld by his or her friends and family members [54].

In general, decision-making in regard to cancer is a highly difficult task. First, it involves the need to consider many different aspects, each with its own background, implications, and assessment characteristics. Secondly, it refers to options that are characterized by uncertainty, involve risks, and are often ambiguous. These features become particularly relevant in view of the fact that many people have an uncertainty aversion to the extent that they may prefer a worse but less risky option [55]. Thirdly, the situation includes strong emotional reactions that may be opposed to the rational cognitive considerations. It requires self-control and expertise to deal with decisions that involve both cognitive and emotional connotations which may not always match [56]. The three mentioned features combine with others to render decision-making in cancer into a highly complicated problem.

Decisions Regarding Nonmedical or Personal Issues

This section is designed to complement the first section of the chapter which dealt with "Decisions regarding medical issues." However, the title of this second section is ambiguous. On the one hand, it is expected to focus on nonmedical issues, but on the other hand, it is evident that in the present context even apparently personal issues are in fact determined and evoked by the medical issues. Still, the situation in regard to personal issues is often more complicated because both the particular characteristics of the personal preexisting situation and the characteristics of the medical situation interact to produce in most cases a unique medico-personal issue.

Decisions Relating to Interpersonal Issues

Some of the major personal decisions that face many patients concern interpersonal relations. The most common questions are: Should I tell my family about my disease? And, if yes, to whom in my family? And how much should I tell them? Questions of these kinds may not arise at all in cases when the initial disclosure of the diagnosis has taken place in the presence of several family members. But when only the closest member, such as a parent or husband/wife, was present, the decision of further disclosure rests with the patient. The questions about disclosure have different versions in the different stages of the disease. They may be relatively simple in the initial stage of diagnosis and turn into more complicated issues when the possibility of death becomes a closer reality. On the one hand, the patient would like to enjoy the support, help, and kind of defense that come with sharing the problems with one's family. However, sharing the news of one's disease may mean extra worrying for the family and a disruption of the daily life routine for all family members. Yet, on the other hand, patients may be reluctant to compromise their freedom of action and decision through the sharing, and to avoid extra care and attention on the part of the family. Most importantly, many patients would like to protect their family from worrying, avoid changes in their role and status in the family, and maintain as much as possible the daily life routine of the family. Be it as it may, not telling one's family or not telling everyone or not everything means that the patient has opted for the secretive approach. Unfortunately, this may often imply less support and more loneliness, and sometimes it may necessitate deviations from telling the truth.

Telling one's family about the disease is often a difficult task for the patient. The information about one's diagnosis may imply, for example, that the patient may not be able at present or in the future to help or contribute to the family as before or that the patient may be in need for help from family members, a fact which may increase their load of work and obligations. Some patients feel ashamed, while others feel guilty at having let the family down or disappointed their expectations of reliance on him or her; still others may feel angry that they have landed in this improbable spot of becoming sick. The difficulty of the task depends also on the communication style of the family. Some families do not have the habit of discussing issues openly. In such cases the task of disclosure to the family may become even harder. There are several possibilities of action for helping the patient that may be adopted instead of holding a family meeting devoted to the news. The disclosure of the news to the family may be done by a health professional or in the presence of a doctor, nurse, social worker, or psychologist. Alternately, the patient may talk to several family members separately or ask one of them to talk to the others [57].

Telling one's family about the cancer diagnosis raises also the issue of telling one's children. When the children are still young, disclosure of this kind of information needs to be done with special attention to the children's emotional reactions so as to control their anxiety. The information about the parent's sickness may be of crucial importance for the children's future and should be discussed with special attention and care [58, 59].

Disclosure about one's cancer in the family may also have implications about the genetic risk of specific family members. In the case of at least some cancers, such as breast cancer, ovarian cancer, colorectal cancer, and lung cancer, the state of information already at present is such that the genetic information is of paramount importance for the risk of other family members. Hence, informing the family about a diagnosis of cancer may be important not only for the patient but also for the family members who may be potentially at risk. It is not surprising that at least some of the family members who unexpectedly discover that they are potentially at risk react with stress and even anger [60].

Similar questions may be raised in regard to friends, acquaintances, and colleagues. Here too patients are caught in the dilemma defined by sharing versus withholding information. While sharing enables getting help and support from one's friends, but also getting their pity as a weak and needy person, withholding means withdrawing from one's social circle, lying, and fighting alone without too much support.

In any case, in regard to disclosure to one's family and to friends and other acquaintances, there exists the possibility that one will not get the expected response. They may react with indifference, or even withdrawal, which may hurt the patient who sometimes needed to mobilize courage in order to break the news. Friends and acquaintances may be scared by the news about cancer either because they are afraid to even think about the disease or because they are reluctant to help the patient in case he or she would need it.

Decisions Relating to Personal Issues

One common personal issue that bothers patients concerns getting help. The dilemma consists in choosing the option of getting help when it is offered or even soliciting it or the option of managing as far as possible on one's own. The options involve different lifestyles. Some people may interpret the decision to get help as indicating readiness to present oneself as weak and of possibly compromising in regard to one's independence. Others however may consider it as an indication of readiness to support one's strength optimally regardless of the means applied for this end.

Another common dilemma bothering many patients focuses on the issue whether and to what extent to maintain one's original lifestyle or to change it. The involved issues may be quite varied. Lifestyle may include one's work, marriage partner, place of residence – apartment, city, or country – friends, financial management, major occupation, hobbies, entertainment, traveling, health, and body. All these and other similar issues constitute themes that may preoccupy cancer patients and about which they feel forced or tempted to decide. A crisis such as cancer brings up to the surface issues which prior to the diagnosis have not been at all formulated or not sufficiently clear or important to evoke interest. Issues of the mentioned kind have the capacity to evoke anxiety, uncertainty, and confusion. Dealing with these issues may be one of the major causes for the bewilderment and loss of confidence and self-esteem that cancer patients may experience in the initial post-diagnosis period and to some extent also later.

The psychological tendencies involved in dealing with the mentioned issues are often based on the awareness that the remaining or available time is limited. Hence the desire to use it as best as one can. However, it is not very clear what is the best use for the time – is it devoting the time to having as much fun as possible, experiencing things one has not experienced before or not enough, or in short living life to the extreme. This direction would involve changing one's lifestyle, diminishing the time devoted to work, and sometimes even changing one's marriage partner. However, if one's life is satisfactory, then the implication of living life to the extreme would be to maintain as much as possible the prevailing conditions, going on with one's work, and maintaining one's marriage and social life. Sometimes maintaining the status quo implies increasing the pace of doing something that belongs to one's existing style of life. For example, a scientist or artist may devote all one's resources to completing as fast as possible some project that would have been accomplished anyway but at a slower pace. Another example along the same lines concerns attempts to solve family conflicts of long-standing that have been put aside for many years, (e.g., concerning property, old fights, assumed insults). Cancer patients sometimes turn their attention to these issues in an attempt to solve them at least to some extent so as to contribute to the well-being and harmony in the family.

Managing financial affairs may involve some of the more complicated issues bothering cancer patients. Some of the dilemmas may arise, on the one hand, from the desire to be fair to all inheritors while trying, on the other hand, to provide special donations to specific members who may deserve consideration because of past wrongs, needy status, or other special characteristics. Managing financial issues is often related to preparing a testament, which is a problematic theme in its own right. Some patients prefer to keep the testament only within strictly objective factual limits, mentioning only items of property or jewelry bequeathed to one or another person. Others feel obliged to refer to feelings, attitudes, blessings, remorse, forgiveness, and other highly personal issues they may experience in regard to several persons, the family, or life in general. Some patients may consider even preparing a document or video will that would function as a kind of spiritual legacy, summarizing their thoughts and experiences about life and existence. Testaments of the former kind may be discussed with lawyers, whereas those of the latter kind may be discussed if at all only with individuals with whom one feels special intimacy.

There is a special set of problems that is likely to bother an increasing number of patients when their disease proceeds. These are the issues that concern dying and death. There may be several common aspects concerning dying. One problem concerns whether to think about that issue at all. It is admittedly a scary issue, regardless of the disease, and there are patients who tend to think that if they at all think about it they kind of turn it from a possibility to a reality and render it into a proximal actuality. Since getting the diagnosis, many patients have been fighting the tendency to think about death, and it is only with quite great difficulty that they have avoided it. It is however barely possible to go on avoiding it when the disease proceeds. Death is usually a theme that evokes fear, anxiety, and even dread or panic. Thus, health professionals with expertise in regard to this domain try to discuss the issue with the patients only when they consider it as a likely eventuality or they notice preoccupation on the part of the patient. Themes that are being raised or considered in this context include how to deal with suffering preceding death, where to spend the last period of one's life, and how to spend that period (e.g., to what to devote it). A special issue that may occur to at least some patients concerns the possibility of suicide. This and all related these are discussed at length in Chap. 13 [61, 62].

Dealing with decisions concerning one's personal life differs from dealing with medical issues. The differences consist mainly in the reliance on oneself, which is mostly larger in regard to personal issues, and in the urgency, which is mostly larger in regard to medical issues. Greater reliance on oneself means that it is easier to discard the suggestions of others, with the result that one has fewer inputs from others and needs actually to decide by oneself. Decisions of that kind may be expected to be more personal, reflecting one's emotions to a greater extent, and often being more difficult to reach.

References

1. Ziegler, L., Newell, R., Stafford, N., & Lewin, R. (2004). A literature review of head and neck cancer patients information needs, experiences and views regarding decision-making. *European Journal of Cancer Care, 13*(2), 19–26.
2. Ha, J., & Longnecker, N. (2010). Doctor-patient communication: A review. *Ochsner Journal, 10*(1), 38–43.
3. Hawley, S. T., & Jagsi, R. (2015). Shared decision making in cancer care: Does one size fit all? *JAMA Oncology, 1*(1), 58–59.
4. Keating, N. L., Guadagnoli, E., Landrum, M. B., Borbas, C., & Weeks, J. C. (2002). Treatment decision making in early-stage breast cancer: Should surgeons match patients' desired level of achievement? *Journal of Clinical Oncology, 20*(6), 1473–1479.
5. Sawka, A. M., Straus, S., Rodin, G., Heus, L., Brierley, J. D., Tsang, R. W., Rotstein, L., Ezzat, S., Segal, P., Gaffni, A., Thorpe, K. E., & Goldstein, D. P. (2015). Thyroid cancer patient

perceptions of radioactive iodine treatment choice: Follow-up from a decision-aid randomized trial. *Cancer, 121*(20), 3717–3726.
6. Verbrugge, M., & Van Hecke, A. (2017). Factors influencing the process of medication (non-) adherence and (non-) persistence in breast cancer patients with adjuvant antihormonal therapy: A qualitative study. *European Journal of Cancer Care, 26*(2), 1365–2354.
7. Fischer, S., Gillessen, S., & Rothermundt, C. (2015). Sequence of treatment in locally advanced and metastatic renal cell carcinoma. *Translational Andrology and Urology., 4*(3), 310–325.
8. Bighin, C., Dozin, B., Poggio, F., Ceppi, M., Bruzzi, P., D'Alonzo, A., Levagg, A., Giraudi, S., Lambertini, M., Miglietta, L., Vaglica, M., Fontana, V., Iacono, G., Pronzato, P., & Mastro, L. D. (2017). Hormonal therapy followed by chemotherapy or the reverse sequence as first-line treatment of hormone-responsive, human epidermal growth factor receptor-2 negative metastatic breast cancer patients: Results of an observational study. *Oncotarget, 18*, 1949–2553.
9. El Shayeb, M., Scarfe, A., Yasui, Y., & Winget, M. (2012). Reasons physicians do not recommend and patients refuse adjuvant chemotherapy for stage III colon cancer: A population based chart review. *BMC Research Notes, 5*, 269.
10. Clarke, G., Johnston, S., Corrie, P., Kuhn, I., & Barclay, S. (2015). Withdrawal of anticancer therapy in advanced disease: A systematic literature review. *BMC Cancer, 15*, 892.
11. Barak, F., Livshits, S., Kaufer, H., Netanel, R., Siegelman-Danieli, N., Alkalay, Y., & Kreitler, S. (2015). Where to die? This is the question: A study of cancer patients in Israel. *Palliative and Supportive Care, 13*, 165–170.
12. Fuchs, T., Hanaya, H., Seilacher, E., Koester, M. J., Keinki, C., Liebl, P., & Huebner, J. (2017). Information deficits and second opinion seeking – A survey on cancer patients. *Cancer Investigation, 35*(1), 62–69.
13. Sherman, K. A., Shaw, L. K., Winch, C. J., Harcourt, D., Boyages, J., Cameron, L. D., Brown, P., Lam, T., Elder, E., French, J., & Spillane, A. (2016). Reducing decisional conflict and enhancing satisfaction with information among women considering breast reconstruction following mastectomy: Results from the BRECONDA randomized controlled trial. *Plastic and Reconstructive Surgery, 138*(4), 592e–602e.
14. American Society of Clinical Oncology. (2003). American society of clinical oncology policy statement update: Genetic testing for cancer susceptibility. *Journal of Clinical Oncology, 21*, 2397–2406.
15. Cameron, L. D., Sherman, K. A., Marteau, T. M., & Brown, P. M. (2009). Impact of genetic risk information and type of disease on perceived risk, anticipated affect, and expected consequences of genetic tests. *Health Psychology, 28*, 307–316.
16. Lee, J. S., Schover, L. R., Partridge, A. H., Patrizio, P., Wallace, W. H., Hagerty, K., Beck, L. N., Brennan, L. V., & Kutluk, O. (2006). American Society of Clinical Oncology recommendations on fertility preservation in cancer patients. *Journal of Clinical Oncology, 24*(18), 2917–2931.
17. Kim, S. I., Lee, Y., Son, Y., Jun, S. Y., Yun, S., Bae, H. S., Lim, M. C., Jung, S. Y., Joo, J., & Lee, E. S. (2015). Assessment of breast cancer patients' knowledge and decisional conflict regarding tamoxifen use. *Journal of Korean Medical Science, 30*, 1604–1610.
18. van den Berg, L., Lobatto, R. M., Zuurmond, W. W., de Lange, J. J., Wagemans, M. F., & Bezemer, P. D. (1997). Patients' refusal to participate in clinical research. *European Journal of Anaesthesiology, 14*, 287–289.
19. Cartmell, K. B., Bonilha, H. S., Matson, T., Bryant, D. C., Zapka, J., Bentz, T. A., Ford, M. E., Hughes-Halbert, C., Simpson, K. N., & Albeerg, A. J. (2016). Patient participation in cancer clinical trials: A pilot test of lay navigation. *Contemporary Clinical Trials Communications, 3*, 86–93.
20. Nappo, S., Iafrate, G. B., & Sanchez, Z. M. (2013). Motives for participating in a clinical research trial: A pilot study in Brazil. *BMC Public Health, 13*, 19.
21. Stunkel, L., & Grady, C. (2014). More than the money: A review of the literature examining healthy volunteer motivations. *PLoS One, 9*(6), e100435.
22. Biedrzycki, B. A. (2010). Decision making for cancer clinical trial participation: A systematic review. *Oncology Nursing Forum, 37*(6), E387–E399.

23. Mills, E. J., Seely, D., Rachlis, B., Griffith, L., Wu, P., Wilson, K., Ellis, P., & Wright, J. R. (2006). Barriers to participation in clinical trials of cancer: A meta-analysis and systematic review of patient-reported factors. *The Lancet Oncology, 7*(2), 141–148.
24. Bell, J. A., & Balneaves, J. G. (2015). Cancer patient decision making related to clinical trial participation: An integrative review with implications for patients' relational autonomy. *Supportive Care and Cancer, 23*(4), 1169–1196.
25. Jenkins, V., Fallowfield, L., & Saul, J. (2001). Information needs of patients with cancer: Results from a large study in UK cancer centres. *British Journal of Cancer, 84*(1), 48–51.
26. Degner, L. F., & Sloan, J. A. (1992). Decision making during serious illness: What role do patients really want to play? *Journal of Clinical Epidemiology, 45*, 941–950.
27. Magee, M. (2003). *Relationship-based health care in the United States, United Kingdom, Canada, Germany, South Africa, and Japan. A comparative study of patient and physician perceptions worldwide*. Ferney–Voltaire: World Medical Association. [Available online; cited June 10, 2010].
28. Davison, B. J., Gleave, M. E., Goldenberg, S. L., Degner, L. F., Hoffart, D., & Berkowitz, J. (2002). Assessing information and decision preferences of men with prostate cancer and their partners. *Cancer Nursing, 25*, 42–49.
29. Stacey, R. N., Paquet, L., & Samant, R. (2010). Exploring cancer treatment decision-making by patients: A descriptive study. *Current Oncology, 17*(4), 85–93.
30. Kehl, K. L., Landrum, M. B., Arora, N. K., Ganz, P. A., Van Rynn, M., Mack, J. W., & Keating, N. L. (2015). Association of actual and preferred decision roles with patient-reported quality of care shared decision making in cancer. *JAMA Oncology, 1*(1), 50–57.
31. Kiesler, D. J., & Auerbach, S. M. (2006). Optimal matches of patient preferences for information, decision-making and interpersonal behaviour: Evidence, models and interventions. *Patient Education and Counselling, 61*, 319–341.
32. O'Connor, A. M. (1995). Validation of a decisional conflict scale. *Medical Decision Making, 15*, 25–30.
33. Vogel, B. A., Leonhart, R., & Helmes, A. W. (2009). Communication matters: The impact of communication and participation in decision making on breast cancer patients' depression and quality of life. *Patient Education and Counseling, 77*(3), 391–397.
34. Chien, C. H., Chuang, C. K., Liu, K. L., Li, C. L., & Liu, H. E. (2014). Changes in decisional conflict and decisional regret in patients with localised prostate cancer. *Journal of Clinical Nursing, 23*(13–14), 1959–1969.
35. Sim, J. A., Shin, J. S., Park, S. M., Chang, Y. J., Shin, A., Noh, D. Y., Han, W., Yang, H. K., Lee, H. J., Kim, Y. W., Kim, Y. T., Jeong, S. Y., Yoon, J. H., Kim, Y. J., Heo, D. S., Kim, T. Y., Oh, D. Y., Wu, H. G., Kim, H. J., Chie, E. K., Kang, K. W., & Yun, Y. H. (2015). Association between information provision and decisional conflict in cancer patients. *Annals of Oncology, 26*(9), 1974–1980.
36. Goh, A. C., Kowalkowski, M. A., Bailey, D. E., Jr., Kazer, M. W., Knight, S. J., & Latini, D. M. (2012). Perception of cancer and inconsistency in medical information are associated with decisional conflict: A pilot study of men with prostate cancer who undergo active surveillance. *British Journal of Urology International, 110*(2 Pt 2), E50–E56.
37. Miller, S. M., Hudson, S. V., Egleston, B. L., Manne, S., Buzaglo, J. S., Devarajan, K., Fleisher, L., Millard, J., Solarino, N., Trinastic, J., & Meropol, N. J. (2013). The relationships among knowledge, self-efficacy, preparedness, decisional conflict, and decisions to participate in a cancer clinical trial. *Psycho-Oncology, 22*(3), 481–489.
38. Harvey, A., Amsellem, M., & Suarez, R. (2015). Factors influencing treatment decisions among cancer patients: Results from national patient education workshops. *Cancer Support Community*, Washington, DC. Presented at the 2015 world congress of pyscho-oncology.
39. Davison, B. J., & Breckon, E. (2011). Factors influencing treatment decision making and information preferences of prostate cancer patients on active surveillance. *Patient Education and Counselling, 87*, 368–374.

40. Legare, F., Ratte, S., Gravel, K., & Graham, I. D. (2008). Barriers and facilitators to implementing shared decision-making in clinical practice: Update of a systematic review of health professionals' perceptions. *Patient Education and Counselling, 73*, 526–535.
41. Castel, P., Negrier, S., & Boissel, J.-P. (2006). Why don't cancer patients enter clinical trials? A review. *European Journal of Cancer, 42*(12), 1744–1748.
42. Hajjaj, F. M., Salek, M. S., Basra, M. K. A., & Finlay, A. Y. (2010). Non-clinical influences on clinical decision-making: A major challenge to evidence-based practice. *Journal of the Royal Society of Medicine, 103*(5), 178–187.
43. Politi, M. C., Kuzemchak, M. D., Kaphingst, K. A., Perkins, H., Liu, J., & Byrne, M. M. (2016). Decision aids can support cancer clinical trials decisions: Results of a randomized trial. *The Oncologist, 21*(12), 1461–1470.
44. Sherman, K. A., Winch, C. J., & Spillane, A. J. (2016). Reducing decisional conflict and enhancing satisfaction with information among women considering breast reconstruction following mastectomy: Results from the BRECONDA randomized controlled trial. *Plastic Reconstructive Surgery, 138*(4), 592e–602e.
45. Song, H., Omori, K., Kim, J., Tenzek, K. E., Morey Hawkins, J., Lin, W. Y., Kim, Y. C., & Jung, J. Y. (2016). Trusting social media as a source of health information: Online surveys comparing the United States, Korea, and Hong Kong. *Journal of Internet Research, 18*(3), e25.
46. Sinnenberg, L., Buttenheim, A. M., Padrez, K., Mancheno, C., Ungar, L., & Merchant, R. M. (2017). Twitter as a tool for health research: A systematic review. *American Journal of Public Health, 107*(1), e1–e8.
47. Tariman, J. D., Berry, D. L., Cochrane, B., Doorenbos, A., & Schepp, K. (2010). Preferred and actual participation roles during health care decision making in persons with cancer: A systematic review. *Annals of Oncology, 21*(6), 1145–1151.
48. Hubbard, G., Kidd, L., & Donaghy, E. (2008). Preferences for involvement in treatment decision making of patients with cancer: A review of the literature. *European Journal of Oncology Nursing, 12*, 299–318.
49. Gattellari, M., Butow, P. N., & Tattersall, M. H. N. (2001). Sharing decisions in cancer care. *Social Science & Medicine, 52*, 1865–1878.
50. Levy, S. M., Herberman, R. B., Lee, J. K., Lippman, M. E., & d'Angelo, T. (1989). Breast conservation versus mastectomy: Distress sequelae as a function of choice. *Journal of Clinical Oncology, 7*(3), 367–375.
51. Tani, Y., Nagai, T., Koida, K., Kitazaki, M., & Nakauchi, S. (2014). Experts and novices use the same factors–but differently–to evaluate pearl quality. *PLoS One, 9*(1), e86400.
52. Isaacs, E. A., & Clark, H. H. (1987). References in conversation between experts and novices. *Journal of Experimental Psychology: General, 116*(1), 26–37.
53. Fong Ha, J., & Longnecker, N. (2010). Doctor-patient communication: A review. *Ochsner Journal, 10*(1), 38–43.
54. Hobbs, G. S., Landrum, M. B., Arora, N. K., Ganz, P. A., van Ryn, M., Weeks, J. C., Mack, J. W., & Keating, N. L. (2015). The role of families in decisions regarding cancer treatments. *Cancer, 121*(7), 1079–1087.
55. Fraenkel, L., Peters, E., Charpentier, P., Olsen, B., Errante, L., Schoen, R. T., & Reyna, V. (2012). Decision tool to improve the quality of care in rheumatoid arthritis. *Arthritis Care Research, 64*(7), 977–985.
56. Charpentier, C. J., De Neve, J.-E., Xinji, L., Charpentier, C. J., De Neve, J.-E., Li, X., Rosier, J. P., & Sharot, T. (2016). Models of affective decision making: How do feelings predict choice? *Psychological Science, 27*, 763–775.
57. Zhang, A. Y., & Siminoff, L. A. (2003). Silence and cancer: Why do families and patients fail to communicate? *Health Communication, 15*(4), 415–429.
58. Swick, S. D., Martin, A. S., & Rauch, P. (2012). When a parent has cancer: Supporting healthy child development during challenging times. In S. Kreitler, M. W. Ben-Arush, & A. Martin

(Eds.), *Pediatric psycho-oncology: Psychosocial aspects and clinical interventions* (2nd ed., pp. 246–259). Chichester: Wiley-Blackwell.
59. Ashbury, N., Lalayiannis, L., & Walshe, A. (2014). How do I tell the children? Women's experiences of sharing information about breast cancer diagnosis and treatment. *European Journal of Oncology Nursing, 18*(6), 564–570.
60. Gallo, A. M., Angst, D. B., & Knafl, K. A. (2009). Disclosure of genetic information within families. *American Journal of Nursing, 109*, 65–69.
61. Kreitler, S. (2012). The psychological point of view: The individual facing death and dying. In S. Kreitler (Ed.), *Confronting dying and death* (pp. 89–102). Hauppauge: Nova Publishers.
62. Kreitler, S. (2018). Dying from cancer: The four tracks. In H. S. Watanabe (Ed.), *Horizons in cancer research* (Vol. 69, pp. 145–172). Hauppauge: Nova Publishers.

Chapter 8
Treatments and Interventions in Cancer

Three Kinds of Treatments

Treatments constitute the major focus of the narrative of cancer for the patients and their families. Originally treatments for cancer referred mainly to specific medical procedures including surgery, radiotherapy, and medication, adjuvant or non-adjuvant. With time these medical options have been developed and greatly expanded to include additional medical procedures, as well as further kinds of nonmedical treatments. The major nonmedical kinds of treatments at present are various complementary or alternative treatments and psychosocial interventions. The presentation of each of the three kinds of treatments includes a major section which consists of the standard treatments and an additional section including less standard ones, which have been more recently developed, are sometimes still experimental, and are often less strictly defined.

The three kinds of treatments differ in several major aspects:

1. *The goal of the treatment*. The goal of the medical treatments is improvement of the patient's state of health. Improvement may have different forms, such as reducing or eliminating the tumor, reducing or eliminating metastases, extending the disease-free interval, or stopping the spread of the disease. The goal of the complementary or alternative treatments is often to alleviate the physical suffering due mostly to the side effects of the medical treatments. Sometimes the stated goal is to engage or activate the self-healing energies of the body. The goal of the psychological interventions is mainly to alleviate the patients' psychological suffering, improve their coping with the difficulties, promote their quality of life, and to some extent support physical survival. The three kinds of treatment are however far from strictly differentiated in terms of goals. Some of the medical treatments are devoted to alleviating physical suffering of the side effects of the treatments or providing palliative care; the complementary treatments often focus on improving quality of life and sometimes strive toward promoting physical recovery and even survival; the psychological treatments often focus on alleviating physical suffering in addition to the psychological one.

S. Kreitler, *Psycho-Oncology for the Clinician*,
https://doi.org/10.1007/978-3-030-06126-5_8

2. *The performers or agents of the treatment.* Medical treatments are carried out only by certified doctors. Alternative treatments are carried out by individuals who claim expertise on the basis of studies or experience, such as naturopaths, holistic healers, osteopaths, or acupuncture experts. Psychosocial treatments are carried out mostly by certified psychologists, psychotherapists, or medically trained social workers.
3. *The means of the treatments.* Medical treatments use medical means, such as surgery, radiation therapy, and medical procedures and medications of different kinds. The means applied by complementary and alternative treatments are quite variegated. They include, for example, herbs, manual manipulations, energy therapy, exerting pressure or inserting thin needles in certain bodily points, verbal means, imagination, electricity and magnetism, bodily movements, exercise, meditating, diets, etc. The means applied by psychologists are mostly exclusively verbal and cognitive.

Despite the differences, all three kinds of treatment share the focus on helping the cancer patient in a variety of ways. The experts of the different treatments approach the cancer patient with different means and from different perspectives which despite the disparities combine their effects in improving the state of the patient in different ways and to different degrees in the different phases of the disease.

The Medical Treatments

The Kinds of Medical Treatments

The list of medical treatments is fairly large [1]. The basic treatment consists of the different protocols of chemotherapy designed to damage or kill cancer cells throughout the body. There are additional treatments which include surgery of different kinds (e.g., open surgery or laparoscopic) and different extents (e.g., mastectomy or lumpectomy; removing one lung or one lobe of the lung); radiotherapy (external beam or internal); stereotactic radiosurgery and stereotactic body radiotherapy; stem cell transplants (autologous or allogeneic); hormonal therapy based on different kinds of medication designed to lower the produced amount of hormones used by the cancer cells or eliminate the receptors on the cells to which the hormones bind; and biological therapy or immunotherapy (e.g., monoclonal antibodies and adoptive cell transfer or cytokines such as interferons and interleukins or antibodies or segments of genetic material) which stimulate the body's immune system to act against cancer cells with or without targeting them directly. A special partly still experimental treatment is gene therapy which consists in the transfer of new genetic material into a cell, for example, for activating the destruction of metastases.

Some of the mentioned treatments are administered only once (e.g., often surgery, although it may also be repeated), some for short-time durations (e.g., radiotherapy) and some for longer-time durations (e.g., chemotherapy). Further, the goals of the treatments may differ to some extent. Some treatments are administered as a major attack on the disease, some with the purpose of maintaining the good response (e.g., hormonal therapy), or as adjuvant therapy. In some cases a medical treatment is designed to alleviate the side effects of the major treatments (e.g., diarrhea, extreme pain). Again, in some cases, the treatment is presented as experimental, for example, gene therapy. Most of the treatment modalities are used in combinations, e.g., radiotherapy after chemotherapy or chemotherapy prior to surgery.

Attitudes Toward the Medical Treatments

Patients are aware of the different medical treatments and may often have quite clear attitudes and preferences in regard to many of them. Patients share with the majority of oncologists the view that chemotherapy is the main tool of treatment. It is considered by many patients as extremely difficult but potent and effective against cancer. The underlying assumption is that since the disease is so strong and difficult, so should also be the treatment. In some cases patients consider chemotherapy as providing the opportunity for undergoing the suffering which is probably necessary for overcoming the disease [2–4].

Radiotherapy is regarded as a much lighter and easier treatment. It is considered as being mainly adjuvant, performing a kind of cleaning up operation following the major treatment, which may be chemotherapy or surgery. Many patients are not aware of side effect of radiotherapy and do not appreciate its role as a major therapeutic tool in its own right. The attitude toward radiotherapy for genital cancers is different and internal-beam radiotherapy is considered to be more painful and harmful [5].

Surgery is considered by many patients as the optimal treatment both because it is short and incisive and attacks the disease headlong and because it is a radical scooping the tumor out of its site and thus eradicating the core of the cancer at the root. Patients expect surgery to take out the whole tumor without leaving any remnants behind. They tend to feel safe and saved when the tumor is no longer inside the body. However, they are very disappointed when it turns out that surgery could not take out the whole of the tumor and that larger or even smaller parts have stayed behind.

Determinants of the Patients' Attitudes Toward Treatments

Studies show that the major determinants of the patient' attitudes toward the treatments are based on considerations of duration, side effects, degree of toxicity, modernity, location of treatment, form of administration, extent of foreseen harm or damage the treatments may cause, and probabilities characterizing their likely contribution to recovery [6, 7].

In general, patients prefer treatments that are of short *duration* (e.g., surgery) or injections that are administered in intervals of, say, once a month rather than more prolonged treatments. The often proffered reason is that short treatments may act against the disease in a more forceful and concentrated manner and additionally enable the patient to consider the disease for as short a time as possible. Concerning *side effects*, patients are aware of the fact that they are unavoidable, and when they start a treatment with side effects, they would usually like to know ahead of time what the side effects are and especially how they can be controlled, e.g., which medications should or could be used for lowering nausea [8]. *Degree of toxicity* of medications is an issue for many patients. It is a major concern which generates quite a lot of resistance to chemotherapy which is generally considered as a basic treatment. Patients sometimes merge the negative effects of the disease with the negative effects of the toxicity to which they are exposed.

The *modernity* of the treatment is considered as a favorable characteristic by many patients who assume that the more recently developed treatments are more advanced and therefore more effective and in the very least are expected to cause fewer side effects. However, many patients feel that more modern treatments may be less safe because of the short time that has elapsed since they have been approved for use. Hence, it is still unknown as to whether after a certain number of years these treatments may cause some negative results [9]. Moreover, some patients conclude that the more modern treatments are less effective because they cause fewer or weaker side effects than the older treatments [10].

Concerning *location of getting the treatments*, there has been a growing tendency in recent years to move the treatment of chemotherapy and similar treatments from the hospitals to the home or at least to local clinics closer to the home of the patients. It is of course more convenient to get the treatment at home or in a clinic close to home which is familiar and often small rather than in the hospital which is a public place and often far from one's residential location. Getting the treatment at home is less time-consuming and less stressful and obviates the need of traveling and parking, as well as finding someone to accompany the patient to the hospital. On the other hand, some patients feel insecure in regard to taking care of themselves if they don't feel well following the ingestion of the drugs at home. Additionally, they sometimes feel afraid that they might be mistaken in selecting the adequate drugs or in their form of ingestion.

The location in which the treatment takes place is related to the issue of the *form of administration* of the medications. The traditional form through infusion has been replaced in recent years in many cases by tablets or pills or by injections. Although these modern forms of administering the drugs are easier and less stressful for the patient, some patients still have their doubts concerning the efficacy and safety of the drugs administered in these new forms. Notably, it is not uncommon for patients to find the swallowing of pills or tablets to be a difficult task either for physical reasons (e.g., they have undergone radiotherapy in the esophagus, mouth, or throat) or for psychological reasons. Also injections may be difficult for some patients who may suffer from fear of injections (trypanophobia) or from a tendency to faint following an injection (e.g., due to a vasovagal response of a drop in blood pressure).

The extent of *the foreseen damage* that the treatment may cause is an issue of major concern for many patients. It may relate to all types of medical treatment. In regard to surgery, the foreseen damage may be the loss of an organ or a limb (e.g., a breast), distortion of external appearance (e.g., in the case of facial surgery), and impairment of some function (e.g., difficulties in mobility following orthopedic surgery, in digestion following stomach surgery, or in bowel management after colorectal surgery). Following colorectal cancer surgery, a patient may need colostomy, which is difficult for many patients to accept [11]. Following prostatectomy not all patients recover full urinary, bowel, and sexual function [12].

In regard to radiotherapy, the foreseen damage is expected to be mostly transitory, e.g., fatigue, damaged skin in the radiated area, difficulty in swallowing if radiotherapy was administered in the chest or oral area, and pain if radiotherapy focused on the cervix. The damage may be more lasting and disturbing in case radiotherapy was administered to the brain as prophylaxis or for treatment of a tumor or metastasis. Following brain radiotherapy the impairment in different executive functions and memory may last for years [13, 14]. Problems in the lungs, liver, bones, glands, teeth, vision, and heart may persist for a long time, depending on the irradiated area. Permanent loss of hair in the scalp following radiotherapy is worrisome for many patients [15].

In regard to chemotherapy, patients are concerned about losing vitality and muscular strength; hair; memory, concentration, and other cognitive abilities [16]; as well as losing emotional control, positive mood, and fertility. Long-lasting impairments following chemotherapy can be expected in the nerves (e.g., neuropathy, loss of sensation), lungs, liver, endocrine system, dental and oral health, heart, and blood pressure, depending on the duration of the treatment and nature of the drugs applied. The range of physical, cognitive, and emotional impairments is so broad that patients are often concerned about losing too much in terms of their quality of life through chemotherapy. When the benefit of chemotherapy is relatively large and certain, patients are mostly ready to the before disease trade in their quality of life, at least for a certain limited period of time, for the benefit of improving their chances of survival, relying on their hope that after termination of chemotherapy, they would be able to reconstruct their quality of life. However, if the chances of recovery become minimal or uncertain because of the nature of the disease, the kind of drugs, previous experience, or one's overall physical state, the patient may be reluctant to trade in one's quality of life, or whatever still survives of it, for an additional round of chemotherapy with the involved suffering it may entail. This choice and this kind of decisions are most frequent in the palliative stage, but they are not limited exclusively to this stage [7].

Finally, the last determinant shaping one's attitudes to the diverse medical treatments is the *probabilities characterizing their likely contribution to recovery*. Studies showed that people in general, patients included, often do not understand adequately statements of probabilities. For example, they do not quite identify the difference between 60% and 80% chances of improvement due to a certain treatment or the meanings of absolute risk, synergistic risk, attributable risk, and relative risk of smoking [17, 18]. Even clinicians and other health professionals may need clarification of meanings of probability [19–21]. Since probability information seems to be a generally difficult issue for understanding and transmitting [22], not a few patients tend to rely on their experiences or private opinions overlooking stated probabilities [23].

Complementary and Alternative Treatments

Kinds of Complementary and Alternative Treatments

CAM is a group of diverse medical and healthcare systems, practices, and products that are not generally considered part of *conventional medicine*. There are a great many different treatments and practices included under this title. They can be grouped into several classes:

1. Treatments based on *applying psychological means and processes*, e.g., hypnosis
2. Treatments based on *specific diets or foods*, e.g., vitamins, herbal supplements, dietary supplements, herbs, green tea, nutrition, specific diets such as macrobiotics, Gerson's, Atkin's diet, vegetarian, zone diet (for reducing diet-induced inflammation), purely organic food; or natural nonvitamin and nonmineral products, or enzymes; special foods, such as garlic, fish oil/omega 3, glucosamine, echinacea, or flaxseed; and specialities, such as milk of female camels and shark cartilage
3. Treatments based on *physical interventions*, e.g., yoga, acupuncture, deep breathing, exercise, rowing, chiropractic or osteopathic care, ring muscle exercises, biofeedback, different kinds of massage (deep massage, external massage), tai chi, Qigong (qi gong, chi kung, or chi gung) which is a holistic system of coordinated body posture and movement, breathing, Alexander technique, Feldenkrais, Pilates, and physical exercise interventions
4. Treatments based on *detoxification*, for example, through fasting and chelation therapy
5. *Treatments based on energy manipulations*, for example, through healers, Reiki, shamans, therapeutic touch, and acupressure (pressure point therapy)
6. *Treatments based on relaxation* – through progressive muscle relaxation or cue-controlled relaxation [24, 25] as well as laughter and dissociation, for example, by removing oneself from one's habitual surroundings and keeping silent for certain periods of time
7. *Treatments based on contact with specific materials*, for example, crystals, magnets, special waters, natural oils, and aromatherapy
8. *Treatments based on contact nature*, for example, by living or spending time close to water sources, forests, and green planes
9. Treatments based on temperature *changes*, mainly cryotherapy and hyperthermia

The above list of CAM represents most of the currently practiced procedures. The list is by no means complete, mainly because it is continuously expanding. Also the categorization used above may not be acceptable to every CAM practitioner, first, because the means used in the practice are not always identical to the underlying goal and, second, because in some cases a practice that started out with one explicit goal tends to add or absorb other goals. Additionally, some practices are designed to serve more than one goal, such as meditation which may be applied in the contexts of spirituality or relaxation or energy manipulations. Admittedly, the boundaries between the different practices are in some cases quite fluid.

Application of the CAM Practices

It has become common to distinguish between three kinds of approaches to these therapeutic means. The first, *complementary medicine*, is often used to refer to treatments applied along with standard medical treatments but are not considered to be standard treatments, for example, using massage, ginger, and relaxation for suppressing nausea and vomiting due to chemotherapy [26]. The second, *alternative medicine*, often refers to treatments that replace standard medical treatments, for example, using a special diet or hyperthermia instead of the standard medical treatment [27]. Finally, *integrative medicine* represents a third approach which is becoming increasingly common and consists in applying standard medical practices along with different complementary and alternative practices considered as safe and efficient [28, 29].

Most of the CAM practices are applied singly out of their original cultural or contextual framework, regardless of whether they have been developed initially in some comprehensive medical or other system (e.g., martial arts). Some CAM practices are applied within their original context, such as Ayurveda or Chinese medicine. An in-between approach consists in applying several selected practices out of the whole cluster of practices that are presented as belonging together, for example, in regard to naturopathy, Qigong, or Trager psychophysical integration.

Notably, some CAM practices need the involvement of a practitioner, for example, a healer (who may exert his or her impact sometimes from a distance). In some cases the patient needs to be instructed only once or not at all. CAM is often practiced on one's own, but in other cases patients practice or discuss CAM in groups.

The goals professed for the different CAM practices refer to a broad range of objectives, including relaxation, prevention or mitigation of side effects of the medical treatments, enhanced action of the medical treatments, strengthening one's physical and mental stamina and health, engaging one's healing forces for recovery, and even attaining full recovery. Not all goals are attached to all practices or pursued by all CAM practitioners. Thus, the expected result ranges from some improvement in quality of life to full survival.

It is not easy to assess the prevalence of the use of CAM by cancer patients because many, probably at least about 50% [26, 30], do not confess to applying CAM due to the declared or feared negative attitude of their doctors or simply their lack of interest [30, 31]. It is not to be excluded that some patients conceal their use of CAM because they are ashamed. An early publication reporting a systematic review of surveys on the use of CAM among cancer patients in 13 countries found an average of 31.4% (range of 7–64%) of CAM users among the adult cancer population [32]. One survey with different cancer patients found that 35.9% (range 14.8–73.1%) used CAM [33]; another study reported that 48.9% of the patients (range 12.5–73%) used CAM [34]; and a third study found 40% in the USA [35]. The broad ranges may be due to differences between countries, cancer centers, cancer diseases, definitions relating to CAM, and even the date of the survey. The latter may play a role in view of the increasing popularity of CAM usage [36]. A survey based on 18 countries showed that the use of CAM in cancer was increasing steadily from 25% in the 1970s to 49% after 2000 [37]. Additionally, reporting the percentage of patients who use a certain CAM practice overlooks the fact that quite a few apply more than one practice at a time. So the reported number of users may be overrated [38].

Determinants and Reasons for Applying CAM

Several surveys dealt with the reasons stated by patients for applying CAM practices (e.g., [26, 39–41]). Surprisingly the reasons reported in the different surveys are quite similar. Major reasons mentioned for addressing CAM are the following:

1. CAM is a completely different kind of treatment approach to cancer than the conventional standard medicine. The underlying principle for many CAM practices is to mobilize the hidden self-healing potentials of the human body, which are neglected by the standard treatments. Thus, CAM depends on the individuals' self-activation of the recovery program [42]. The mentioned features of CAM promote the patient's empowerment which may also contribute to recovery [43]. Since standard medical treatment does not promise full recovery from cancer, it is important not to miss out on the chance that using CAM may contribute to one's state of health.
2. CAM enables the patient to recover some control over one's health and the undertaken treatments. CAM is based on a free choice by the patient, and it is easily available and may be discontinued at any time. This contrasts with the frustrating situation of standard medical treatment in which the patient who has accepted the treatment has given up all kind of control over undergoing the treatment and the conditions of its application [44].
3. CAM is safe, natural, and nontoxic. In these respects CAM differs from standard medical treatments which are toxic, involve side effects, and may be harmful for different organs in the body and mind [30, 42].
4. CAM is a holistic approach. It addresses the body, the mind, and the spirit in all their parts. This approach seems superior to any standard medical treatment which deals exclusively with one specific sector of the human system. Since the disease affects the whole system – body, mind, and spirit – the best approach to healing should be based on addressing all these aspects at the same time [28].
5. CAM often provides the chance of closer relations with the practitioner providing the treatment than with the standard medical doctor. This relationship promises to provide a certain degree of support for the patient which may contribute to healing [45].
6. CAM may be expected to provide improvement to the patient's quality of life mainly by alleviating the suffering from side effects of the standard medical treatments and mitigating or limiting the harm they may cause [46–50]. A major expectation of the patients is that CAM may provide help in the relief of pain [51]. The hope of alleviation of psychological distress through CAM plays an important role [52, 53]. Thus, CAM may contribute to standard medical treatments [33].
7. CAM does not rely as much as psychosocial treatments on verbal communication and discussions that may be difficult for many patients [54].
8. CAM is used by healthy people for enhancing their physical and mental health. By applying CAM cancer patients assert the fact that they do not differ essentially from the rest of the population [45].

Scientific Support for CAM

There are studies which examined the outcomes of different practices of CAM. Some studies were devoted to examining the impact of CAM on the tumors or the metastases. Most of these studies had negative results. For example, healing touch did not prove to be effective in regard to the tumor [55], nor did combined immunotherapy with dendritic cells and cytokine-induced killer cells [56] or the Gerson's diet, according to reviews by the National Cancer Institute and the New York County Medical Society [57]. Some effect of neem leaf extract on inhibiting mammary carcinogenesis in rats was found [58]. Patients who used only CAM but not any standard medical treatment fared worse from a medical point of view than those who used medical treatment [59, 60].

These examples demonstrate that most of the different CAM practices that have been studied did not prove efficacious in regard to minimizing the tumor itself or the metastases. However, some studies showed that different CAM practices affected positively specific aspects of the patients' quality of life, for example, massage reduced distress, pain and sleeping difficulties [61], or pain, fatigue, and anxiety [62]. Acupuncture was found to be efficacious in the treatment of different symptoms, such as nausea, neuropathic pain, depression and anxiety, and leukocytosis [63, 64]. However, some of these results were found to be controversial, mainly due to risk of bias [65]. There is empirical evidence for the benefits of yoga in regard to reducing pain, fatigue, and sleeping difficulties [66, 67]. Further, there is evidence for the beneficial effects of physical exercise on physical fitness and overall health especially in cancer survivors [68].

It is evident that the scientific support for the efficacy of CAM is not optimal. There are not enough empirical studies with well-selected samples and matched control groups. Yet, on the basis of the existing studies and the reports of patients, it is generally accepted that CAM can help patients in regard to symptom control, reduce side effects, improve patients' well-being, and enhance their strength to undergo the standard treatments [46].

In regard to the use of herbs in the framework of CAM, there is some uncertainty on the part of physicians about the safety of the medications and about possibly harmful clinically relevant CAM-drug interactions [69]. The problem is exacerbated by the fact that many patients conceal from their physicians their use of CAM (e.g., [26]). Another often mentioned negative effect of CAM is that it may cause delay in starting standard medical treatment of even stopping it [70].

Psychosocial Interventions

Kinds of Psychosocial Interventions

The diversity of psychosocial interventions is no less than that of CAM practices. The diversity is further increased through the flexibility in the manner in which the different kinds of intervention are applied. The major kinds of psychosocial interventions are:

A. *Standard psychotherapy*. Psychotherapy is being applied in different contexts outside cancer. There are many versions of this procedure ranging from classical dynamic psychotherapy to short-term therapy. The different versions vary in duration, theoretical background, and means. Yet they all share several major components: using verbal means; providing empathic listening; creating an accepting warm environment where the patient may feel secure and safe; providing the patient insight into one's behavior and feelings; addressing cognitions, emotions, and behaviors; offering a theoretical framework which enables the patient to get a deeper understanding of one's problems and reactions; helping the patient gain strength and insight through the relationship with the therapist; keeping full privacy and confidentiality; keeping standard time and place for a given number of sessions; and targeting improvement in the patient's well-being [71, 72].

   There are different kinds of psychotherapy, based on different theoretical frameworks:

   (a) *Psychodynamic analytical psychotherapies*. They are sometimes called depth or insight therapies. The approach was developed originally by Freud and his followers (e.g., Anna Freud, Steckel) and is based primarily on the constructs of drives, superego, and unconsciousness, emphasizing the importance of gaining insight into one's hidden motivations for behavior and emotions. A different theoretical approach characterizes the Jungian therapy based on the constructs of the archetypes and the collective unconscious and the Adlerian therapy based on the constructs of control, style of life, and inferiority. Other versions grounded in psychodynamic approach are ego psychology, object relations theory, and self-psychology [72].
   (b) *Humanistic psychotherapies*. These forms of therapy derive from approaches such as existentialism and phenomenology and have been inspired by Maslow and Carl Rogers. They are based primarily on the constructs of self-actualization, creativity, and authenticity. The major goals are to broaden one's awareness and develop one's conception of oneself as a whole human being. This implies encompassing all of one's needs and abilities and relying on one's personal tendencies to find fulfillment, happiness, and health within oneself, in a comprehensive context of community and culture. Versions of this approach have been called positive psychology [73].

B. *Cognitive behavioral therapy (CBT)*. Cognition is a major resource in psychotherapy and promotes a variety of interventions. They may involve change in one's thoughts, beliefs, or the manner of thinking, acquiring new conceptions and constructs, and learning to cope and to apply new skills and problem-solving means. CBT is a major kind of cognitive therapy, based on a general cognitive coping model [74, 75]. It is defined as a structured cognitive intervention that is focused on changing or eliminating consciously accessible thoughts which play a role in producing the patient's problems. The negative thoughts are, for example, "I am vulnerable," "No one can help me," "The bad situation will turn soon into worse," "I am helpless," and "I cannot cope." It is assumed that they are grounded in striving for perfectionism and overcontrol. The intervention targets improving the patients' adjustment in general and in regard to specific responses (e.g., anxiety, depression) by training the patient to respond with helpful or positive thoughts to the negative ideas that may often occur in his/her mind. In a stepwise graded process, the patient is taught more adequate responses (e.g., "I can cope") or behaviors that could prevent or mitigate depression and other responses of the helplessness-hopelessness kind. CBT consists of a systematic training program, based on teaching specific cognitive responses and particular behaviors. The patient is taught to identify the negative ideas and the situations in which they occur and to replace them by specific positive ideas [75]. The standard classical CBT has been applied mainly for reducing anxiety and depression in cancer patients. The efficacy of CBT in these domains has been proven in several large-scale controlled trials (e.g., [76–78]). However, there is evidence for a steady decline in the effectiveness of CBT in treatment from 1977 onward [79].

CBT has become a kind of umbrella term for a great number of cognitive therapies [80]. Three major versions of CBT are discussed here:

(a) *Cognitive therapy* is one of the versions of CBT, based on Beck's approach (1995) [81, 82]. It shares with the general CBT model the emphasis on suppressing or replacing negative inadequate conscious thoughts by more adequate thoughts and by applying problem-solving skills that promote coping. Cognitive therapy is specifically focused on cancer patients and their major symptoms, mainly depression, anxiety, fatigue, and insomnia [83, 84]. It considers specifically the realistic basis of their fears and emotional reactions to the disease. The therapy also takes into account the possible tendencies of patients to apply in regard to cancer inadequate responses that have been acquired and applied earlier in life in only apparently similar situations and are not effective in regard to cancer. The patient is confronted with his/her inadequate cognitive and behavioral responses and is encouraged to explore alternatives cognitively or in action so as to attain better adjustment [85]. There is empirical evidence about improvement of quality of life following the application of this model [74] (see also Chap. 9).

(b) *Cognitive analytic therapy (CAT)* is another version of CBT [86]. It is an integrative model of psychotherapy emphasizing relational aspects of development potentially responsible for psychological distress. Major theoretical constructs are reciprocal roles that constitute a repertoire of relational styles based on earlier experiences with key figures, e.g., threatened or trapped, and reciprocal role procedures which are habitual behavioral coping responses designed to avoid or manage the unbearable emotions evoked by the roles, e.g., feeling humiliated. The reformulation brings together the roles and the responses as internalized by the individual and enacted in the real-life situation. Probing into the experience of early childhood sheds light on the reactions to the cancer situation and highlights the responses that need to be changed for taking control and identifying effective coping behaviors. CAT provides understanding of the patient, listening to him/her and the potential for changing.

(c) *Acceptance and commitment therapy (ACT)* is a third recent version of CBT whose target is to change the function of problematic or distressing thoughts for the individual rather than changing or adapting or eliminating them [87]. Thus, distressing thoughts or expressions are viewed as normal in case of a challenging situation, and therapy should help the patient to accept them and live with them. Thus, the treatment consists in teaching the patients to recognize the disturbing thoughts and their concomitant emotions and to realize that having a thought does not mean that it will necessarily turn into reality. Moreover, the patient is taught to continue functioning in life and promoting one's goals and values despite the changes in the situation due to cancer. Some evidence about the positive effects of this treatment in regard to quality of life is available [88, 89].

C. *Cognitive orientation therapy*. Cognitive orientation (CO) is a theory, research methodology, and treatment procedure that enables understanding, predicting, and changing specific psychological and physiological outputs, e.g., behavior, disease, symptoms, etc. The approach has been developed, applied, and tested since 1972 [90, 91]. The basic assumption of the CO approach is that each output is a function of a motivational disposition implemented by a behavioral program. Both components are affected by cognition but in different ways. The motivational disposition is composed of particular cognitions that represent four types of beliefs referring to contents relevant for the output in question. The four types of beliefs are beliefs that refer to oneself, beliefs that refer to rules and norms, beliefs that refer to goals and wishes, and general beliefs that refer to others and reality. The beliefs refer to contents representing deeper underlying meanings (called "themes") of the behavior of interest rather than to the surface behavior itself. The relevant themes are identified by means of a structured meaning-based systematic procedure of stepwise interviewing of pretest subjects. Thus, for example, some themes for a stress reaction are taking responsibility for everything occurring around oneself even if not done by oneself, no prioritizing of tasks, high demands of oneself, and acting without considering limitation of resources. Themes representing the underlying meanings of a behavior are not known to a patient. When four or at least three belief types referring to themes of a certain behavior orient toward that behavior, it can be predicted that that behavior will actually occur, if there is an adequate behavioral program for its implementation [92].

There are three conditions that need to be met to guarantee the success of the procedure of predicting a behavior by the CO approach: (1) there is a motivational disposition for that behavior defined by four or three belief types referring to themes representing the underlying meanings of the behavior in question; (2) there is an adequate behavioral program for implementing the motivational disposition; and (3) the specific behavior in question is clearly identified.

The CO methodology may be applied for predicting a broad range of different outputs including behaviors, emotions, or psychopathological reactions [93]. Of special interest and importance is the application of the CO approach for identifying the themes supporting health disorders and cancer diseases [75, 94–97]. These themes are disease specific [98] and function as risk factors for the disease, increasing the chances of its occurrence in the presence of a pathogen (see Chap. 5).

In order to change a behavior, it may be necessary to change the relevant beliefs. The process of changing the relevant beliefs is structured and already largely computerized. It consists of mobilizing in the patient support for the relevant themes each separately, in terms of beliefs related meaningfully to that theme in the four belief types. After a basic preliminary training, most patients can continue on their own, with minimal guidance by the therapist which must not require face-to-face contact. In order to guarantee the occurrence of the desired behavior, it is necessary to attain support for that behavior by a sufficient number of themes, though not necessarily of all relevant themes. Training of a relevant behavioral program is recommended when necessary. The success of the training depends on establishing a stable and well-grounded motivational disposition representing four belief types in regard to a sufficient number of relevant themes. In the case of outputs referring to specific behaviors, it is necessary also to guarantee the existence of an adequate behavioral program for implementing the motivational disposition and a clear definition of the specific behavior in question [99].

Evidence in support of the CO therapy approach is available in regard to behaviors supporting health, e.g., smoking cessation [100] and positive reactions to acupuncture treatment of pain [101] and side effects of chemotherapy [102] and cancer [103].

D. *Acquiring problem-solving skills*. Problem-solving skills may seem to belong primarily to the behavioral domain because they provide answers to the question "how to do it." But it belongs no less to the cognitive domain because identifying problems and problem solutions and applying the solutions in the adequate manner require a host of cognitive processes. It is evident that cancer patients are confronted with different problems which they have not faced before nor were required to solve. Problems that are frequently encountered by cancer patients concern, for example, making decisions (see Chap. 7), integrating the goals or requirements of different areas of activity (e.g., family, work, treatments), sequencing of tasks, multitasking, prioritizing, changing perspectives or plans, avoiding overload, adapting to fast changing conditions, adjusting the tempo of performance to one's abilities and state at present, and taking into account information that has not been considered before (e.g., one's physical resources). Patients may use faulty or inadequate solutions to the problems they face because of lack of experience or information, lack of flexibility, and emotional distress.

A therapy based on problem-solving focuses on identifying the major types of problems which confront patients. This includes describing the main causes and situations for the occurrence of these problems, analyzing the main components of the problems, devising means for finding solutions for the problems, outlining procedures for selecting the right solutions, as well as applying them in an adequate manner. In problem-solving therapy, patients learn to identify their specific problems, set realistic goals, give up faulty solutions, change major assumptions which may have led them astray, analyze different alternative possibilities, and improve their cognitive functioning under stress and emotional unrest [104, 105].

E. *Meaning-based interventions*. Since meaning is an integral component of cognition, it is evident that meaning-based interventions are actually cognitive therapies. The major special characteristic of these interventions is that they focus on helping the patient find meaning or a new meaning for their life in their problematic and difficult situation. The major assumptions underlying these interventions are, first, that many cancer patients suffer from different existential concerns, such as "why me," "why do I deserve all this suffering," or "what is the meaning of my remaining life," and, second, that enhancing or reconstructing the meaningfulness of life would contribute to reducing their despair and distress. There are several meaning-based interventions, and many of them target specifically patients with metastatic disease or in the palliative stage when existential concerns become particularly salient. The meaning-centered psychotherapy [106, 107] is the best known and most successful of these interventions. Other interventions are the dignity therapy [108], "the healing journey" [109], "re-creating your life" [110], cognitive-existential therapy [111], meaning-making intervention [112], cognitive-existential intervention [113], supportive-expressive group psychotherapy [114], increasing meaningfulness of life [115], narrative therapy [116], Managing Cancer and Living Meaningfully (CALM) therapy [117], and life review therapy [118].

These interventions share several characteristics. They use psychotherapeutic means, mainly verbal discussions; they consist of several consecutive sessions; they are often based on group psychotherapy; they are basically cognitive; and they focus on issues of meaning of life which consist mainly in finding meaning in and despite the adversities of the patients' life. There are also differences between the interventions. For example, in some cases, the focus is on managing the dying process [108] while in other cases on redefining one's identity (see Chap. 7) or improving one's quality of life in the relatively short period prior to dying [117]. In one case the verbal discussion on meaning is replaced by an online training designed to increase the meaningfulness of life in general rather than in regard to cancer in a brief session activated by the patient at will [115]. Despite differences in criteria, reviews show that most of the interventions are at least to some degree efficacious in helping cancer patients in the palliative stage.

F. *Guided imagery*. Guided imagery has a long history as a procedure for improving the well-being of individuals. It has been used in one or another version for thousands of years in different cultures. It is based on the principle that an individual can direct to some extent physiological processes in a desired direction if the procedure is enacted adequately. The criteria of adequate implementation include using only images (of any sensory channel), stating the directions in a syntactically positive manner (e.g., "a sponge should absorb all the pain" rather than "the pain should be no more"), being precise and specific in all formulations (e.g., "I will be free of pain in my leg when I go to bed tonight" rather than "I will be free of pain"), and adjusting the instructions presented through the image preferably in a psychologically and physiologically adequate manner (i.e., being free of pain should be expressed through an image that is meaningful for the individual and should be in accord with physiological processes).

There are various versions of guided imagery. Sometimes it is restricted only to images, or even to particular images; at other times words are also used. Sometimes the individual practices the procedure alone; at other times, there is a guiding mentor. Often guided imagery is applied in the context of other CAM or psychosocial interventions. The main advantages of guided imagery are that it is cheap, it is constantly available, it is accessible to everyone, it can be practiced on one's own without the intervention of other agents, it has apparently no negative effects, and it is widely used for a broad range of domains including sports, physical disorders, psychological symptoms, distress, and everyday-life problems. There is evidence about its frequent use by cancer patients of all kinds, including children. Many though not all studies reported positive results for improving stress, pain, and even wound healing [119].

G. *Mindfulness interventions*. This procedure is most often related to stress reduction or meditation. It is based on two major components: self-regulating attention and acceptance of the experienced. The procedure consists in training of focusing attention on purpose on the immediate experience and accepting it nonjudgmentally. A set of skills, including sitting meditation, body scan, breathing, and mindfulness exercises, are applied for training the style of attention and the attitudes of acceptance and openness to experience. There is empirical evidence about the positive effects of mindfulness interventions on psychological distress, sense of control, and overall well-being of cancer patients [120, 121]. Related practices with similar positive results for cancer patients are the practice of yoga and of meditation [66, 122, 123].

H. *Religion and spirituality*. Cancer patients of different religions often turn to religion when they are in distress. This has been reported about patients who may be described as observant of religious ways of life and others who may simply be in spiritual distress or have spiritual needs. There are various ways in which religion and spirituality can be involved, for example, through prayer, joining a religious community, contact with holy personages, visiting sacred sites, using amulets, practicing meditation or kabala, learning religious philosophy, or enhancing one's faith. The potential contributions of religion and spirituality to cancer patients may be affective, behavioral, cognitive, and others (e.g., social) [124]. Several comprehensive meta-analyses showed that overall religiosity/spirituality scores were significantly associated with social health [125] and with better patient-reported physical health [126] and moderately associated with mental health of the cancer patients [127]. Several reviews showed that the impact of religion on cancer patients may not be always beneficial [128, 129]. When coping by means of religion is of a positive nature (e.g., patients consider God as their partner and source of help), their quality of life and adherence to the treatments are affected positively. If however they expect God to help them without medicine or they are angry with God for having let them down or consider the disease as a punishment by God, the impact of religion on cancer patients may be negative [126, 130, 131]. These findings suggest that when practicing psychosocial support in the context of religiosity and spirituality, psychosocial care professionals should support the patients in choosing the track of positive coping by religion rather than the negative track.

I. *Art and expressive therapy*. There are several different forms of art therapy, such as literature or visual arts (see below). Some therapeutic versions are active and involve production by the patient, and some are passive, involving primarily exposure to art products. This kind of therapy is practiced sometimes individually and sometimes in groups or in the presence of others, who may be, for example, patients, friends, or family members. It may be practiced in clinics, in hospitals, at home, in the course of treatments, or in waiting rooms. Sometimes the products of art therapy are shared, even with strangers, and sometimes they are kept private. The sharing may be by concrete presentation of the products or by the Internet. The contact with art may be accompanied by therapeutic conversations with a therapist or not. It may form the major core of the therapy or serve as background promoting a supportive atmosphere for another therapy or occupation. There is empirical evidence about the positive impact of contact with art on the quality of life, stress level, and coping of patients [132–137]. The beneficial effects of dealing with the arts are based on increase in insight, relaxation, catharsis, identification, self-expression, and projection that active and passive contact with art provides in different forms. The following are the major kinds of art therapy:

Bibliotherapy. This form of therapy may take the active forms, such as writing poetry, narrative therapy [116], written emotional disclosure [138], and writing or telling stories about oneself or other themes. In addition to the active forms, there are the more passive ones of reading or listening to stories, myths, poetry, legends, biographies, philosophy, etc. or to relevant materials about problems in relationships or life in general [139, 140].

Music therapy. This form of therapy is highly variegated. It includes playing musical instruments of all kinds by patients who have learned how to play the instruments as well as by those who did not or are just starting to learn. Sometimes it involves simply producing tones or sounds by touching chords or different objects. An important part consists of listening to music of all kinds, recording one's own music, as well as singing known melodies or melodies, rhythms, or simply sounds expressive of one's state or mood [141, 142].

Visual art therapy. This kind of art therapy may focus on drawing, painting, producing collages and other designs, or observing paintings of all kinds in museums, at home, or on the Internet [133, 143].

Dance and movement therapy. This kind of therapy may be practiced in many forms, both formal and informal. It may be practiced by improvisation or in line with learned movements, alone or together with others, with or without music. It is used for improving body image, freedom of movement, self-esteem, communication with others, and overall sense of well-being. There is no empirical support for the utility of dance and movement therapy for cancer patients, but a review still states that the findings of individual studies suggest that dance/movement therapy may have a beneficial effect on quality of life, somatization, and vigor [144, 145].

Drama, theater, and acting. This kind of therapy includes psychodrama and different kinds of role playing in line with different kinds of literary or dramatic texts or improvisation. It may be practiced together with dance and movement therapy, mostly in groups (e.g., [146]).

J. *Supportive and psychoeducational psychotherapy*. It is controversial whether this kind of intervention should be identified as psychotherapy, but it is not controversial that it is being practiced, although often not systematically, and that it is helpful for patients. The major components of this kind of therapeutic approach are offering the patients support of different kinds, listening to their stories and reports, and providing guidance and instruction in solving their basic problems that concern management of treatment, communication with others, and their daily life in general.

This approach is based on the assumption that cancer patients are essentially inexperienced in the kind of problems and daily hassles they confront and some help in providing information about basic issues may be beneficial. This kind of support can be provided by psychooncologists, social workers, and nurses and other healthcare professionals, friends, acquaintances, and other patients. It may play an important role in different phases of the disease. Providing support and general information may be helpful particularly for newly diagnosed patients, who may benefit from being introduced to the complexities of treatments, clinics, and keeping daily routines [71]. Guidance and support of a different type are helpful for patients in the transition from treatments to survival, who may be anxious about reconstructing their life. Empowering the patient and training for self-management figure as salient components [147]. Again, a different kind of support is needed for patients in the palliative phase, when the fears of deteriorating, weakening, and approaching death dominate the scene. In sum, the characteristics of supportive and psychoeducational psychotherapy are flexibility, constant adjustment to the patient's needs, continuous consideration of the current situation, and readiness to apply interchangeably provision of information, guidance, and support. It is adapted to cancer patients differing in diagnosis, gender, age, stage of disease, and focal issues (e.g., financial, marital relations, communication with children, medical information). Accordingly, also the goals of the psychotherapeutic procedure may differ, ranging from providing information and support, listening to the patient's problems, or expressing empathy to counseling in diverse practical affairs engendered by the disease. On the whole, supportive psychoeducational psychotherapy was shown to have positive effects on the patients' quality of life, mood level, and overall functioning [148–150].

Some Summative Remarks

The fact that there are many treatment options of different kinds for cancer does not make things much easier for the patient. Although it could be expected that the diversity of options would exert a calming and reassuring impact, it also creates embarrassment and confusion attended by anxiety and worry. This is due not merely to lack of expertise and low level of understanding in regard to health issues on the part of the innocent nonprofessional patient, nor to the oppressive need to make choices, which may sometimes or for some patients be quite difficult. Rather, the multiplicity of treatments suggests to many patients that there is actually no treatment for cancer but only a great number of attempts at treatment none of which is conclusive or completely reliable. A plausible implication is that it is necessary to apply several if not many or all treatments so as not to miss out on any chance for recovery. The attempt not to miss out on any treatment chance produces a lot of stress for the patients. One possible implication of the multiplicity of treatments is the need to refer to a second opinion to one's doctor, which may be embarrassing for many patients.

An additional difficulty arises from the problem that many of the suggested or available treatments are not purely medical but rather complementary or psychosocial. This discourages many patients who assume that the disease may be psychologically determined, which may indicate – though erroneously – that they are to blame for getting the disease. Further, many patients are not sure how to manage or deal with these nonmedical treatments. All too often they avoid consulting their doctors about these additional treatments, or they are ashamed to admit to their use. In that case they are often conflicted about whether using the additional treatments may not be harmful or may not diminish the therapeutic impact of the medical treatment.

In general, selecting specific treatments is difficult and problematic for many patients, actually not less so than the attempt to combine several treatments or apply an integrated approach.

On the other hand, the multiplicity of approaches and their variety suggest to the patients that there are many treatment options, so that even if one fails or does not culminate in the expected recovery, there are always other options that can be applied.

References

1. Van de Velde, C. J., Baumann, M., Kerr, D. J., Haller, D. G., & Saijo, N. (2016). *Oxford textbook of oncology*. Oxford, UK: Oxford University Press.
2. Kacen, L., Madjar, I., Denham, J., Ackland, S., & Ariad, S. (2005). Patients deciding to forgo or stop active treatment for cancer. *European Journal of Palliative Care, 12*, 113–116.
3. Citrin, D. L., Bloom, D. L., Grutsch, J. F., Mortensen, S. J., & Lis, C. G. (2012). Beliefs and perceptions of women with newly diagnosed breast cancer who refused conventional treatment in favor of alternative therapies. *The Oncologist, 17*(5), 607–612.
4. Madjar, I., Kacen, L., Ariad, S., & Denham, J. (2007). Telling their stories, telling our stories: Physicians' experiences with patients who decide to forgo or stop treatment for cancer. *Qualitative Health Research, 17*(4), 428–441.
5. Rodriguez, J., & Hart, W. R. (1982). Endometrial cancers occurring 10 or more years after pelvic irradiation for carcinoma. *International Journal of Gynecological Pathology, 1*(2), 135–144.

6. Voogt, E., van der Heide, A., Rietjens, J. A., van Leeuwen, A. F., Visser, A. P., van der Rijt, C. C., & van der Maas, P. J. (2005). Attitudes of patients with incurable cancer toward medical treatment in the last phase of life. *Journal of Clinical Oncology, 23*(9), 2012–2019.
7. Slevin, M. L., Stubbs, L., Plant, H. J., Wilson, P., Gregory, W. M., Armes, P. J., & Downer, S. M. (1990). Attitudes to chemotherapy: Comparing views of patients with cancer with those of doctors, nurses, and general public. *BMJ, 300*(6737), 1458–1460.
8. Ankem, K. (2015). Assessing cancer patients' health information needs: a standardised approach. *Information Research, 20*(2), paper 668. Retrieved from http://InformationR.net/ir/20-2/paper668.html.
9. Dean, L. T., Moss, S. L., McCarthy, A. M., & Armstrong, K. (2017). Healthcare system distrust, physician trust, and patient discordance with adjuvant breast cancer treatment recommendations. *Cancer Epidemiology and Prevention Biomarkers, 26*(12), 1745–1752.
10. Barak, F., Kreitler, S., Kovner, F., & Inbar, M. (2003, January). *Adjuvant chemotherapy for breast cancer patients: Patients' expectations and physicians' attitudes*. Poster presented at the 2nd conference of the Israeli society for clinical oncology and radiation therapy (ISCORT-2), Eilat, Israel.
11. Engida, A., Ayelign, T., Mahteme, B., Aida, T., & Abreham, B. (2016). Types and indications of colostomy and determinants of outcomes of patients after surgery. *Ethiopian Journal of Health Sciences, 26*(2), 117–122.
12. Resnick, M. J., Koyama, T., Fan, K. H., Albertsen, P. C., Goodman, M., Hamilton, A. S., Hoffman, R. M., Potosky, A. L., Stanford, J. L., Stroup, A. M., Van Horn, R. L., & Penson, D. F. (2013). Long-term functional outcomes after treatment for localized prostate cancer. *The New England Journal of Medicine, 368*(5), 436–445.
13. Kreitler, S., Krivoy, E., & Toren, A. (2012). Psychosocial aspects of radiotherapy in pediatric cancer patients. In S. Kreitler, M. W. Ben-Arush, & A. Martin (Eds.), *Pediatric psycho-oncology: Psychosocial aspects and clinical interventions* (2nd ed., pp. 62–70). Oxford: Wiley-Blackwell.
14. Kreitler, S., Ben-Arush, M. W., Kriboy, E., Golan, H., Kreitler, M., & Toren, A. (2010). Psychosocial aspects of radiotherapy for the child and family with cancer. In E. C. Halperin, L. S. Constine, N. J. Tarbell, & L. E. Kun (Eds.), *Pediatric radiation oncology* (5th ed., pp. 447–456). Philadelphia: Lippincott, Williams & Wilkins.
15. Ali, S., & Singh, G. (2010). Radiation-induced alopecia. *International Journal of Trichology, 2*(2), 118.
16. Hutchinson, A. D., Hosking, J. R., Kichenadasse, G., Mattiske, J. K., & Wilson, C. (2012). Objective and subjective cognitive impairment following chemotherapy for cancer: A systematic review. *Cancer Treatment Reviews, 38*(7), 926–934.
17. Dawson, I. G., Johnson, J. E., & Luke, M. A. (2013). Helping individuals to understand synergistic risks: An assessment of message contents depicting mechanistic and probabilistic concepts. *Risk Analysis, 33*(5), 851–865.
18. Hanoch, Y. (2004). Improving doctor-patient understanding of probability in communicating cancer-screening test findings. *Journal of Health Communication, 9*(4), 327–335.
19. Krosnick, J. A., Malhotra, N., Mo, C. H., Bruera, E. F., Chang, L., Pasek, J., & Thomas, R. K. (2017). Perceptions of health risks of cigarette smoking: A new measure reveals widespread misunderstanding. *PLoS One, 12*(8), e0182063.
20. Kazem, M. A. (2017). Predictive models in cancer management: A guide for clinicians. *The Surgeon, 15*(2), 93–97.
21. Mahon, S. M. (2006). What are the chances? Risk in the real world. *Clinical Journal of Oncology Nursing, 10*(1), 99–101.
22. O'Quigley, J. (2017). Faulty BRCA1, BRCA2 genes: How poor is the prognosis? *Annals of Epidemiology, 27*(10), 672–676.
23. Holmberg, C., Waters, E. A., Whitehouse, K., Daly, M., & McCaskill-Stevens, W. (2015). My lived experiences are more important than your probabilities: The role of individualized risk estimates for decision making about participation in the Study of Tamoxifen and Raloxifene (STAR). *Medical Decision Making, 35*(8), 1010–1022.

24. Benson, H., & Klipper, M. Z. (1992). *The relaxation response*. New York: Harper Collins.
25. Jacobsen, E. (1929). *Progressive relaxation*. Chicago: University of Chicago Press.
26. Downer, S. M., Cody, M. M., McCluskey, P., Wilson, P. D., Arnott, S. J., Lister, T. A., & Slevin, M. L. (1994). Pursuit and practice of complementary therapies by cancer patients receiving conventional treatment. *BMJ, 309*(6947), 86–89.
27. Dewhirst, M., Stauffer, P. R., Das, S., Craciunescu, O. I., & Vajaskovic, Z. (2016). Hyperthermia. In L. L. Gunderson & J. E. Tepper (Eds.), *Clinical radiation oncology* (4th ed.). Philadelphia: Elsevier.
28. White, M. A., Verhoef, M. J., Davison, B. J., Gunn, H., & Cooke, K. (2008). Seeking mind, body and spirit healing-why some men with prostate cancer choose CAM (Complementary and Alternative Medicine) over conventional cancer treatments. *Integrative Medicine Insights, 3*, 1–11, IMI-S377.
29. Deng, G. (2008). Integrative cancer care in a US academic cancer centre: The Memorial Sloan–Kettering experience. *Current Oncology, 15*(Suppl 2), s108–es68.
30. Bott, J. (2007). An analysis of paper-based sources of information on complementary therapies. *Complementary Therapies in Clinical Practice, 13*(1), 53–62.
31. Richardson, M. A., Mâsse, L. C., Nanny, K., & Sanders, C. (2004). Discrepant views of oncologists and cancer patients on complementary/alternative medicine. *Supportive Care in Cancer, 12*(11), 797–804.
32. Ernst, E. (2000). The role of complementary and alternative medicine in cancer. *The Lancet Oncology, 1*(3), 176–180.
33. Molassiotis, A., Fernadez-Ortega, P., Pud, D., Ozden, G., Scott, J. A., Panteli, V., Margulies, A., Browall, M., Magri, M., Selvekerova, S., Milovics, L., Bruyns, I., Gudmundsdottir, G., Hummerston, S., Ahmad, A. M.-A., Platin, N., Kearney, N., Patiraki, E., & Madsen, E. (2005). Use of complementary and alternative medicine in cancer patients: A European survey. *Annals of Oncology, 16*(4), 655–663.
34. Berretta, M., Della Pepa, C., Tralongo, P., Fulvi, A., Martellotta, F., Lleshi, A., Fisichella, R., Romano, C., De Divitiis, C., Fiorica, F., Di Francia, R., Di Mari, A., Del Pup, L., Crispo, A., De Paoli, P., Santorelli, A., Quagliariello, V., Iaffaioli, R. V., Tirelli, U., Facchini, G., & Taibi, R. (2017). Use of complementary and alternative medicine (CAM) in cancer patients: An Italian multicenter survey. *Oncotarget, 8*(15), 24401.
35. Eisenberg, D. M., Davis, R. B., Ettner, S. L., Appel, S., Wilkey, S., Van Rompay, M., & Kessler, R. C. (1998). Trends in alternative medicine use in the United States, 1990–1997: Results of a follow-up national survey. *JAMA, 280*(18), 1569–1575.
36. Adams, M., & Jewell, A. P. (2007). The use of complementary and alternative medicine by cancer patients. *International Seminars in Surgical Oncology*, 4, 10.
37. Horneber, M., Bueschel, G., Dennert, G., Less, D., Ritter, E., & Zwahlen, M. (2012). How many cancer patients use complementary and alternative medicine: A systematic review and metaanalysis. *Integrative Cancer Therapies, 11*(3), 187–203.
38. Scott, J. A., Kearney, N., Hummerston, S., & Molassiotis, A. (2005). Use of complementary and alternative medicine in patients with cancer: A UK survey. *European Journal of Oncology Nursing, 9*(2), 131–137.
39. Wortmann, J. K., Bremer, A., Eich, H. T., Wortmann, H. P., Schuster, A., Führer, J., Büntzel, J., Muecke, R., Prott, F. J., & Huebner, J. (2016). Use of complementary and alternative medicine by patients with cancer: A cross-sectional study at different points of cancer care. *Medical Oncology, 33*(7), 78.
40. Vyas, T., Hart, R. D., Trites, J. R., Philips, T. J., Archibald, K. E., Phillips, J. E., & Taylor, S. M. (2010). Complementary and alternative medicine use in patients presenting to a head and neck oncology clinic. *Head & Neck, 32*(6), 793–799.
41. Richardson, M. A. (1999). Research of complementary/alternative medicine therapies in oncology: Promising but challenging. *Journal of Clinical Oncology, 17*(11), 38–43.
42. Begbie, S. D., Kerestes, Z. L., & Bell, D. R. (1996). Patterns of alternative medicine use by cancer patients. *The Medical Journal of Australia, 165*(10), 545–548.

43. Wilkinson, S. (2002). Complementary therapies-patient demand. *International Journal of Palliative Nursing, 8*, 468.
44. Ernst, E., & Fugh-Berman, A. (2002). Complementary and alternative medicine: What is it all about? *Occupational and Environmental Medicine, 59*(2), 140–144.
45. Ernst, E. (1998). The prevalence of complementary/alternative medicine in cancer. *Cancer, 83*(4), 777–782.
46. Risberg, T., Kaasa, S., Wist, E., & Melsom, H. (1997). Why are cancer patients using non-proven complementary therapies? A cross-sectional multicentre study in Norway. *European Journal of Cancer, 33*(4), 575–580.
47. Roberts, D., McNulty, A., & Caress, A. L. (2005). Current issues in the delivery of complementary therapies in cancer care—Policy, perceptions and expectations: An overview. *European Journal of Oncology Nursing, 9*(2), 115–123.
48. Kaasa, S. (2001). Assessment of quality of life in palliative care. *Journal of Palliative Medicine, 4*(3), 413–416.
49. Balneaves, L. G., Kristjanson, L. J., & Tataryn, D. (1999). Beyond convention: Describing complementary therapy use by women living with breast cancer. *Patient Education and Counseling, 38*(2), 143–153.
50. Shumay, D. M., Maskarinec, G., Gotay, C. C., Heiby, E. M., & Kakai, H. (2002). Determinants of the degree of complementary and alternative medicine use among patients with cancer. *Journal of Alternative and Complementary Medicine, 8*(5), 661–671.
51. Harris, P., Finlay, I. G., Cook, A., Thomas, K. J., & Hood, K. (2003). Complementary and alternative medicine use by patients with cancer in Wales: A cross sectional survey. *Complementary Therapies in Medicine, 11*(4), 249–253.
52. Richardson, M. A., Sanders, T., Palmer, J. L., Greisinger, A., & Singletary, S. E. (2000). Complementary/alternative medicine use in a comprehensive cancer center and the implications for oncology. *Journal of Clinical Oncology, 18*(13), 2505–2514.
53. Lengacher, C. A., Bennett, M. P., Kip, K. E., Gonzalez, L., Jacobsen, P., & Cox, C. E. (2006). Relief of symptoms, side effects, and psychological distress through use of complementary and alternative medicine in women with breast cancer. *Oncology Nursing Forum, 33*(1), 97–104.
54. Paltiel, O., Avitzour, M., Peretz, T., Cherny, N., Kaduri, L., Pfeffer, R. M., Wagner, N., & Soskolne, V. (2001). Determinants of the use of complementary therapies by patients with cancer. *Journal of Clinical Oncology, 19*(9), 2439–2448.
55. Cancerbacup. (2000). *Cancer and complementary therapies*. UK: Ashford Colour Press.
56. Chen, R., Deng, X., Wu, H., Peng, P., Wen, B., Li, F., & Li, F. (2014). Combined immunotherapy with dendritic cells and cytokine-induced killer cells for malignant tumors: A systematic review and meta-analysis. *International Immunopharmacology, 22*(2), 451–464.
57. Cassileth, B. (2010). Gerson regimen. *Oncology (Williston Park, NY), 24*(2), 201–201.
58. Arumugam, A., Agullo, P., Boopalan, T., Nandy, S., Lopez, R., Gutierrez, C., Narayan, M., & Rajkumar, L. (2014). Neem leaf extract inhibits mammary carcinogenesis by altering cell proliferation, apoptosis, and angiogenesis. *Cancer Biology & Therapy, 15*(1), 26–34.
59. Chang, E. Y., Glissmeyer, M., Tonnes, S., Hudson, T., & Johnson, N. (2006). Outcomes of breast cancer in patients who use alternative therapies as primary treatment. *American Journal of Surgery, 192*(4), 471–473.
60. Sheldon, T. (2004). Netherlands to crack down on complementary medicine. *BMJ: British Medical Journal, 328*(7438), 485.
61. Smith, M. C., Kemp, J., Hemphill, L., & Vojir, C. P. (2002). Outcomes of therapeutic massage for hospitalized cancer patients. *Journal of Nursing Scholarship, 34*(3), 257–262.
62. Cassileth, B. R., & Vickers, A. J. (2004). Massage therapy for symptom control: Outcome study at a major cancer center. *Journal of Pain and Symptom Management, 28*(3), 244–249.
63. Dean-Clower, E., Doherty-Gilman, A. M., Keshaviiah, A., Baker, F., Kaw, C., Lu, W., Manola, J., Penson, R. T., Matulonis, U. A., & Rosenthal, D. S. (2010). Acupuncture as palliative therapy for physical symptoms and quality of life cancer patients. *Integrative Cancer Therapies, 9*(2), 158–167.

64. Lu, W., Dean-Clower, E., Doherty-Gilman, A., & Rosenthal, D. S. (2008). The value of acupuncture in cancer care. *Hematology/Oncology Clinics, 22*(4), 631–648.
65. Garcia, M. K., McQuade, J., Haddad, R., Patel, S., Lee, R., Yang, P., Palmer, J. L., & Cohen, L. (2013). Systematic review of acupuncture in cancer care: A synthesis of the evidence. *Journal of Clinical Oncology, 31*(7), 952.
66. Banasik, J., Williams, H., Haberman, M., Blank, S. E., & Bendel, R. (2011). Effect of Iyengar yoga practice on fatigue and diurnal salivary cortisol concentration in breast cancer survivors. *Journal of the American Association of Nurse Practitioners, 23*(3), 135–142.
67. Rosenbaum, E., Gautier, H., Fobair, P., Neri, E., Festa, B., Hawn, M., Andrews, A., Hirshberger, N., Selim, S., & Spiegel, D. (2004). Cancer supportive care, improving the quality of life for cancer patients. A program evaluation report. *Supportive Care in Cancer, 12*(5), 293–301.
68. Stene, G. B., Helbostad, J. L., Balstad, T. R., Riphagen, I. I., Kaasa, S., & Oldervoll, L. M. (2013). Effect of physical exercise on muscle mass and strength in cancer patients during treatment—A systematic review. *Critical Reviews in Oncology/Hematology, 88*(3), 573–593.
69. McCune, J. S., Hatfield, A. J., Blackburn, A. A., Leith, P. O., Livingston, R. B., & Ellis, G. K. (2004). Potential of chemotherapy–herb interactions in adult cancer patients. *Supportive Care in Cancer, 12*(6), 454–462.
70. Bozza, C., Agostinetto, E., Gerratana, L., & Puglisi, F. (2015). Complementary and alternative medicine in oncology. *Recenti Progressi in Medicina, 106*(12), 601–607.
71. Lederberg, M. S., & Holland, J. C. (2011). Supportive psychotherapy in cancer care: An essential ingredient of all therapy. In M. Watson & D. Kissane (Eds.), *Handbook of psychotherapy in cancer care* (pp. 1–14). Hoboken: Wiley-Blackwell.
72. Prochaska, J. O., & Norcross, J. C. (2018). *Systems of psychotherapy: A transtheoretical analysis*. New York: Oxford University Press.
73. Lebow, J. L. (Ed.). (2012). *Twenty-first century psychotherapies: Contemporary approaches to theory and practice*. Hoboken: Wiley.
74. Daniels, S. (2015). Cognitive behavior therapy for patients with cancer. *Journal of the Advanced Practitioner in Oncology, 6*(1), 54.
75. Horne, D., & Watson, M. (2011). Cognitive-behavioral therapies in cancer care. In M. Watson & D. Kissane (Eds.), *Handbook of psychotherapy in cancer care* (pp. 15–26). Hoboken: Wiley-Blackwell.
76. Telch, C. F., & Telch, M. J. (1986). Group coping skills instruction and supportive group therapy for cancer patients: A comparison of strategies. *Journal of Consulting and Clinical Psychology, 54*(6), 802.
77. Lejuez, C. W., Hopko, D. R., & Hopko, S. D. (2001). A brief behavioral activation treatment for depression: Treatment manual. *Behavior Modification, 25*(2), 255–286.
78. Hopko, D. R., Funderburk, J. S., Shorey, R. C., McIndoo, C. C., Ryba, M. M., File, A. A., & Vitulano, M. (2013). Behavioral activation and problem-solving therapy for depressed breast cancer patients: Preliminary support for decreased suicidal ideation. *Behavior Modification, 37*(6), 747–767.
79. Johnsen, T. J., & Friborg, O. (2015). The effects of cognitive behavioral therapy as an anti-depressive treatment is falling: A meta-analysis. *Psychological Bulletin, 141*(4), 747–768.
80. Dobson, K. S., & Dozois, D. J. A. (2008). Historical and philosophical bases of the cognitive-behavioral therapies. In K. S. Dobson (Ed.), *Handbook of cognitive-behavioral therapies* (3rd ed., pp. 3–39). New York: Guilford Press.
81. Beck, A. T. (1967). *Depression: Clinical, experimental, and theoretical aspects*. Philadelphia: University of Pennsylvania Press.
82. Beck, J. S. (1995). *Cognitive therapy: Basics and beyond*. New York: Guilford Press.
83. Gielissen, M. F., Verhagen, S., Witjes, F., & Bleijenberg, G. (2006). Effects of cognitive behavior therapy in severely fatigued disease-free cancer patients compared with patients waiting for cognitive behavior therapy: A randomized controlled trial. *Journal of Clinical Oncology, 24*(30), 4882–4887.

84. Savard, J., Simard, S., Ivers, H., & Morin, C. M. (2005). Randomized study on the efficacy of cognitive-behavioral therapy for insomnia secondary to breast cancer, part I: Sleep and psychological effects. *Journal of Clinical Oncology, 23*(25), 6083–6096.
85. Moorey, S., & Greer, S. (2011). *Oxford guide to CBT for people with cancer*. New York: Oxford University Press.
86. Pitceathly, C., Tolosa, I., Kerr, I. B., & Grassi, L. (2011). Cognitive analytic therapy in psycho-oncology. In M. Watson & W. D. Kissane (Eds.), *Handbook of psychotherapy in cancer care* (pp. 27–38). Hoboken: Wiley-Blackwell.
87. Hayes, S. C., Strosahl, K. D., & Wilson, K. G. (2011). *Acceptance and commitment therapy: The process and practice of mindful change*. New York: Guilford Press.
88. Ruiz, F. J. (2010). A review of Acceptance and Commitment Therapy (ACT) empirical evidence: Correlational, experimental psychopathology, component and outcome studies. *International Journal of Psychology and Psychological Therapy, 10*(1), 125–162.
89. Feros, D. L., Lane, L., Ciarrochi, J., & Blackledge, J. T. (2013). Acceptance and Commitment Therapy (ACT) for improving the lives of cancer patients: A preliminary study. *Psycho-Oncology, 22*(2), 459–464.
90. Kreitler, H., & Kreitler, S. (1976). *Cognitive orientation and behavior*. New York: Springer Publishing Company.
91. Kreitler, H., & Kreitler, S. (1982). The theory of cognitive orientation: Widening the scope of behavior prediction. In B. Maher & W. B. Maher (Eds.), *Progress in experimental personality research* (Vol. 11, pp. 101–169). New York: Academic.
92. Kreitler, S., & Kreitler, M. M. (2014). Changing attitudes and beliefs. In C. Pracana (Ed.), *InPACT international psychological applications conference and trends* (pp. 99–102). Lisbon: W.I.A.R.S.
93. Kreitler, S. (2015). Psychopathology: The cognitive orientation approach. In C. Pracana (Ed.), *InPACT international psychological applications conference and trends* (pp. 58–63). Lisbon: W.I.A.R.S.
94. Kreitler, S. (2016). The motivation for health: What is it and how to assess it. In C. Pracana & M. Wang (Eds.), *InPACT international psychological applications conference and trends: Proceedings* (pp. 172–176). Lisbon: W.I.A.R.S.
95. Kreitler, S., & Kreitler, H. (1991). Cognitive orientation and physical disease or health. *European Journal of Personality, 5*(2), 109–129.
96. Kreitler, S., & Kreitler, H. (1998). Cognitive orientation and disease in cancer patients. *Psycho-Oncology, 1*, 174.
97. Kreitler, S., Kreitler, M. M., Len, A., Alkalay, Y., & Barak, F. (2008). Psychological risk factors for colorectal cancer? Facteurs de risque psychologiques du cancer colorectal? *Psycho-Oncologie, 2*(3), 131–145.
98. Kreitler, S., Kreitler, M. M., & Barak, F. (2013). Psychosocial risk factors of cancer diseases: How specific are they? *Open Journal of Social Sciences, 1*(6), 81–86.
99. Kreitler, H., & Kreitler, S. (1990). Cognitive primacy, cognitive behavior guidance, and their implications for cognitive therapy. *Journal of Cognitive Psychotherapy, 4*(2), 155–173.
100. Kreitler, S., Shahar, A., & Kreitler, H. (1976). Cognitive orientation, type of smoker and behavior therapy of smoking. *Psychology and Psychotherapy: Theory, Research and Practice, 49*(2), 167–175.
101. Kreitler, S., Kreitler, H., & Carasso, R. (1987). Cognitive orientation as predictor of pain relief following acupuncture. *Pain, 28*(3), 323–341.
102. Kreitler, S., & Richkov, V. (2015). Cognitive orientation of health as a moderator of side effects of chemotherapeutic treatment. *Psycho-Oncology, 24*, 267.
103. Kreitler, S., & Inbar, M. (2000). Cognitive orientation variables as predictors of survival in cancer. *Psycho-Oncology, 9*(5), S2.
104. Nezu, A. M., Nezu, C. M., & D'Zurilla, T. (2012). *Problem-solving therapy: A treatment manual*. New York: Springer Publishing Company.

105. Nezu, A. M., Nezu, C. M., Houts, P. S., Friedman, S. H., & Faddis, S. (1999). Relevance of problem-solving therapy to psychosocial oncology. *Journal of Psychosocial Oncology, 16*(3–4), 5–26.
106. Breitbart, W. S., & Poppito, S. R. (2014). *Individual meaning-centered psychotherapy for patients with advanced cancer: A treatment manual*. New York: Oxford University Press.
107. Breitbart, W., & Poppito, S. R. (2014). *Meaning-centered group psychotherapy for patients with advanced cancer: A treatment manual*. New York: Oxford University Press.
108. Chochinov, H. M., Kristjanson, L. J., Breitbart, W., McClement, S., Hack, T. F., Hassard, T., & Harlos, M. (2011). Effect of dignity therapy on distress and end-of-life experience in terminally ill patients: A randomised controlled trial. *The Lancet Oncology, 12*(8), 753–762.
109. Cunningham, A. J. (2002). *Bringing spirituality into your healing journey*. Toronto: Key Porter Books.
110. Cole, B., & Pargament, K. (1999). Re-creating your life: A spiritual/psychotherapeutic intervention for people diagnosed with cancer. *Psycho-Oncology, 8*(5), 395–407.
111. Kissane, D. W., Love, A., Hatton, A., Bloch, S., Smith, G., Clarke, D. M., & Snyder, R. D. (2004). Effect of cognitive-existential group therapy on survival in early-stage breast cancer. *Journal of Clinical Oncology, 22*(21), 4255–4260.
112. Creamer, M., Burgess, P., & Pattison, P. (1992). Reaction to trauma: A cognitive processing model. *Journal of Abnormal Psychology, 101*(3), 452–459.
113. Gagnon, P., Fillion, L., Robitaille, M. A., Girard, M., Tardif, F., Cochrane, J. P., Le Moignan Moreau, J., & Breitbart, W. (2015). A cognitive–existential intervention to improve existential and global quality of life in cancer patients: A pilot study. *Palliative & Supportive Care, 13*(4), 981–990.
114. Spiegel, D., & Spira, J. (1991). *Supportive-expressive group therapy: A treatment manual of psychosocial intervention for women with recurrent breast cancer*. Palo Alto: Psychosocial Treatment Laboratory, Department of Psychiatry, Stanford University.
115. Kreitler, S. (2018). Meaningfulness of life and existential distress. *Advances in Clinical and Experimental Psychology, 1*(1), 1–10.
116. Borman, S. (2011). Narrative therapy. In M. Watson & D. W. Kissane (Eds.), *Handbook of psychotherapy in cancer care* (pp. 69–77). Hoboken: Wiley- Blackwell.
117. Lo, C., Hales, S., Rydall, A., Panday, T., Chiu, A., Malfitano, C., Jung, J., Li, M., Nissim, R., Zimmermann, C., & Rodin, G. (2015). Managing cancer and living meaningfully: Study protocol for a randomized controlled trial. *Trials, 16*, 391. Published online 2015 Sep 3. https://doi.org/10.1186/s13063-015-0811-1.
118. Keall, R. M., Clayton, J. M., & Butow, P. N. (2015). Therapeutic life review in palliative care: A systematic review of quantitative evaluations. *Journal of Pain and Symptom Management, 49*(4), 747–761.
119. Kreitler, S. (2012). Guided imagery: A psychological tool in the service of health psychology. In K. R. Carter & G. E. Murphy (Eds.), *Alternative medicine: Practices, health benefits and controversies* (pp. 1–26). Hauppauge: Nova Publishers.
120. Baer, R. A. (Ed.). (2015). *Mindfulness-based treatment approaches: Clinician's guide to evidence base and applications*. New York: Elsevier and Academic Press.
121. Ledesma, D., & Kumano, H. (2009). Mindfulness-based stress reduction and cancer: A meta-analysis. *Psycho-Oncology, 18*(6), 571–579.
122. Buffart, L. M., Van Uffelen, J. G., Riphagen, I. I., Brug, J., van Mechelen, W., Brown, W. J., & Chinapaw, M. J. (2012). Physical and psychosocial benefits of yoga in cancer patients and survivors, a systematic review and meta-analysis of randomized controlled trials. *BMC Cancer, 12*(1), 559.
123. Speca, M., Carlson, L. E., Goodey, E., & Angen, M. (2000). A randomized, wait-list controlled clinical trial: The effect of a mindfulness meditation-based stress reduction program on mood and symptoms of stress in cancer outpatients. *Psychosomatic Medicine, 62*(5), 613–622.
124. Salsman, J. M., Fitchett, G., Merluzzi, T. V., Sherman, A. C., & Park, C. L. (2015). Religion, spirituality, and health outcomes in cancer: A case for a meta-analytic investigation. *Cancer, 121*(21), 3754–3759.

125. Sherman, A. C., Merluzzi, T. V., Pustejovsky, J. E., Park, C. L., George, L., Fitchett, G., Jim, H. S., Munoz, A. R., Danhauer, A. C., Snyder, M. A., & Salsman, J. M. (2015). A meta-analytic review of religious or spiritual involvement and social health among cancer patients. *Cancer, 121*(21), 3779–3788.
126. Jim, H. S., Pustejovsky, J. E., Park, C. L., Danhauer, S. C., Sherman, A. C., Fitchett, G., Merluzzi, T. V., Munoz, A. R., George, L., Snyder, M. A., & Salsman, J. M. (2015). Religion, spirituality, and physical health in cancer patients: A meta-analysis. *Cancer, 121*(21), 3760–3768.
127. Salsman, J. M., Pustejovsky, J. E., Jim, H. S., Munoz, A. R., Merluzzi, T. V., George, L., Park, C. L., & Fitchett, G. (2015). A meta-analytic approach to examining the correlation between religion/spirituality and mental health in cancer. *Cancer, 121*(21), 3769–3778.
128. Schreiber, J. A., & Brockopp, D. Y. (2012). Twenty-five years later—What do we know about religion/spirituality and psychological well-being among breast cancer survivors? A systematic review. *Journal of Cancer Survivorship, 6*(1), 82–94.
129. Park, C. L., Sherman, A. C., Jim, H. S., & Salsman, J. M. (2015). Religion/spirituality and health in the context of cancer: Cross-domain integration, unresolved issues, and future directions. *Cancer, 121*(21), 3789–3794.
130. Thuné-Boyle, I. C. V., Stygall, J., Keshtgar, M. R. S., Davidson, T. I., & Newman, S. P. (2011). Religious coping strategies in patients diagnosed with breast cancer in the UK. *Psycho-Oncology, 20*(7), 771–782.
131. Herbert, R., Zdaniuk, B., Schulz, R., & Scheier, M. (2009). Positive and negative religious coping and well-being in women with breast cancer. *Journal of Palliative Medicine, 12*(6), 537–545.
132. Boehm, K., Cramer, H., Staroszynski, T., & Ostermann, T. (2014). Arts therapies for anxiety, depression, and quality of life in breast cancer patients: A systematic review and meta-analysis. *Evidence-Based Complementary and Alternative Medicine, 2014, 2014*, 103297. https://doi.org/10.1155/2014/103297. Epub 2014 Feb 26.
133. Bozcuk, H., Ozcan, K., Erdogan, C., Mutlu, H., Demir, M., & Coskun, S. (2017). A comparative study of art therapy in cancer patients receiving chemotherapy and improvement in quality of life by watercolor painting. *Complementary Therapies in Medicine, 30*, 67–72.
134. Lee, J., Choi, M. Y., Kim, Y. B., Sun, J., Park, E. J., Kim, J. H., Kang, M., & Koom, W. S. (2017). Art therapy based on appreciation of famous paintings and its effect on distress among cancer patients. *Quality of Life Research, 26*(3), 707–715.
135. Archer, S., Buxton, S., & Sheffield, D. (2015). The effect of creative psychological interventions on psychological outcomes for adult cancer patients: A systematic review of randomized controlled trials. *Psycho-Oncology, 24*(1), 1–10.
136. Kreitler, S., Oppenheim, D., & Segev-Shoham, E. (2004). Fantasy, art therapies, humor and pets as psychosocial means of intervention in pediatric cancer patients. In S. Kreitler & M. W. Ben-Arush (Eds.), *Psychosocial aspects of pediatric oncology* (pp. 351–388). Hoboken: Wiley.
137. Kreitler, S., Oppenheim, D., & Segev-Shoham, E. (2012). Fantasy, art therapies, and other expressive and creative psychosocial interventions. In S. Kreitler, D. M. W. Ben-Arush, & A. Martin (Eds.), *Pediatric psycho-oncology: Psychosocial aspects and clinical interventions* (2nd ed., pp. 143–159). Hoboken: Wiley-Blackwell.
138. Stanton, A. L., Danoff-Burg, S., Sworowski, L. A., Collins, C. A., Branstetter, A. D., Rodriguez-Hanley, A., Kirk, S. B., & Austenfeld, J. L. (2002). Randomized, controlled trial of written emotional expression and benefit finding in breast cancer patients. *Journal of Clinical Oncology, 20*(20), 4160–4168.
139. Pardeck, J. T. (1992). Bibliotherapy and cancer patients. *Family Therapy, 19*(3), 223–232.
140. Roberts, N., & Lee, V. (2016). Acceptability of bibliotherapy for patients with cancer: A qualitative, descriptive study. *Oncology Nursing Forum, 43*(5), 588–594.
141. Zhang, J. M., Wang, P., Yao, J. X., Zhao, L., Davis, M. P., Walsh, D., & Yue, G. H. (2012). Music interventions for psychological and physical outcomes in cancer: A systematic review and meta-analysis. *Supportive Care in Cancer, 20*(12), 3043–3053.

142. Bradt, J., Dileo, C., Magill, L., & Teague, A. (2011). Music interventions for improving psychological and physical outcomes in cancer patients. *Cochrane Database Systematic Review, 8*, CD006911. https://doi.org/10.1002/14651858.CD006911.pub2. Lee, J., Choi, M. Y., Kim, Y. B., Sun, J., Park, E. J., Kim, J. H., Kang, M., & Koom, W. S. (2017). Art therapy based on appreciation of famous paintings and its effect on distress among cancer patients. *Quality of Life Research, 26*(3), 707–715.
143. Bräuninger, I. (2014). Specific dance movement therapy interventions—Which are successful? An intervention and correlation study. *The Arts in Psychotherapy, 41*(5), 445–457.
144. Bradt, J., Shim, M., & Goodill, S. W. (2015). Dance/movement therapy for improving psychological and physical outcomes in cancer patients. *Cochrane Database of Systematic Reviews, 1*, CD007103. https://doi.org/10.1002/14651858.CD007103.pub3.
145. Basting, A. (2004). Handle with care? And standing ovation: Performing social science research about cancer. *Gerontologist, 44*(4), 579–581.
146. Moyer, A., Goldenberg, M., Hall, M. A., Knapp-Oliver, S. K., Sohl, S. J., Sarma, E. A., & Schneider, S. (2012). Mediators of change in psychosocial interventions for cancer patients: A systematic review. *Behavioral Medicine, 38*(3), 90–114.
147. Daniels, J., & Kissane, D. W. (2008). Psychosocial interventions for cancer patients. *Current Opinion in Oncology, 20*(4), 367–371.
148. Guo, Z., Tang, H. Y., Li, H., Tan, S. K., Feng, K. H., Huang, Y. C., Bu, Q., & Jiang, W. (2013). The benefits of psychosocial interventions for cancer patients undergoing radiotherapy. *Health and Quality of Life Outcomes, 11*(1), 121.
149. Raingruber, B. (2011). The effectiveness of psychosocial interventions with cancer patients: An integrative review of the literature (2006–2011). *ISRN Nursing, 2011, 2011*, 638218. Published online 2011 Nov 16. https://doi.org/10.5402/2011/638218.
150. Semple, C., Parahoo, K., Norman, A., McCaughan, E., Humphris, G., & Mills, M. (2013). Psychosocial interventions for patients with head and neck cancer. *Cochrane Database of Systematic Reviews*, (7), CD009441. https://doi.org/10.1002/14651858.CD009441.pub2.

Chapter 9
Coping with Cancer

Introducing Coping

Coping is the major term that brings together the patient and the disease situation, from the point of view of the patient. It is a response or set of responses of any person who feels he or she is in trouble or experiences stress, regardless of the cause which may be cancer, bereavement, financial loss, or some other problem. Thus, any individual may engage in coping. Coping may be a behavior, a thought, an attitude, or a feeling. It is difficult to describe coping in terms of its characteristics, because these may vary. It has many faces and can assume many forms. Coping can be external, such as an act of flight or fight, or it may be internal, such as recalling a melody or the hand wave of a beloved person. It can be imitated or learned from the coping of another individual encountered, for example, in a therapeutic group session or invented by the individual himself or herself. Coping can be an act or event of short duration, such as going to a music festival, or it can be of long duration, such as renovating one's apartment. Coping can be a one-time event, such as going to a party, or some behavior engaged in sporadically, such as attending lectures from time to time, or a continuous undertaking, such as changing one's occupation. Notably, coping is a flexible construct: different kinds or processes of coping can be applied concurrently. This implies that any individual may apply several or even many coping mechanisms and may change or exchange them when any of them does not prove to be satisfactory [1].

Hence, the most important characteristic of coping is that it may vary in its success and usefulness, namely, in how much respite and relief it provides.

S. Kreitler, *Psycho-Oncology for the Clinician*,
https://doi.org/10.1007/978-3-030-06126-5_9

What Kind of a Response Is Coping?

In general terms coping is a response evoked in circumstances involving suffering, physical or psychological or both, experienced by the individual as difficult or distressing. Following the well-known model of coping by Lazarus and Folkman [2], situations of this kind may be conceptualized in terms of the balance between the demands of the situation, namely, the resources required by the situation and the resources available to the individual in that situation. The amount of both kinds of resources depends on the estimate of the individual, which is in fact a function of the overall appraisal of the situation by the individual. The appraisal refers evidently also to the harm or loss expected by the individual and the extent of involved threat. Notably, it is not the situation or event as such that evoke the different responses by the individual. An event or object becomes a threat or stressful only through the meaning assigned to it by the individual.

Both the required resources and the available resources are the result of the subjective evaluations by the individual. If the two kinds of resources – the required and the available – are approximately equal, or the gap between them is minimal, the options of *adaptation or adjustment* are likely, possible and applicable. The gap is barely noticed and may be expected to disappear on its own. If however the required resources are evaluated as higher than those available to the individual, the gap between them could be characterized as small, in which case the situation may require some effort on the part of the individual. This may be called the response of *challenge*. It involves mobilization of extra internal or external resources on the part of the individual who feels that he or she can overcome the difficulty if they try hard enough or differently than before. The challenge response may also end in adaptation, but the way is more difficult than when the required and available resources are equal.

A more difficult situation arises when the resources required by the situation are much more than those available to the individual. In cases of this kind, the individual feels that engaging more effort on his or her side, trying harder, or devoting more resources than regularly would probably not solve the problem or lead to a significant improvement. The gap between the required and available resources may be characterized as medium, and the distress is too large to be expected to disappear on its own or due to applying merely some effort. This specifically defines the state in which *coping* is called for. Coping is not merely an approach or attitude but involves applying different coping mechanisms or strategies for handling the situation (see Different Coping Mechanisms).

A worse situation arises when the gap between the required and available resources is grasped right from the beginning as large, so large that the individual feels there may be no way or means for handling the problem. It is in situations of this kind when despair engendered by hopelessness-helplessness may set in. The individual is in danger of giving up even before trying anything to overcome the problem or despair.

Despair may set in also if the patient tried applying one or more coping mechanisms but became convinced sooner or later that these coping mechanisms were not efficient in handling the situation. Due to the failure, distress may even increase.

Hence, coping may be conceived as the set of responses applied by a cancer patient or anyone in distress when the gap between the required and available resources as evaluated by the individual is about medium, so that special means of handling the situation are called for, but the gap is not so very large or not so exceedingly large that it may seem futile and hopeless to try anything at all. A shorter characterization would be that coping is evoked when the individual concludes that something needs to be done and can be done. This description may serve as a preliminary definition to be amplified in the course of this chapter.

What Coping Is NOT?

A clearer definition of coping would benefit from pointing out the differences between coping and other apparently similar kinds of responses. First in line are problem-solving strategies [3]. In distinction from regular problem-solving strategies that are applicable to problems of any kind, regardless of the accompanying emotions, coping mechanisms target mainly issues of personal significance, specifically in circumstances that involve suffering and distress.

Then one may wonder whether coping mechanisms are traits or personality tendencies. Many studies show that coping is affected to some extent by personality, both in the sense that groups of coping mechanisms and specific coping mechanisms are related to personality dispositions and traits [4] (see section "Determinants of Coping"). Also, some tendencies like optimism may count both as personality tendencies and coping mechanisms. Nevertheless it is evident that coping and personality are different concepts, especially since personality is a much broader and more basic construct than coping, affecting the behavior, cognition, emotions, and even physiological functioning of individuals under all conditions. Moreover, coping mechanisms do not have the breadth of effects and the stability characterizing personality traits [5].

Defense mechanism is another construct that needs to be distinguished from coping [6]. The distinction is important for cancer patients and their caretakers because coping mechanisms are much more under the control of the patient than defenses. Further, since defense mechanisms are often considered as related to psychopathology, binding coping to defenses may cause cancer patients to avoid coping as a psychiatric symptom. The issue may be confusing because some defenses, e.g., projection or repression, may be used in the function of coping mechanisms, and some like denial may be used with different degrees of pathology [7]. Some authors graded defenses on levels of pathology. The best known is the scale that differentiates between pathological defenses (e.g., psychotic denial), immature defenses (e.g., passive aggression, acting out), neurotic defenses (e.g., displacement, reaction formation), and mature defenses (e.g., humor, sublimation). However, even the defenses in the highest level do not resemble coping [8, 9].

The differences between defenses and coping mechanisms are very clear. Defenses are essentially processes activated unconsciously designed to deal primarily with internal threats of the kind represented by drives and ethical demands, conflicting with each other and with reality, evoking anxiety, and decreasing the individuals' well-being [10]. Defenses are often of a pathological nature either because of the triggers or because of the results that may involve divergencies from reality, for example, in the form of regression and projections [11]. Further, defenses may involve responses harming the individual, such as hurting oneself psychologically or physically. In contrast, coping is a response activated consciously, mostly under the control of the individual, in order to deal with situations in reality involving pain, suffering, or distress, bringing about improvement in one's situation psychologically and often physically too, and has little if anything to do with mental pathology.

It is possible that cancer patients may have psychological problems preceding their disease and in parallel to it, in which case they may be using defense mechanisms in addition to coping.

Different Coping Mechanisms

There are a great many coping mechanisms that have been identified in individuals in distress. The list is so long that there are different kinds of grouping of the coping mechanisms into types. One well-known grouping distinguishes between emotion-focused coping mechanisms, such as self-soothing, relaxation, expression of negative emotions, or avoidance, and problem-focused coping mechanisms, such as reducing the occasions that evoke stress and anxiety or using pain medication [2]. Another classification distinguishes between engagement coping that deals directly with the stressor and disengagement coping that involves distancing oneself from the stress source, for example, by avoidance and denial [12, 13]. A different pair of coping mechanisms is accommodative coping, which is based on changing oneself in ways that render it possible to survive with the stressor on a long-run basis, for example, by acceptance, cognitive restructuring, and reducing one's goals [14], and meaning-focused coping, which consists in finding meaning and benefits in adversity [15, 16].

The taxonomies of coping mechanisms indicate the broad range of coping mechanisms but do not present the actual mechanisms themselves available to those in need [17]. Some examples of the long list are compartmentalization (of the conflicting thoughts), compensation (of weakness in one domain by strength in another), displacement, dissociation, helping others, intellectualization, passive aggression, regression, trivializing, blaming others, projection, fantasy, idealization, identification, provocation, substitution, acting-out, suppression, somatization, denial, and social support. Some coping mechanisms are considered as negative, for example, self-harm, constant anger, violent behavior, excessive avoidance of others, self-negligence, and absorption in a dangerous addiction.

The examples of common coping mechanisms suggest that almost any behavior may function as coping if used with that intention. This does not mean that all coping mechanisms are activated intentionally and purposefully by the individual. Possibly some are not completely under the individual's control all through, but when they occur, the individual may use them for the sake of coping. Notably, each coping mechanism may be used for coping in different ways. For example, regression may serve coping by setting the patient in a time period preceding the disease occurrence, by behaving as a helpless child justifying the requirement for help, and by setting oneself in an early age slot with limited cognitive abilities denying the implications of disease and death.

Some studies focused specifically on coping mechanisms in cancer patients. One of the studies came up with the following very well-known list of coping mechanisms of cancer patients making up the Mental Adjustment to Cancer scale [18]: Fighting spirit, Obsessive preoccupation, Stoic acceptance, Hopelessness-helplessness, and Denial. The following five dimensions are used in several coping mechanisms scales: positive problem-solving (seeking information, fighting against the illness), self-reliance (developing a lay explanation for the disease, not necessarily that offered by the doctors), emotional availability (not withdrawing from others), distress (brooding, self-pity), and solace (through drugs or alcohol) [19]. The following five patterns of coping were identified in a large-scale study of cancer patients: seeking or using social support, focusing on the positive, distancing, cognitive escape-avoidance, and behavioral escape-avoidance [20]. A more detailed and concrete list was defined on the basis of a study with cancer patients of different kinds [21]. The first stage of interviewing resulted in identifying 48 coping mechanisms, such as fighting the disease, humor, religiosity, self-improvement, and overall strengthening of one's health. Factor analyses led to defining 21 primary-level groups (factors) of coping mechanisms: fighting the disease, searching for new solutions, strengthening one's health in general, preoccupation with the disease, coming to terms with the situation, humor, drawing practical conclusions, denial, dissociation, distraction, focusing on others, looking for support, religiosity, relying on experts, changing oneself and one's personality, strengthening one's spirituality, focusing on emotions, enhancing self-understanding, wish fulfillments, self-improvement, despair, and helplessness. A finer cluster analysis of these 21 factors led to identifying the following six second-level coping tendencies: focusing on the disease and strengthening one's health, coming to terms with the situation, denial, strengthening oneself and seeking support, psychological change, and helplessness.

Special Coping Mechanisms

Two coping mechanisms of those listed above stand out as most important and salient: denial and social support. Their importance is based on the ubiquity of their use and on their psychological role and determinants.

Denial

Denial is one of the most frequently mentioned and most commonly applied coping mechanisms [7]. It is listed both under the title Denial but also under other titles, such as suppression, repression, distraction, blunting, distancing, escape, as well as in the general coping mechanisms of disengagement or of avoidance. It is likely that it plays some role also as a component in the contexts of other coping mechanisms, such as rationalization, undoing, or trivializing. It is a basic strategy for dealing with threatening and painful situations or thoughts [22], grounded in a fundamental possibly evolutionary tendency to look away from disturbing or annoying stimuli. Research revealed that there may be different forms of denial, varying in manifestations, degree, complexity, reality distortion, motivation, effects, and even function. Thus, Breznitz [23] defined seven kinds of denial: denial of personal relevance, of urgency, of vulnerability or responsibility, of affect, of affect relevance, of threatening information, and of information. Weisman [24] defined three degrees of denial of death referring to disavowal (a) of the primary facts of the person's illness tantamount to the pathological syndrome of "denial of illness" (or anosognosia), (b) of the implications of the illness and its possible extensions, and (c) of the image of death itself, the extinction. Greer [25] differentiated between complete denial, denial of implications of the diagnosis, and denial of affect. Wool and Goldberg [26] distinguished between denial of the physical manifestations of the disease, of the diagnosis, of its implications, and of the evoked affect.

Studies show that denial plays a central role in coping with cancer and affects most domains of life. Its effects are mostly positive, which may seem surprising in view of the controversial reputation of denial grounded in dynamic psychology. However, it seems that as long as denial does not affect the patient' adherence to the medical instructions, it has a great potential in improving their quality of life. A study about head and neck cancer patients showed clearly that survivors who used denial as a coping mechanism had a better quality of life and were better adjusted than those who did not use denial [27]. Also other studies with cancer patients support the conclusion that the use of disengagement coping, including avoidant coping strategies, affects quality of life positively, while emotion coping lowers quality of life [28, 29]. In general, shifting attention away from the threatening stimuli has beneficial effects on adjustment [30]. For example, perceptions of the stressfulness of a cancer-related event or situation were found to be related significantly to more coping through escape-avoidance which is related to less emotional distress [20]. Denial was also found to be related to reduced side effects of chemotherapy and reactions of anxiety and depression to the treatment [31] and to better adjustment in cancer survivors following termination of treatment [32, 33].

Denial seems to be a basic coping strategy, that is often applied in a partial manner, in regard to a specific aspect of the threatening situation and may be in need of strengthening when it starts to weaken [23]. It may be used in an on-and-off manner and also in combination with other coping mechanisms. Its use varies in line with the issues and the situation of the disease.

Research shows that it is used in different forms in the different phases of cancer, for example, it may be a means for combatting anxiety in the first phase following diagnosis, and it serves for overcoming fear of death in the terminal stage prior to death. It seems to be applied particularly by patients in advanced stages of the disease or those considered as incurable [34].

There is almost general support for the conclusion that disengagement coping, including behavioral disengagement, avoidance, and denial, should be targeted to mitigate cancer-related distress [28]. However, there is also some evidence that does not support this conclusion. For example, the use of avoidant coping strategies (cognitive and behavioral escape) was related to lower overall quality of life in pretreatment head-and-neck cancer patients [35], to more perceived stress and depressive symptoms in patients after total laryngectomy [36] or among gynecologic cancer patients [37], and to higher emotional distress in gynecologic patients in stages 3–4 undergoing chemotherapy [38].

Thus, denial may also have negative effects. Some of the reasons may be, for example, that denial may interfere with getting treatment (e.g., delay in going to the doctor, not showing up for follow-ups, noncompliance), may disrupt the process of assimilating the stressful event by avoiding emotional elaboration, may affect adversely interpersonal relations by limiting communication, and constitutes a cumulative stressor depressing even immunocompetence [7, 39].

Social Support

Social support is one of the most common sources of support for cancer patients, and its effects have been widely studied. Several kinds of social support have been identified. The major ones are emotional support which consists in providing empathy, affection, and encouragement, sometimes also by appraisal or esteem support that enhances one's self-confidence; instrumental support which provides material assistance, for example, in the form of money, purchases, or transfer; informational support by providing advice, guidance, explanation of medical facts, and sometimes additional information; and companionship support by spending time with the patient and providing accompaniment for entertainment [40]. The mentioned kinds of support may be provided in a face-to-face manner, by phone or online [41], in individual contact or in group settings, by family members, acquaintances, and friends as well as by community members who belong to social networks to which the patient belongs. The relation between social support and coping has been often noted [42, 43]. Both from the theoretical and the applied points of view, social support and coping mechanisms may be considered as sharing the same overall function which is to serve as stress-buffers. Further, several social support manifestations, such as providing distraction or a new cognitive interpretation of the situation, could be considered as coping mechanisms, and some coping mechanisms such as joining a religious community may be categorized as a means of social support.

However, it needs to be emphasized that in some cases social support may affect the application of coping. One way would be by turning the patient's attention to the possibility or availability of specific coping mechanisms [44]. Another possibility consists in strengthening the patient to the level where he or she feel empowered and confident enough to start coping, or he or she reach the point of considering the situation as calling for coping rather than for hopelessness-helplessness. Yet, despite the benefits and relative accessibility of social support, its effects are not ubiquitous. For some patients the message of social support is that they are too weak and incapacitated to the degree that they cannot manage without the help of others. Other considerations that may cause patients to withdraw from social support are fear of losing one's independence and of intrusion into one's privacy [45].

Religion and Spirituality

This is one of the most interesting and powerful coping mechanisms. It may take the form of embracing one's religion, sometimes a religion which differs from the one into which one was born and often choosing just spirituality. It may be attended by practicing the religion in the traditional way or in some nontraditional way or focusing only on the faith. There are many reports of cancer patients who find comfort and strength through religion or spirituality [46–48]. The benefits of religion have been noted in patients differing in gender, age, diagnoses, and culture [49–51]. Joining a religion by becoming a member of a community or getting closer to God and other superior powers in other ways may provide the patient confidence, peace of mind, and often a sense of harmony with oneself and the surrounding world. Sometimes the help that religion provides is in letting go of control through reliance on higher powers. Further aspects of religion that patients mention are that by evoking memories of early childhood when one visited the church or synagogue with one's family, religion lets oneself feel protected as a child. Additionally, one may feel empowered by the prayers for oneself by people whom one has never met but belong to the same community or religion. Be it as it may, religion often enhances hope, sometimes by expecting a miracle, at other times by becoming worthy of help from God through forgiveness and undergoing other forms of purification [52].

Finding Meaning

This is a coping strategy that has been mentioned increasingly in publications in recent years [53–55]. It consists in the individuals' efforts to identify the meaning of the situation of stress and pain in which they find themselves. Meaning finding addresses issues such as: "Why me?" "What does this disease mean for me and what should I make of it?" "Is there some message for me or my beloved ones hidden in this situation?" "Why am I exposed to all this suffering?" "What kind of purpose can I find in this misfortune or crisis that has befallen me?" "Am I being tested?" "Have I been chosen?" "What could be the goal of my life now?" Notably meaning finding may be a coping strategy in itself but can also lead to other specific coping strategies, such as helping others, joining a religious community, enjoying nature, and expressing oneself through some act of creativity. This coping mechanism leads patients to psychotherapy where the issue of meaning finding may be discussed, especially in the framework of cancer interventions devoted to meaning [56, 57] (see Chap. 8). Meaning finding or rather the search for meaning may be considered as beneficial for patients even beyond the benefit finding in the disease which may contribute to reducing the stress and even anger of patients [56, 58]. The positive impact of dealing with meaning is that the patients get involved actively in considering their life at large and their situation at present, struggling cognitively and emotionally with problems, elaborating experiences from different stages in their life, and possibly getting to a comprehensive overall conception of living which is seldom attained in the regular course of life.

Posttraumatic Growth

Posttraumatic growth is another possible outcome of undergoing the trauma and difficulties of cancer diagnosis and treatments. While some individuals invest their efforts in maintaining the situation as is or reinstating their former life prior to the disease, some patients may discover new possibilities and strive to attain a higher or better level of existence and functioning than they had before. Hence their coping consists precisely in developing a new life course and uncovering new skills which they have not applied prior to the disease [59, 60]. Thus, posttraumatic growth may be considered either as a coping mechanism in its own right or rather as a tendency born out of the despair and suffering and leading the person towards new coping mechanisms designed to establish new venues of life and creativity (see section "Determinants of Coping") [61–63]. The tendency toward posttraumatic growth is grounded in a set of beliefs of four types – about oneself, about goals, about norms and general beliefs, and about others and reality – that were identified as orienting towards it, in line with the cognitive orientation theory. Major among them are beliefs in the possibility and utility of change, high self-demands from oneself, sharing feelings and experiences with others, reliance on improvisation, and perseverance in pursuing one's goals [64].

Determinants of Coping

There are multiple factors affecting coping. Major ones are the patient's personality and the patient's situation. Each of these factors includes several components that contribute to the activation and shaping of coping.

Personality

Personality refers to the dispositional tendencies of the individual, including traits, emotions, and motivational factors. Three phases can be identified in the theoretical approach to the relation of personality to coping. According to the early psychoanalytic approach, personality and coping were equated. According to the second transactional approach, personality affected coping less than cognition and motivation, and in the third phase, it is considered as affecting coping in a differentiated manner [65]. Meta-analyses showed broad-range relations between personality and coping: optimism, extraversion, conscientiousness, and openness are related to more engagement coping; neuroticism to more disengagement coping; and optimism, conscientiousness, and agreeableness to less disengagement coping [4]. Extraversion and conscientiousness were related more to problem-solving and cognitive restructuring, whereas neuroticism was related to a lower degree to wishful thinking, withdrawal, and emotion-focused coping and support seeking [66].

Of the different personality traits related to coping, *optimism* stands out as one of the most important ones. Some investigators consider optimism as a coping mechanism, which is often viewed as affiliated with positive thinking. As such its effect on the patient's well-being is positive. More often however optimism is viewed as a personality disposition which affects the selection and application of coping mechanisms. Several studies found that optimism is related positively to the use of coping mechanisms that are beneficial for combatting distress, for example, minimization, suppression, seeking succor, substitution, and reversal [67]. Optimism was also found to be affiliated to approach coping strategies aiming to eliminate, reduce, or manage stressors or emotions. As such it is negatively associated with avoidance coping strategies promoting tendencies to ignore, avoid, or withdraw from stressors [68]. Thus, greater optimism and self-efficacy were associated with less negative illness appraisal, less avoidant coping, and decreased mood disturbance [38]. The finding that hope is related positively with coping [69] suggests that patients in a mood of optimism or hope feel strong and motivated enough to apply coping and thus improve their subjective and objective situation. Accordingly, optimism may be considered as a coping mechanism in its own right or as a mediator for other coping mechanisms.

There are other personality tendencies that may play a role as mediators for coping mechanisms. *Pessimism*, for example, is related to the choice of avoidance coping mechanisms, including denial, distancing, and disengagement from the goal with which the stressor was interfering [70]. *Anxiety* is a personality disposition that also affects coping. For example, in head and neck cancer patients, anxiety was found to be correlated with the coping strategies of giving up and intake of medication, alcohol, and smoking (nicotine) [71]. Breast cancer patients high on trait anxiety tended to use the coping strategies of denial, avoiding the problem-focused approach [72]. Patients with symptoms of *depression* scored significantly higher in behavioral disengagement and self-blame as their coping strategies compared to those who were not depressed [73]. Depression was found to be related to avoidant coping [22], coping through religion [74], and in hematological patients getting BMT coping through acceptance-resignation and cognitive avoidance [75]. Depression in breast cancer patients was found to be related to coping through obsessive preoccupation with the disease and to hopelessness-helplessness but not to fighting spirit [76].

Resilience is another personality tendency which may affect coping. For example, resilient individuals tend to apply cognitive coping strategies such as risk perception, accepting change [77], and problem-solving strategies [78]. According to the cognitive orientation approach, the problem-solving approach of resilience relies mainly on focusing on change, perseverance, accepting limitations, reliance on improvisation, high self-demands, and sharing feelings and experiences [79].

Some of the effects of personality on coping may depend on the cultural background of the individual. A large cross-cultural study [80] showed that cultural values predicted coping by religion, and this relation was not accounted fully by personally valuing tradition, cultural norms, or by perceived difficulty of adapting. Cultural values predicted emotion-focused/avoidant coping more than neuroticism and predicted seeking social support better than extraversion [50, 80]. Culture may affect coping by influencing the patients' attitudes toward treatment, for example, avoiding surgery or chemotherapy as dangerous and hiding information about symptoms in specific organs like the cervix which may be considered taboo, or by reinforcing and enhancing spirituality and reliance on religion, which may be beneficial for the patients [50].

Personality may be related to coping also through motivational tendencies. These tendencies are manifested in the form of beliefs of four types – about oneself, about reality, about rules and norms, and about goals – grounded in deep-lying meanings related to coping [81]. The meanings that orient an individual to apply coping refer to different themes. The major ones are:

- Beliefs in the possibility and utility of changes in oneself.
- Viewing life as a continuous development.
- Considering development as a nonlinear process, namely, development may consist in undertaking steps that are not determined fully by former steps or situations.
- The possibility and need to realize one's potential.
- The constant existence of options, even beyond those expected.
- There may be benefits to suffering.
- There are hidden possibilities and undiscovered skills in every person, which means that every person is stronger and more capable than he or she assumes.
- It is never too late to embark on an adventure in life by doing new things.

Studies showed that if a patient accepts at least four of the eight described themes, in terms of beliefs of four or three types, he or she is likely to apply coping mechanisms when in need or distress [21].

Patient's Situation

The patient's situation is a second important determinant of coping. The patient's situation includes a host of factors. Some factors are of a more external nature, such as the habitat of the patient, the support of the family, and social support in general which may depend on the patient's social network and his or her community. Other factors are of a more internal nature focused on the disease and its effects, such as the diagnosis, the stage of disease, the treatments the patient gets, and the overall physical and emotional state of the patient.

Patients who stay at home, with their family, and enjoy the benefits of support of their family and of others would be inclined to engage in coping rather than sink into the despair abyss of hopelessness-helplessness. Factors that lower the patient's overall state or render it difficult and painful, such as the absence of support, scarcity of available help, loneliness, the need to undergo many treatments for long time periods, financial difficulties in the family, and depressed mood and physical pain, may contribute to rendering coping difficult. Patients in such states may wonder whether coping is of any use at all. Family support may provide the information, encouragement, and the means for applying specific kinds of coping [82]. It is likely that also demographic factors such as age, gender, education, and income play a role in determining coping – engaging in coping and the kind of coping applied.

Research findings show that both the diagnosis and the phase of the disease play a role in regard to coping. A body of studies deals with examining the effects of various coping mechanisms in different groups of patients. For example, women diagnosed with breast cancer tend to cope by means of positive cognitive restructuring, wishful thinking, emotional expression, disease acceptance, increased religious practice, family and social support, and yoga and physical exercise [83]. The coping of colon and rectal cancer patients who were practically cured appears to be more confrontational toward the diagnosis, applying more fighting spirit and less anxious preoccupation, and hopeless/helplessness, while the non-cured patients coped more by avoidance of aversive thoughts [34]. Patients with head and neck cancer used a great variety of coping strategies, with social support seeking being the most salient [35]. However, there is also evidence that regardless of their diagnosis, patients scoring high on perceived stress tend to cope more through social support and different and more forms of escape and avoidance [20].

Studies of this kind provide evidence for the common use of coping mechanisms by cancer patients of different kinds. Although only few studies checked the salience and appropriateness of particular coping mechanisms for specific cancer disease, it is likely that the cancer diagnosis is the only one determinant of the selection of coping mechanisms in a given situation. The phase of the disease and the state of the patient seem to be no less important factors in activating different coping mechanisms. For example, in the first phase of the encounter with cancer, the situation may not even call for coping. But further down the road, the need for coping becomes increasingly evident. In the advanced stages of cancer, denial and the avoidant coping strategies seem to be more frequent than in the previous stages of the disease.

Finally, when dealing with the determinants of coping, it is necessary to emphasize that in addition to the major ones mentioned earlier, there may be several further factors which need to be considered but about whose effect not much is known. There are indications that psychological interventions focused on providing group support [44] or mindfulness training [84] may lead to increased coping on the part of the patient.

The Effects of Coping

The impact of coping on the patients' physical health is an issue of major interest. There are only few studies showing positive effects of coping on the patients' physical health. The effects are mostly based on reports of the patients themselves [85]. Some studies report reduction in side effects due to coping. The findings need to be interpreted with caution because it is unclear whether there are actually fewer side effects or the rate of occurrence is the same but they disturb less, are noticed less, or are simply reported less. Another study showed that fighting spirit did not affect the side effects but anxious preoccupation increased the occurrence of a whole range of physical symptoms [86] and a monitoring or information-gathering coping style increased anticipatory anxiety and nausea before and during chemotherapy [31].

The commonly cited effects of coping are improvement in the patients' quality of life, which mostly reflects a reduction in the patients' difficulties and less suffering from the disease and treatments. A study about the effects of different coping mechanisms in cancer patients with different diagnoses and in different stages of the disease was done by using the multidimensional inventory of quality of life [21, 87]. This tool provides scores for 15 different subscales in addition to the total score of quality of life. Major findings referred to the domains of life affected by the different coping mechanisms. Thus, the use of denial was correlated with higher scores in the overall quality of life and in the following scales: positive feelings, cognitive functioning, friends and social ties, body image, sense of mastery and independence, self-image, and meaningfulness of life. Additionally, it was related to lower scores in negative feelings, confusion and bewilderment, pain, health worries, and stress. The two domains unrelated to denial were sexuality and family life.

The use of humor as a coping mechanism was related to higher scores in overall quality of life, as well as in the scales of positive feelings, friends and social ties, and self-image. There were however no negative effects.

The use of wish fulfillment as a coping mechanism was related to a higher scores in overall quality of life, as well as in the scales of positive feelings, friends and social ties, body image, sense of mastery, self-image, and meaningfulness of life. Additionally, there were lower scores in the scales of confusion, health worries, and stress.

The use of religiosity as a coping mechanism was related only to lower scores in negative feelings, health worries, pain, and stress. The use of changing oneself and one's personality as coping mechanisms was related to lower scores in negative feelings, confusion and bewilderment, pain, stress, as well as overall quality of life score and in the following scales: positive feelings, cognitive functioning, sexuality, mastery and independence, self-image, and meaningfulness of life.

The use of the triad fighting the disease, preoccupation with the disease, and focusing on the disease as coping mechanisms was related to higher scores in negative feelings, confusion and bewilderment, health worries, pain, and stress and lower scores in overall score of quality of life and in the scales of positive feelings, cognitive functioning, sexuality, sense of mastery and independence, and self-image. The two unrelated scales were friends and social relations and meaningfulness of life.

Finally, not surprisingly, the use of hopelessness-helplessness as a coping mechanism seems to indicate a negative state of affairs. Higher scores in this approach were related to higher scores in negative feelings, confusion and bewilderment, pain, health worries, and stress and lower scores in overall score of quality of life, as well as in the scales of positive feelings, cognitive functioning, friends and social ties, body image, sense of mastery and independence, self-image, meaningfulness of life, family, and sexuality.

In sum, quality of life in general and in the specific domains is related to the patient's coping strategies. Denial is a potent coping strategy that contributes positively to quality of life and many of its domains. The findings show that in regard to quality of life, denial and defensiveness are preferable to preoccupation with the disease. The utility of denial in regard to quality of life sheds light also on three further findings about coping mechanisms that may seem surprising. One is the finding that fighting the disease, preoccupation with the disease, and a headlong attack on the disease affect quality of life negatively. The reason is probably that these coping mechanisms involve minimum denial. The same applies to the finding that emotional coping increases distress [28, 29]. Again, the reason may be because it involves confronting the issues openly. Similarly, changing oneself and one's personality, in the framework of psychotherapy or on one's own, may also lead to negative results in regard to quality of life due to the reduction in denial which these coping mechanisms involve.

In addition to denial, other coping strategies with positive contributions to quality of life are humor and wish-fulfillments. Coping strategies which contribute negatively to quality of life are fighting the disease, preoccupation with the disease, helplessness, and changing oneself.

Notably, it seems that the specific cancer-related issues, including type of cancer, time since diagnosis, and whether a person was currently in treatment, had few relationships to coping, which confirms previous findings [20]. Further analyses of the findings showed that coping strategies reflecting activity are not related to quality of life in the case of cancer. Additionally, also the mere number of coping strategies used by the patient is not related to the patient's quality of life.

The more general conclusions about the relations of coping and quality of life are that there exist many coping strategies affecting quality of life, each with specific effects in specific domains of quality of life. So, which coping mechanisms are best for the patient? In view of the large range and variety of coping mechanisms, it is to be expected that not all of the identified coping mechanisms are equally successful or useful for all patients. It is evident that some coping mechanisms may be more adequate for some patients than for others in view of their personality and situation. Further, the usefulness of coping mechanisms needs to be evaluated in terms of different criteria. For example, some coping mechanisms may improve specific aspects of the patient's quality of life, such as his/her emotional state but not her/his functional state. Additionally, it is important to keep in mind that coping is not a win-win strategy. This indicates that coping may not always result in a positive outcome but may sometimes even lead to deterioration of the patient's state [81, 88–90]. Further, the effects of coping may not persist. Hence, it may become necessary to change coping mechanisms, replace less useful ones, and acquire new ones.

How Is Coping Acquired? The General Principles of Learning to Become a Coper

Coping is not always an easy task for the patient. There are three major phases in the process of learning to become a coper. The first phase may best be called Getting Started, the second Learning about Coping Mechanisms, and the third Management of Coping. Each of the three phases can be performed by the patient on one's own without any help, with partial help, or with a lot of support and professional intervention.

Getting Started

For many patients there is the issue of whether to cope at all. Some patients have no problem to start coping right away when the diagnosis or any difficulty shows up on the horizon. Others may have some hesitation or difficulty, but for many of them personality factors, such as optimism on the one hand and encouraging support from others, on the other hand, may play a role in igniting hope in these patients and setting them on the course of coping.

However, in the initial stages of the process of dealing with the disease, it is not uncommon for patients to consider the option of giving up because they are anxious, depressed, and bewildered. Many do not believe anything can be done for them or that an improvement in their situation is at all possible. Patients of this kind need to undergo an intervention aimed at preparing them for coping. In line with our experience [21], the intervention should include two parts.

One part is to be devoted to helping the patient perceive and assess adequately the gap between the evaluations of the resources required by the situation and those available to him or her. Some patients need to become at all aware of the gap and its significance. As stated above (see section "What Kind of a Response Is Coping?"), when the gap is too large, the patient is liable to fall prey to a sense of hopelessness-helplessness which is antagonistic to coping. Means that can be applied for reducing the gap are based on changing the evaluation of the resources the patient has: increasing the evaluation of the resources the patient has available or reducing the evaluation of the resources the patient assumes is required or both. The gap between the evaluation of resources can be minimized regardless of which kind of evaluation is changed more or first. Thus, striving toward both goals is advisable. Means that can be used for increasing the evaluation of the resources available to the patient are, for example, encouraging the patient to engage in some physical activity or doing some actions or recalling some behavior from one's past that may convince the patient that he or she are more capable than they had assumed. Means that can be used for decreasing the evaluation of the resources required for handling the situation may include, for example, comparing oneself to other patients in the waiting room or in a group session who are doing well in that situation, or analyzing precisely what is actually needed for overcoming the difficulties perceived in the situation. The comparison with other patients and the analysis of the situation may help the patient to conclude that maybe he or she actually possess or could mobilize the resources that may enable them to cope, even if some special efforts would be required.

Another part of the preparatory intervention for coping may deal with mobilizing the patient's support for the themes identified as orienting toward coping [21]. The major ones are focus on change, on viewing life as a continuous development, belief in the possibility to achieve change at any point in life, belief in the existence of options, trying to realize one's potential, and expecting that even suffering can produce some benefits (see "Personality" in section "Determinants of Coping"). Mobilizing support on the part of the patient entails evoking in the patient beliefs about oneself, about rules and norms, about reality, and about goals that support the listed themes, for example, by providing for the themes examples, stating their implications and manner of operation, and devising for them convincing arguments.

Learning About Coping Mechanisms

In order to engage in coping, it is necessary to find out about coping mechanisms. Where or how can the patient become exposed to coping mechanism or learn about what is available or possible? There are three major possibilities. The first and most common one is *learning about coping mechanisms from others – lay persons or nonprofessionals.* The frequent source are other patients with whom the patient comes in contact in waiting rooms, treatment clinics, self-help groups, focus groups, and group psychotherapies. Similar second sources are blogs and the Internet, where patients often describe coping mechanisms. A third source of information about coping refers to the disclosures and stories about the coping of celebrities of different kinds, e.g., fashion, financial, academics, artists, or actors, which are often publicized in the Internet and the media. Literature, novels, and films are another source that may inspire people about coping. A fifth source of learning from others is the family, neighbors, and other acquaintances, even concerning situations and difficulties that are not related to cancer.

The second major possibility is *learning about coping through health professionals*, i.e., physicians, nurses, social workers, and psychologists who may encourage patients toward coping informally or formally, in systematic sessions or educational interventions.

The third major possibility of leaning about coping is *invention by the patients themselves*, mostly ad hoc or on the basis of their observations of others and their own experience or analysis of the situation.

General Principles of Applying Coping

After choosing to cope and being exposed to several coping mechanisms, it is necessary for the patient to choose the coping approach or mechanism he or she responds to and to adopt them. Adopting a coping mechanism is the preparatory phase for applying the coping mechanism. The patient needs to consider required changes in the coping mechanism so that it can be adequately applied in his or her case. For the coping mechanism to work for the patient, it needs often to be adapted, specialized, and adequately adjusted. Take "wish fulfillment," for example. The patient needs to decide which wish or wishes he or she will focus on and how to realize them in a manner that will attain the goals so that they will get integrated adequately with the rest of one's life.

Coping involves often acquiring a new attitude or behavior. Only few patients and even professionals are aware of the need to train that attitude or behavior. The training may involve binding the coping strategy to the adequate cues in one's environment or life space, or adapting it to the prevailing conditions, or combining it with other strategies.

Settling on a coping mechanism requires repeated monitoring whether it works for one, and whether it continues to fulfill the expectations. It is not uncommon that an adopted coping mechanism turns out to be inadequate, so that it is necessary to change it or even completely replace it, especially when the situation of the patient or of the disease changes. The setting in of depression or distress is often the sign that implies the need to refresh coping. Hence, coping requires learning to switch between coping strategies, giving up those strategies that do not work for one, and selecting those strategies that one likes or fulfill the expectations, considering thereby mainly what pleases oneself rather than others.

Some Afterthoughts About Coping

Coping is a major means for enabling the patient to continue to function and live with the disease and despite the attendant difficulties. Regardless of whether it boils down to small change in attitude or behavior or whether it involves a major change in life, it is of major importance for continued functioning and often of survival. It is an expression of real empowerment on the part of the patient and consists in mobilizing what is necessary for survival. For the success of coping, it is necessary to be aware of the two major features of coping: that it is a learning process and that it is a dynamic evolving way of life.

References

1. Lazarus, R. S. (1993). Coping theory and research: Past, present, and future. *Psychosomatic Medicine, 55*, 234–247.
2. Lazarus, R. S., & Folkman, S. (1984). *Stress, appraisal, and coping*. New York: Springer.
3. Davidson, J. E., & Sternberg, R. J. (Eds.). (2003). *The psychology of problem solving*. New York: Cambridge University Press.
4. Carver, C. S., & Connor-Smith, J. (2010). Personality and coping. *Annual review of psychology, 61*, 679–704.
5. Hewitt, P. I., & Flett, G. L. (1996). Personality traits and the coping process. In M. Zeidner & N. S. Endler (Eds.), *Handbook of coping: Theory, research and applications* (pp. 410–433). New York: Wiley.
6. Cramer, P. (1998). Coping and defense mechanisms: What's the difference? *Journal of Personality, 66*(6), 919–946.
7. Kreitler, S. (1999). Denial in cancer patients: Psychosocial issues. *Cancer Investigation, 17*(7), 514–534.
8. Vaillant, G. E. (2000). Adaptive mental mechanisms: Their role in a positive psychology. *American Psychologist, 55*(1), 89.
9. Vaillant, G. E. (1995). *The wisdom of the ego*. Cambridge, MA: Harvard University Press.
10. Freud, A. (1937). *The ego and its mechanisms of defense*. London: Hogarth.
11. Freud, S. (1933). *New introductory lectures on psychoanalysis*. London: Hogarth.
12. Moos, R. H., & Schaefer, J. A. (1993). Coping resources and processes: Current concepts and measures. In L. Goldberger & S. Breznitz (Eds.), *Handbook of stress: Theoretical and clinical aspects* (2nd ed., pp. 234–257). New York: Free Press.
13. Skinner, E. A., & Zimmer-Gembeck, M. J. (2007). The development of coping. *Annual Reviews in Psychology, 58*, 119–144.
14. Morling, B., & Evered, S. (2006). Secondary control reviewed and defined. *Psychological Bulletin, 132*(2), 269.
15. Folkman, S. (2008). The case for positive emotions in the stress process. *Anxiety, Stress, and Coping, 21*(1), 3–14.
16. Tennen, H., Affleck, G., Armeli, S., & Carney, M. A. (2000). A daily process approach to coping: Linking theory, research, and practice. *American Psychologist, 55*(6), 626.
17. Krohne, H. W. (1996). Individual differences in coping. In M. Zeidner & N. S. Endler (Eds.), *Handbook of coping: Theory, research and applications* (pp. 381–409). New York: Wiley.
18. Watson, M., & Homewood, J. (2008). Mental adjustment to cancer scale©: Psychometric properties in a large cancer cohort. *Psycho-Oncology, 17*(11), 1146–1151.
19. Ben-Tovim, D. I., Dougherty, M. L., Stapleton, A. M., & Pinnock, C. B. (2002). Coping with prostate cancer: A quantitative analysis using a new instrument, the centre for clinical excellence in urological research coping with cancer instrument. *Urology, 59*(3), 383–388.
20. Dunkel-Schetter, C., Feinstein, L. G., Taylor, S. E., & Falke, R. L. (1992). Patterns of coping with cancer. *Health Psychology, 11*(2), 79.
21. Kreitler, S. (2005). Coping and quality of life in the context of physical disease. In A. V. Lee (Ed.), *Coping with disease* (pp. 81–120). New York: Nova Biomedical Books.
22. Ness, D. E., & Ende, J. (1994). Denial in the medical interview: Recognition and management. *JAMA, 272*(22), 1777–1781.
23. Breznitz, S. (1983). The seven kinds of denial. In S. Breznits (Ed.), *The denial of stress* (pp. 257–280). New York: International Universities Press.
24. Weisman, A. D. (1972). *On dying and denying: A psychiatric study of terminality*. New York: Behavioral Publications.
25. Greer, S. (1992). The management of denial in cancer patients. *Oncology, 6*(12), 33–36.
26. Wool, M. S., & Goldberg, R. J. (1987). Assessment of denial in cancer patients: Implications for intervention. *Journal of Psychosocial Oncology, 4*(3), 1–14.

27. Kreitler, S., Chaitchik, S., & Kreitler, H. (1993). Repressiveness: Cause or result of cancer? *Psycho-Oncology, 2*(1), 43–54.
28. Langford, D. J., Cooper, B., Paul, S., Humphreys, J., Keagy, C., Conley, Y. P., & Miaskowski, C. (2017). Evaluation of coping as a mediator of the relationship between stressful life events and cancer-related distress. *Health Psychology, 36*(12), 1147.
29. Shakeri, J., Kamangar, M., Ebrahimi, E., Aznab, M., Shakeri, H., & Arman, F. (2015). Association of coping styles with quality of life in cancer patients. *Indian Journal of Palliative Care, 21*(3), 298.
30. Sharpe, L., Butow, P., Smith, C., McConnell, D., & Clarke, S. (2005). Changes in quality of life in patients with advanced cancer: Evidence of response shift and response restriction. *Journal of Psychosomatic Research, 58*(6), 497–504.
31. Lerman, C., Rimer, B., Blumberg, B., Cristinzio, S., Engstrom, P. F., MacElwee, N., & Seay, J. (1990). Effects of coping style and relaxation on cancer chemotherapy side effects and emotional responses. *Cancer Nursing, 13*(5), 308–315.
32. Kreitler, S., Shaked, S., Chaitchik, S., Shaked, T., & Kaufman, Z. (1997). Medical characteristics, control and anxiety as determinants of adjustment to cancer. *Personality Psychology in Europe*, *6*, 1–3.
33. Kreitler, S., Chaitchik, S., Rapoport, Y., & Algor, R. (1995). Psychosocial effects of level of information and severity of disease on head-and-neck cancer patients. *Journal of Cancer Education, 10*(3), 144–154.
34. Nordin, K., & Glimelius, B. (1997). Psychological reactions in newly diagnosed gastrointestinal cancer patients. *Acta Oncologica, 36*(8), 803–810.
35. List, M. A., Lee Rutherford, J., Stracks, J., Haraf, D., Kies, M. S., & Vokes, E. E. (2002). An exploration of the pretreatment coping strategies of patients with carcinoma of the head and neck. *Cancer, 95*(1), 98–104.
36. Eadie, T. L., & Bowker, B. C. (2012). Coping and quality of life after total laryngectomy. *Otolaryngology—Head and Neck Surgery, 146*(6), 959–965.
37. Siwik, C., Hicks, A., Phillips, K., Rebholz, W. N., Zimmaro, L. A., Weissbecker, I., Cash, E., & Sephton, S. E. (2017). Impact of coping strategies on perceived stress, depression, and cortisol profiles among gynecologic cancer patients. *Journal of Health Psychology*. https://doi.org/10.1177/1359105317740737.
38. Sumpio, C., Jeon, S., Northouse, L. L., & Knobf, M. T. (2017). Optimism, symptom distress, illness appraisal, and coping in patients with advanced-stage cancer diagnoses undergoing chemotherapy treatment. *Oncology Nursing Forum, 44*(3), 384–392.
39. Mulder, C. L., & Antoni, M. H. (1992). Psychosocial correlates of immune status and disease progression in HIV-1 infected homosexual men: Review of preliminary findings, and commentary. *Psychology and Health, 6*(3), 175–192.
40. Thoits, P. A. (1995). Stress, coping, and social support processes: Where are we? What next? *Journal of Health and Social Behavior, 35*(Extra Issue), 53–79.
41. Winzelberg, A. J., Classen, C., Alpers, G. W., Roberts, H., Koopman, C., Adams, R. E., & Taylor, C. B. (2003). Evaluation of an internet support group for women with primary breast cancer. *Cancer, 97*(5), 1164–1173.
42. Dukes Holland, K., & Holahan, C. K. (2003). The relation of social support and coping to positive adaptation to breast cancer. *Psychology and Health, 18*(1), 15–29.
43. Taylor, S. E. (2011). Social support: A review. In M. S. Friedman (Ed.), *The handbook of health psychology* (pp. 189–214). New York: Oxford University Press.
44. Richardson, M. A., Post-White, J., Grimm, E. A., Moye, L. A., Singletary, S. E., & Justice, B. (1997). Coping, life attitudes, and immune responses to imagery and group support after breast cancer treatment. *Alternative Therapies in Health and Medicine, 3*, 62–71.
45. Kreitler, S. (2012). *Who is afraid of social support?* Presented at the 26th conference of the European Health Psychology Society. Prague, Czech Republic, August 21–25.
46. Büssing, A., Ostermann, T., & Matthiessen, P. F. (2007). Adaptive coping and spirituality as a resource in cancer patients. *Breast Care, 2*(4), 195–202.

47. Gall, T. L. (2004). The role of religious coping in adjustment to prostate cancer. *Cancer Nursing, 27*(6), 454–461.
48. Thuné-Boyle, I. C., Stygall, J., Keshtgar, M. R., Davidson, T. I., & Newman, S. P. (2013). Religious/spiritual coping resources and their relationship with adjustment in patients newly diagnosed with breast cancer in the UK. *Psycho-Oncology, 22*(3), 646–658.
49. Peteet, J. R., & Balboni, M. J. (2013). Spirituality and religion in oncology. *CA: A Cancer Journal for Clinicians, 63*(4), 280–289.
50. Daher, M. (2012). Cultural beliefs and values in cancer patients. *Annals of Oncology, 23*(suppl. 3), 66–69.
51. Krupski, T. L., Kwan, L., Fink, A., Sonn, G. A., Maliski, S., & Litwin, M. S. (2006). Spirituality influences health related quality of life in men with prostate cancer. *Psycho-Oncology, 15*(2), 121–131.
52. van Laarhoven, H. W., Schilderman, J., Vissers, K. C., Verhagen, C. A., & Prins, J. (2010). Images of god in relation to coping strategies of palliative cancer patients. *Journal of Pain and Symptom Management, 40*(4), 495–501.
53. Harrop, E., Noble, S., Edwards, M., Sivell, S., Moore, B., & Nelson, A. (2017). Managing, making sense of and finding meaning in advanced illness: A qualitative exploration of the coping and wellbeing experiences of patients with lung cancer. *Sociology of Health and Illness, 39*(8), 1448–1464.
54. Campo, R. A., Wu, L. M., Austin, J., Valdimarsdottir, H., & Rini, C. (2017). Personal resilience resources predict post-stem cell transplant cancer survivors' psychological outcomes through reductions in depressive symptoms and meaning-making. *Journal of Psychosocial Oncology, 35*(6), 666–687.
55. Farsi, Z. (2015). The meaning of disease and spiritual responses to stressors in adults with acute leukemia undergoing hematopoietic stem cell transplantation. *Journal of Nursing Research, 23*(4), 290–297.
56. Hales, S., Lo, C., & Rodin, G. (2015). Managing cancer and living meaningfully (CALM) therapy. In J. C. Holland, W. S. Breitbart, P. N. Butow, P. J. Jacobson, M. J. Loscalzo, & R. Mccorkle (Eds.), *Psycho-oncology* (pp. 487–491). New York: Oxford University Press.
57. Lichtenthal, W. G., Applebaum, A. J., & Breitbart, W. S. (2015). Meaning-centered psychotherapy. In J. C. Holland, W. S. Breitbart, P. N. Butow, P. J. Jacobson, M. J. Loscalzo, & R. Mccorkle (Eds.), *Psycho-oncology* (pp. 475–479). New York: Oxford University Press.
58. Pascoe, L., & Edvardsson, D. (2013). Benefit finding in cancer: A review of influencing factors and health outcomes. *European Journal of Oncology Nursing, 17*(6), 760–766.
59. Moreno, P. I., & Stanton, A. L. (2013). Personal growth during the experience of advanced cancer: A systematic review. *The Cancer Journal, 19*(5), 421–430.
60. Greup, S. R., Kaal, S. E., Jansen, R., Manten-Horst, E., Thong, M. S., van der Graaf, W. T., & Husson, O. (2017). Post-traumatic growth and resilience in adolescent and young adult cancer patients: An overview. *Journal of Adolescent and Young Adult Oncology*. https://doi.org/10.1089/jayao.2017.0040.
61. Tedeschi, R. G., & Calhoun, L. G. (1995). *Trauma and transformation: Growing in the aftermath of suffering*. Thousand Oaks: Sage.
62. Shakespeare-Finch, J., & Lurie-Beck, J. (2014). A meta-analytic clarification of the relationship between posttraumatic growth and symptoms of posttraumatic distress disorder. *Journal of Anxiety Disorders, 28*(2), 223–229.
63. Meichenbaum, D., Calhoun, L. G., & Tedeschi, R. G. (2006). Resilience and posttraumatic growth: A constructive narrative perspective. In L. G. Calhoun & R. S. Tedeschi (Eds.), *Handbook of posttraumatic growth: Research and practice* (pp. 355–368). Mahwah: Lawrence Erlbaum.
64. Kreitler, S. (2012). *The cognitive orientation of resilience*. Presented at the 26th conference of the European Health Psychology Society. Prague, Czech Republic, August 21–25.
65. Suls, J., David, J. P., & Harvey, J. H. (1996). Personality and coping: Three generations of research. *Journal of Personality, 64*(4), 711–735.
66. Connor-Smith, J. K., & Flachsbart, C. (2007). Relations between personality and coping: A meta-analysis. *Journal of Personality and Social Psychology, 93*(6), 1080–1107.

67. Rim, Y. (1990). Optimism and coping styles. *Personality and Individual Differences, 11*(1), 89–90.
68. Nes, L. S., & Segerstrom, S. C. (2006). Dispositional optimism and coping: A meta-analytic review. *Personality and Social Psychology Review, 10*(3), 235–251.
69. Herth, K. A. (1989). The relationship between level of hope and level of coping response and other variables in patients with cancer. *Oncology Nursing Forum, 16*(1), 67–72.
70. Scheier, M. F., Weintraub, J. K., & Carver, C. S. (1986). Coping with stress: Divergent strategies of optimists and pessimists. *Journal of Personality and Social Psychology, 51*(6), 1257–1264.
71. De Maddalena, H., & Zenner, H. P. (1991). Anxiety and coping with anxiety in patients with head and neck cancers. *Head and Neck Oncology, 39*(2), 64–69.
72. Silva, A. V. D., Zandonade, E., & Amorim, M. H. C. (2017). Anxiety and coping in women with breast cancer in chemotherapy. *Revista Latino-Americana de Enfermagem, 25*, e2891.
73. Saniah, A. R., & Zainal, N. Z. (2010). Anxiety, depression and coping strategies in breast cancer patients on chemotherapy. *Malaysian Journal of Psychiatry*, *19*(2), 1–6
74. Haghighi, F. (2013). Correlation between religious coping and depression in cancer patients. *Psychiatria Danubina, 25*(3), 236–240.
75. Wells, K. J., Booth-Jones, M., & Jacobsen, P. B. (2009). Do coping and social support predict depression and anxiety in patients undergoing hematopoietic stem cell transplantation? *Journal of Psychosocial Oncology, 27*(3), 297–315.
76. Mitchell, A. M., Pössel, P., Van Voorhees, B. W., & Eaton, W. W. (2017). Associations of depression status and hopelessness with breast cancer: A 24-year follow-up study. *Journal of Health Psychology, 22*(10), 1322–1331.
77. Shaw, D., Scully, J., & Hart, T. (2014). The paradox of social resilience: How cognitive strategies and coping mechanisms attenuate and accentuate resilience. *Global Environmental Change, 25*, 194–203.
78. Molina, Y., Jean, C. Y., Martinez-Gutierrez, J., Reding, K. W., Joyce, P., & Rosenberg, A. R. (2014). Resilience among patients across the cancer continuum: Diverse perspectives. *Clinical Journal of Oncology Nursing, 18*(1.), 93), 93–191.
79. Kreitler, S., & Kreitler, M. M. (2015). Predicting resilience in car accident victims by cognitive orientation. In K. A. Moore, S. Howard, & P. Buchwals (Eds.), *Stress and anxiety: Applications to schools, well-being, coping, and internet use* (pp. 141–152). Berlin: Logos Verlag.
80. Bardi, A., & Guerra, V. M. (2011). Cultural values predict coping using culture as an individual difference variable in multicultural samples. *Journal of Cross-Cultural Psychology, 42*(6), 908–927.
81. Kreitler, S. (2004). The cognitive guidance of behavior. In J. T. Jost, M. R. Banaji, & D. A. Prentice (Eds.), *Perspectivism in social psychology: The Yin and Yang of scientific progress* (pp. 113–126). Washington, DC: American Psychological Association.
82. Aymanns, P., Filipp, S. H., & Klauer, T. (1995). Family support and coping with cancer: Some determinants and adaptive correlates. *British Journal of Social Psychology, 34*(1), 107–124.
83. Al-Azri, M., Al-Awisi, H., & Al-Moundhri, M. (2009). Coping with a diagnosis of breast cancer-literature review and implications for developing countries. *The Breast Journal, 15*(6), 615–622.
84. Witek-Janusek, L., Albuquerque, K., Chroniak, K. R., Chroniak, C., Durazo-Arvizu, R., & Mathews, H. L. (2008). Effect of mindfulness based stress reduction on immune function, quality of life and coping in women newly diagnosed with early stage breast cancer. *Brain, Behavior, and Immunity, 22*(6), 969–981.
85. Kvillemo, P., & Bränström, R. (2014). Coping with breast cancer: A meta-analysis. *PLoS One, 9*(11), e112733.
86. Whitford, H. S., & Olver, I. N. (2012). When expectations predict experience: The influence of psychological factors on chemotherapy toxicities. *Journal of Pain and Symptom Management, 43*(6), 1036–1050.
87. Kreitler, S., & Kreitler, M. M. (2006). Multidimensional quality of life: A new measure of quality of life in adults. *Social Indicators Research, 76*(1), 5–33.

88. Brunault, P., Champagne, A. L., Huguet, G., Suzanne, I., Senon, J. L., Body, G., Rusch, E., Magnin, G., Voyer, M., Revèillère, C., & Camus, V. (2016). Major depressive disorder, personality disorders, and coping strategies are independent risk factors for lower quality of life in non-metastatic breast cancer patients. *Psycho-Oncology, 25*(5), 513–520.
89. Roberts, D., Calman, L., Large, P., Appleton, L., Grande, G., Lloyd-Williams, M., & Walshe, C. (2017). A revised model for coping with advanced cancer. Mapping concepts from a longitudinal qualitative study of patients and carers coping with advanced cancer onto Folkman and Greer's theoretical model of appraisal and coping. *Psycho-Oncology, 27*(1), 229–235.
90. Li, L., Li, S., Wang, Y., Yi, J., Yang, Y., He, J., & Zhu, X. (2017). Coping profiles differentiate psychological adjustment in Chinese women newly diagnosed with breast cancer. *Integrative Cancer Therapies, 16*(2), 196–204.

Chapter 10
Quality of Life

What Is Quality of Life?

Quality of life (QOL) is one of those basic constructs which everyone uses and somehow knows what it is, but it does not lend itself easily to definition. In recent years a serious advance has been made in defining QOL mainly because the initially simplistic attempts to reduce QOL to one-dimensional definitions have been replaced by approaches emphasizing multidimensionality. Thus, instead of definitions equating QOL with general satisfaction or absence of disease or disability, happiness, or well-being in general, the new generation of definitions amplify the unidimensional ones by introducing further meaningful components [1]. Thus, QOL is defined as the individuals' perception of their functioning and well-being in different domains of life [2] or the individuals' evaluation and satisfaction with their current level of functioning compared to what they consider as possible or ideal [3]. The major components recurring in many definitions are the individual's own evaluation of one's state; evaluation of one's functioning, well-being, and state in life; evaluation in terms of one's culture and social community; and evaluation in terms of one's interests. The most encompassing approach is evident in the WHO definition of QOL as the "individuals perception of their position in life in the context of the culture and value systems in which they live and in relation to their goals, expectations, standards and concerns" [4].

Definitions of this kind were previously known as "life satisfaction"or "subjective well-being" and are now referred to as "global QOL" or "overall QOL." They are designed to represent the individuals' overall satisfaction with their state in major domains of life that make up one's QOL or contribute to it rather than only to health-based QOL.

S. Kreitler, *Psycho-Oncology for the Clinician*,
https://doi.org/10.1007/978-3-030-06126-5_10

What Quality of Life Is Not

A more complete characterization of QOL requires specifying those aspects that are not included routinely in the definition of QOL. This includes related constructs and some specific items.

The related constructs refer mainly to the following:

(a) Health status: Health status is the person's relative status of health or illness, considering the presence of physiological dysfunction, symptoms, and functional impairment. Most definitions of health status refer to physical function, sensation, self-care and dexterity, cognition, pain and discomfort, and psychological well-being. The Health Utilities Index (HUI) represents two major multi-attribute health status: classification systems, HUI Mark 2 (HUI2) including seven attributes (sensation, mobility, emotion, cognition, self-care, pain, and fertility) and HUI Mark 3 (HUI3) with eight attributes (vision, hearing, speech, ambulation, dexterity, emotion, cognition, and pain) as reported in subjects' interviews or questionnaires. The HUI indices are common tools for assessing different domains of life insofar as they are affected by one's physical health [5].
(b) Perceived health status: Perceived health status is the patients' subjective ratings of their overall health status. Health means not only the absence of disease or disability but also refers to overall physical and mental well-being. Perceived health status is assessed mostly by a question like the following, in various formulations: How do you assess your health? The requested answers are in terms of choices ranging from very good to very bad [6]. Though health status and perceived health status may coincide, they are not necessarily identical [7].
(c) Health-related quality of life (HRQL): HRQL refers to the individual's evaluation of one's state, function, and well-being insofar as they are affected by one's disease and the related treatments. Most conceptualizations of HRQL refer to the effects of disease in general (generic HRQL) or a particular disease or treatment (condition-specific HRQL) on physical, social, emotional, and cognitive functioning [8]. These domains are the basic ones defined by the European Organization for the Research and Treatment of Cancer (EORTC) [9].

For the sake of clarity, it may be advisable to list the following constructs which are mostly not included in the assessments of QOL:

1. The diagnosis, disease duration, disease severity, and overall health status.
2. Prognosis, expected duration of life, i.e., survival, or "quantity of life."
3. Symptoms due to the disease or the treatments. Admittedly, some QOL scales include a few of the symptoms that are assumed to affect QOL, such as nausea, insomnia, or pain.
4. Functional status: Refers to the individual's ability to perform regular activities required to meet basic needs, fulfill one's roles, and maintain well-being [7, 10]. It is usually based on actual assessment of functional capacity, on the reports of others and often on self-reports as well.
5. The patient's mental or psychiatric state, including major depression and other psychiatric diagnoses.

The list of the aspects usually excluded from QOL includes features that are primarily more medical or physical (mainly Nos. 1. 2 and 5) as well as most of the symptoms (No. 3) and the functional status (No. 4). The latter is often assessed independently of QOL and plays an important role in regard to determining the patients' treatment options, rehabilitation potential, and required intensity of palliative care, e.g., Karnovsky grade which runs from 100 to 0 [11] and ECOG grade which runs from 0 to 5 [12]. The patient's mental state (No. 5) is included in the list because it refers to characteristic psychiatric symptoms that are not transitory or temporal and not emotional reactions to the current state.

In some cases the boundaries between QOL and the five mentioned constructs are difficult to draw and get blurred for theoretical or methodological reasons [7]. As noted, specific symptoms are included in some QOL scales, and emotional responses (e.g., anxiety, depression) are included in many QOL scales.

Major Features Characteristic of Quality of Life

The standard approaches to QOL are based on the following characteristics of QOL which may be considered as the defining features of QOL [13]:

1. QOL is a *subjective* construct, reflecting the individual's view of his or her well-being and functioning.
2. QOL is a *phenomenological* construct, providing a bird's-eye aerial view of the situation, without explaining how or why it arose.
3. QOL is an *experiential or evaluative* construct, which can be expressed in terms of judgments without attempting to relate them to objectively identifiable facts.
4. QOL is a *dynamic* construct, designed to reflect significant changes in the individual's state.
5. QOL is a *quantifiable* construct, which may be assessed so that it may be used for comparing scores across different individuals or across different states or different time points in the same individual.
6. QOL is a *multidimensional* construct, which in addition to a global evaluation of QOL includes evaluations in specific domains that have been identified as major constituents of QOL.

The Multidimensionality of Quality of Life

The early assessments of QOL by an overall evaluation in terms of one inclusive dimension have been replaced or rather amplified in subsequent generations of assessing QOL by specific scales addressing particular domains of QOL. Domains are defined in terms of general constructs describing different aspects of one's life, such as entertainment or social relations. Domains are not to be identified with specific diseases for which particular assessment modules have been devised, in addition to the questionnaire for overall QOL, e.g., breast, lung or lymphoma modules in the framework of the European Organization for Research and Treatment of Cancer (EORTC) questionnaire [14]. Domains have been identified in diverse ways, e.g., judgments of scientific experts (WHOQOL-100) [15], or interviewing of patients [16]. Here are some examples designed to demonstrate both the overlap in the different lists of domains and the relative diversity they represent.

The domains are assessed in one of the best known tools, the WHOQOL-100: the following are the 6 domains including 24 facets: physical health (energy and fatigue, pain and discomfort, sleep and rest), psychological (bodily image and appearance, negative feelings, positive feelings, self-esteem, thinking-learning-memory-concentration), level of independence (mobility, daily life activities, dependence on medical aids, work capacity), social relationships (personal, social support, sexual activity), environment (financial, freedom and security, health and social care, home environment opportunities for acquiring new information, recreation, physical environment, transport), and spirituality (religion). In the abbreviated version of the World Health Organization Quality of Life Assessment (WHOQOL-BREF) [17], only the following four domains are covered: physical health, psychological, social relationships, and environment. The quality-of-life scale (QOLS) [18] covers the following six domains: material and physical well-being; relationships with other people; social, community, and civic activities; personal development and fulfillment; recreation; and independence, the ability to do for yourself.

In the Medical Outcomes Study, Short Form 36 (SF-36 Health Survey) [19], the following eight domains are assessed: physical functioning, role limitations due to physical health, bodily pain, general health perceptions, vitality, social functioning, role limitations due to emotional problems, and mental health.

The European Organization of Research and Treatment for Cancer (EORTC) covers the following nine domains: nine multi-item scales – five functional scales (physical, role, cognitive, emotional, and social); three symptom scales (fatigue, pain, and nausea and vomiting); and a global health and quality-of-life scale. Several single-item symptom measures are also included [9].

The Functional Assessment of Cancer Therapy-General (FACT-G) [20] is based on assessing the following domains: physical, social/family, emotional, and functional well-being.

The multidimensional inventory of QOL for adults [16] assesses the following 16 domains, with 1–3 items per domain: positive feelings, negative feelings, cognitive functioning, friends and social ties, body image, sense of mastery and independence, self-image, meaningfulness of life, confusion and bewilderment, physical health, physical functioning, stress, sexuality, family life, fun and entertainment, and living conditions. The list of domains for the Children's QOL questionnaire (CHQOL) [21] is similar: the number of scales is 15, and the differences are that sexuality is omitted, and health worries are replaced by worries, meaningfulness of life by motivation for doing things, and living conditions by basic needs.

It is evident that the different QOL scales include overlapping domains which speaks for the sharing of the basic conception of QOL by the different investigators. However, a comparison between the EORTC-30 and FACT-G showed that the relations between the comparative scores in the same sample were at best moderate which indicates that despite the overlap in domains, the two tools measured markedly different aspects of QOL [22]. It is likely that the reason for the differences resides in the particular items used for representing the domains. For example, the domain of emotions may be assessed by asking about controlling one's emotions in general or responding with empathy to one's friends. The responses may greatly differ. Again, having a best friend is included in the multidimensional inventory of QOL for adults [16] in the scale of social ties and relations, but in the Children's QOL questionnaire [21], it is included in the scale of basic needs, on the basis of factor analysis.

What Are the Functions of Assessing Quality of Life?

Basically the question is what are the uses of QOL, why is it necessary or recommended to consider it and to assess it? What are its benefits and possibly its drawbacks or even harms? These questions have implications in regard to medical practice, medical research, relations between clinicians and patients, and the role of the patient in the framework of treatment [23].

In the framework of *medical treatment*, an important advantage of QOL is that it may complement the information clinicians get about the effects of treatments administered to patients. While the information usually considered reflects mostly medically significant facts relevant for the cure, QOL provides information about additional effects that reflect outcomes in terms of the patients' overall life, including the costs of possible resulting disabilities and suffering as well as improvement and other positive results. Thus, QOL enables forming a more encompassing basis for evaluating treatments. This may be important for comparing different treatments and for selecting the most appropriate treatment for a particular patient. Moreover, following changes in QOL in the course of treatment may sometimes help the clinician adapt the treatment better to the capacities and state of the patient.

Insofar as *healthcare* is concerned, information about the QOL effects of specific treatments or disease states may help health professionals in planning or preparing ahead of time adequate interventions for moderating or alleviating the foreseen effects. In some cases information about the QOL effects of a treatment may help in preventing deterioration of QOL by administering preventive treatment to all patients or at least to those assumed to be especially vulnerable to the negative effects of the treatment. The intervention may sometimes consist merely in preparing the patient for the likely effects. This in itself may help the patient maintain one's QOL at least to some degree. Hence, QOL may contribute to the shaping and evaluation of health services.

Information about QOL may contribute to *research in medicine* and the development of medications. Knowing about the QOL effects of diverse drugs and other treatments may prompt studies designed to develop treatment options with fewer side effects affecting QOL negatively.

QOL plays an important role in the *relations between clinicians and patients*. Since QOL refers to the general life conditions and responses of the patient, it introduces all these essentially human aspects into the context of the relations between doctor and patient that are otherwise defined primarily in medical terms. QOL contributes to the enrichment of the relationship by blurring the sharp demarcation lines between the doctor as the expert and the patient as the customer. QOL contributes a more personal flavor to the interaction. Patients have often stated their wish for personalizing the interaction with the doctor (see Chap. 12). The patient's QOL becomes a concern shared by doctor and patient, both of whom focus on it with a common intent of improving it.

Finally, addressing the patient's QOL as a theme delivers to the patient the message that he or she is treated by the physician as *a whole person*. Hence, despite the definition of the situation mainly in medical terms, the health professionals do not lose sight of the basic fact that the patient is first and foremost a human being. This message is expressed through the direct reference by means of QOL to the patient's emotions, mood, fears, living conditions, family life, friends, and other basic needs and concerns. By addressing such aspects of QOL, the doctor manifests his or her respect and concern for the patient.

Introducing these personal aspects into the context of treatment may have the effect of motivating the patient to mobilize one's own forces for the goal of recovery. This may result in the patient's empowerment and hence may contribute to improving his or her health.

One important result of the closer relations between doctor and patient is that they may discuss together issues that concern treatment and choice of treatment options. One such issue is in cases of doubt whether to apply a given treatment in view of its minimal or uncertain benefits for the patient's health. The impact of that treatment on QOL gains in importance and may tip the balance in favor of undergoing the treatment or not. The situation is even more loaded emotionally when the suggested treatment with minimal or uncertain advantages for survival involves serious impairment of QOL. In such cases that are not rare in patients with advanced disease, quantity of life is pitted against quality of life. It is not uncommon for patients to choose the venue that supports QOL. A study about preferences of patients at the end of life showed that only a minority (3%) chose only life extension, while the majority prioritized improving QOL, either alone (54%) or QOL together with life extension (39%) [24]. Sometimes the decision patients undertake involves stopping the treatment altogether. In other cases the situation is easier, for example, selecting a treatment option with lower medical value but also less harmful for QOL or delaying the starting of treatment although it may have detrimental medical results but harming less one's QOL. Decisions of this kind are more satisfactory and have often better outcomes for the patient when they are met by both doctor and patient who may consider both quality and quality of life (see Chap. 7).

Determinants of Quality of Life

A patient's QOL is embedded within the overall framework of the individual's general QOL which is affected by social, cultural, economic, physical, physiological, political, psychological, and ecological circumstances. This broad-range variegated set of circumstances affects also the manner in which the patient's QOL is shaped by the disease and treatments. This fact adds to the complexity of the issue of dealing with the determinants of QOL. A further complicating factor is the apparent difficulty of differentiating between the components of QOL and its determinants. Thus, one study found that determinants of QOL in cancer patients included disease stage, spiritual well-being, financial state, mood disorders, and the procedure applied for questionnaire administration [25]. Another study found that for predicting QOL in cancer patients, it is necessary to consider demographic variables (e.g., age, gender, ethnicity, and socioeconomic status), clinical factors (e.g., disease type and stage), and social characteristics (e.g., religious affiliation, relationship with doctor) [26].

Findings of this kind render it necessary to define carefully the determinants of QOL.

A fairly comprehensive survey of the studies about the determinants of QOL leads to the following list of major determinants of QOL:

1. *Diagnosis*. Diagnosis determines QOL in multiple forms. Prognosis is one factor that impacts QOL. As may be expected, good prognosis is related to better QOL and poor prognosis to worse QOL. However, while there is a significant effect of prognosis on the general score of QOL and on physical aspects of QOL, there are only marginal effects of prognosis groups on social and psychological functioning [27]. Further, a more advanced disease stage is often related to lower QOL in different types of cancer [28–30], but in breast cancer 5 years after diagnosis, it is not related any more to QOL [31]. Again, metastases and recurrence of disease are often related to lower QOL [32, 33], as well as the length of a malignant disease, the presence of comorbidities, and the worsening of the health condition in general are correlated with low QOL scores [34].
2. *Different medical treatments*. Medical treatments were often shown to cause a deterioration of QOL. This applies mainly to chemotherapy which despite all developments in this field still causes symptoms which affect QOL negatively [35, 36]. Notably, the effect is less negative when there is at least a partially good response to chemotherapy [35]. The effects of chemotherapy on QOL may persist for long periods after termination of treatment [37]. Differences in the impact on QOL have been found also between two types of treatment. One example is the difference between the effects on QOL of the two kinds of surgery for breast cancer: mastectomy and lumpectomy [38]. Although lumpectomy is mostly related to better QOL, in some cases it may result in lower QOL because the patient is scared of recurrence or that some remnants of the tumor may have remained or because of dissatisfaction with the shape of the breast after surgery. Concerning other treatments, there is evidence that also

radiotherapy affects QOL negatively [30], but when it is applied with the purpose of palliation, it often improves QOL [39]. Radiotherapy causes a decline in QOL also in children [40], but the negative effect may be moderated by adequate psychosocial support [41]. Also children who underwent treatments because of cancer diseases may suffer from deterioration in QOL for long periods after termination of the treatments [42]. Sometimes a mere change in the kind of applied installation as in the case of enterostomy may be related to better QOL [43].

3. *Different alternative treatments or interventions*. Major among these are physical exercise [44], activities designed to maintain or develop physical fitness [45], muscle relaxation techniques [46], qigong [47], art therapies [48], music therapy [49], and mindfulness [50], as well as treatment according to traditional Chinese medicine at least in Chinese patients [51] were shown to affect QOL positively.
4. *Psychosocial interventions*. Several studies and reviews of studies show that positive impact on QOL has been found for different psychological interventions, such as self-regulatory training targeting illness perceptions and coping [52], psychoeducational support [53], cognitive-behavioral therapy [54], counseling [55], creative writing [56], guided self-help [57], psychotherapy [58], participating in supportive-expressive group discussions [59], or hypnosis [60]. Some of the interventions took place individually, face-to-face, and some in group settings. The effects of interventions of this kind on QOL were mostly positive but moderate or limited only to specific aspects of QOL, such as depression or fatigue [60]. In some cases it was found that the effect on QOL depended on the patients' personality tendencies [61] or on the use of additional moderators, such as nutrition or physical exercise [55]. Over 20 years ago, a review reached a similar conclusion that the impact of psychological interventions on QOL seems to be of a medium degree [62]. Further research is needed to clarify the issue and its causes.
5. *Overall physical state of the patient*. The patient's overall physical state was found to affect QOL negatively [31, 63]. Major aspects of the patient's overall state that could have a negative effect on QOL are a long duration of the chronic disease state [64], comorbidities [28, 31], and the patient's nutritional state [65, 66]. A low nutritional state affects QOL negatively both directly and by lowering the patient's physical state [67, 68]. Even a small improvement in the patient's nutritional state leads to a better QOL [69].
6. *Physical symptoms related to disease or treatments*. The symptoms that affect QOL negatively may be caused by the disease itself or they may be side effects of the treatments. The symptoms may appear during the treatments or after their termination. They include abnormal sensations, fatigue, difficulties in mobility [70, 71], pain [34], lack of appetite, nausea [35], cough, breathing difficulties, and sleep problems [72]. There is a negative correlation between the number of symptoms and QOL: The fewer physical symptoms there are, the better QOL is [72].

7. *The patient's functional status.* The functional status was shown to be an important factor of positive QOL in cancer patients. It refers to the overall state of the patient's functioning, which may be based primarily on good performance in the different domains of daily life and performance at work or studies [72]. Notably, the patient's functional state is neither identical nor based exclusively on the patient's physical state. It is not uncommon to observe a patient whose functional state is much higher or much lower than that apparently warranted by his or her physical state. An important contributing factor to the patient's functional state is the degree to which the patient has been able to maintain one's former state of functioning which is manifested in having no significant changes and no particular life events [35], preserving the erectile function despite prostate cancer [73] and fertility despite different cancer treatments [74].
8. *The patient's psychological state.* Trait anxiety and depression [72, 75] and state anxiety symptoms [70] are potent factors that reduce QOL [72, 75] in cancer patients. Further psychologically based factors that affect negatively QOL are, for example, unmet cancer-related information needs and impaired sense of control over life [76], feeling of uncertainty [77], low self-efficacy in regard to cancer-related issues such as taking care of oneself or enterostomy [43], and cognitive impairment manifested in difficulties in regard to concentration and task completion [70]. Notably, patients mentioned also the following two factors as reducing QOL: a negative view of life [70] and the stigma, blame and shame they may feel because of the disease, especially in regard to smoking and lung cancer [78].
9. *Coping by patient.* As can be expected, the coping mechanisms applied by the patient are an important factor affecting QOL. There is empirical evidence that in patients with different tumor sites and disease stage, higher QOL is related to good emotional coping by patient and acceptance of disease [79]; in women with breast cancer, it is related to coping through posttraumatic growth [75] and to coping with anger by cognitive strategies [80]; in prostate cancer patients, it is related to coping by fighting spirit that leads to acceptance of disease and adjustment to life [81]; and in terminally ill patients, it is related to the use of positive framing and active coping or approach-oriented coping and denial in regard to diagnosis [82, 83]. But QOL is low in head and neck cancer patients whose coping focuses on helplessness and fatalism [84].
10. *Patient's satisfaction with care.* Satisfaction with care is a complex construct which includes evaluation of the doctors' technical competence, communication skills, interpersonal approach, as well as of the quality, accessibility, and continuity of overall care, during treatment and following its termination [85]. Studies showed that satisfaction with overall care affects QOL and is related to better QOL especially during treatment [79]. In general, satisfaction with care is a function of the patient's state of health, so that when health deteriorates, the impact of satisfaction with care on QOL is negative [86]. In some cases QOL is affected more by satisfaction with emotional care than with physical care [87]. Communication with doctors is of special importance for maintaining the patients' QOL [44].

11. *Patient's personality.* Cognitive and motivational factors were shown to be related to the patient's QOL [88–90]. Indeed, it is to be expected that the patient's personality affects one's QOL through the manner in which he or she behave, think, what they want to attain, and how they interpret the events and situation. Studies show that optimism affects positively QOL, although not immediately after initial diagnosis [91]. A study in which the impact of the Big Five personality traits on QOL was investigated [92] showed significant relations between neuroticism and pessimism with lower physical function, between optimism and better QOL, and between extraversion and reduced depression and lower severity of GVHD symptoms reported by the patient and physician.

    Information about patient-centered preferences in regard to treatments has become an important component in personalized medicine contributing to improving patients' QOL. Findings showed that personality traits are associated with particular preferences of palliative care in prostate cancer patients at the end of life. Patients scoring high on neuroticism were characterized as service reluctant, while those scoring high on agreeableness were characterized as service accepting patients in regard to receiving life support and palliative care [93]. Other personality tendencies that were found to contribute to improving QOL are resilience [94] and hope [95]. Both promote the patient's ability to handle difficulties successfully.

    Finally, *meaningfulness of life* is another personality-based factor that was found to affect QOL. Its contribution to QOL in cancer patients is optimal under two conditions: first, when its score is in the medium range (i.e., neither too high so that maintaining it does not require too many resources nor too low so that it does not provide any coping support), and second, when it includes components of the different aspects of meaningfulness of life (i.e., sensory-perceptual, experiential-cognitive, actional-dynamic, and contextual-situational). Meeting the two conditions renders meaningfulness of life sufficiently stable, comprehensive, and variegated to provide coping support for improving QOL [96].
12. *Patient's family environment.* network that may provide social support to the patient, a special role is assigned to the impact of social support of the patient's family. Adequate social support from family members was associated with significantly improved quality of life of cancer patients [51, 97, 98]. But discrimination by family members or relatives lowered QOL appreciably [35].
13. *Patient's social environment.* There is a lot of evidence that adequate social support from friends and neighbors is related to improved QOL of cancer patients [51, 99, 100]. Even Internet-based group support improves the patients' QOL [101]. Living alone [71], being socially isolated or rejected, and having no friends are factors reducing the patient's QOL. Notably, in some cases, when the patient interprets the social support as evidence for his or her weakness, the support may reduce one's QOL [35].
14. *Patient's financial state.* Higher income, better household financial situation, and medical insurance guaranteeing lower medical expenses are associated

with higher QOL [51]. Losing money and income because of the disease was shown to lower the QOL, for example, in head and neck cancer patients [102]. Similarly, being unemployed or in a financially insecure position, especially because of the disease, affects QOL negatively [35, 103].

15. *Patient's demographic factors*. Different demographic variables were found to affect the patients' QOL, for example, age, education level, and gender [28, 31, 35]. Mostly, the effects were more negative when the age was younger, the education level lower, and the gender female. In general the demographic factors seem to affect QOL less than chemotherapy [104, 105].

The list of the 15 determinants of QOL demonstrates the complexity of the issue. The determinants are diverse in their content, context, and nature. They include representatives from the major aspects of the patient's life, i.e., medical, psychological, social, and environmental. As a whole, they constitute a complex of objective and subjective factors affecting the subjectively based evaluation of one's QOL. It suggests that in different patients, QOL may be affected to different degrees by different determinants. Thus, demographic factors may have a greater or smaller impact on QOL than the social factors, and the medical factors may have a greater or smaller impact than the psychological ones. The differences may be a function of the disease, the administered treatments, the patient's personality, and the culture which affects expectations, attitudes, and behaviors. Further, the effects of the different determinants may not be identical because some determinants may affect only specific domains of QOL and others may affect other domains, e.g., optimism may affect spiritual well-being, while financial state may affect the sense of safety and security. Again, some determinants may have different even opposite effects in different patients, such as social support may raise QOL or impair it. Additionally, the different determinants may function in different ways, some directly and some in combination or through other determinants, such as personality traits and physical symptoms may affect QOL through coping, while physical symptoms may affect QOL through the patient's functional state. One study showed that different kinds of determinants with negative impact can combine to lower QOL. Thus, women with breast cancer who underwent chemotherapy had lower QOL when they were new immigrants from another country than when they were not immigrants [106]. The outlined possibilities and others indicate that there are many diverse options that may be applied for improving the QOL of a patient if necessary (see Improving the Patient's QOL).

Impact of Quality of Life on the Patient

QOL is constantly present in the life of an individual and enters as a contributing factor into the matrix of determinants that shape the patients' medical, physiological, psychological, social, and economic state. Studies with different types of cancer patients show that QOL is related to survival [28, 107, 108]. Notably, this has been shown concerning QOL in patients after diagnosis [107] as well as in patients with advanced gastric disease [108]. The implication is that patients whose QOL is good live longer. But it may also be that patients whose state promotes longer survival also have a better QOL. Yet the original direction of the relation does not obliterate the complementary interpretation that QOL contributes to the prognosis.

Good QOL enhances the patient's will to live and to engage in actions that promote survival, such as undergoing different treatments even if their benefit for survival may not be especially great. Further, good QOL often involves lower levels of suffering so that the patient is able to invest in activities and plans bound with enhancing joy, vitality, satisfaction, and possibly happiness.

Finally, it is likely that good QOL strengthens the motivation to devise and apply coping mechanisms that could contribute in themselves to maintaining the good QOL. The motivation engendered by good QOL may also contribute to enhancing the patient's social relations with one's family and friends and may even bring about improvement in one's financial state by exploiting venues for earning money or using financial resources that could be made available.

In sum, the constructs of physical state, survival, functional state, and QOL should not be considered as identical. Survival as well as functional state may be better or worse than those expected in view of the patient's physical state and diagnosis. For example, one cancer patient in stage IV may live longer than predicted by the health professionals, while another cancer patient in stage II may be in a functional state lower than that expected for his or her physical state. In both cases, the reason may be found at least partly in the patient's QOL. It seems that in many cases, a good QOL may prompt higher achievements in function and survival than warranted on purely medical bases or may bring about lower achievements than would be normally expected in view of the patient's medical state.

Improving the Patient's Quality of Life

One of the major goals of treatment of cancer patients is to improve, maintain, or at least not lower their QOL. There are a great many factors that could impair the QOL of a cancer patient. The diagnosis, the treatments, the break in the routine of one's life, the anxiety about the future, and the unclarity about what could happen are just a few of the factors threatening to impair one's QOL. A decline in QOL bothers the patient both because it is low and because it deviates from ones habitual level. Hence, a decline in the level of QOL calls for a response on the part of the individual. This response is the function of two tendencies. One consists in the attempt simply to raise the QOL level so as to improve it. This tendency is grounded in the common drive for development. The other tendency consists in the attempt to reinstate the former state of QOL that characterized one's usual level. This tendency is grounded in the common drive for maintaining homeostasis.

There are two ways for improving one's QOL. One focuses on the determinants of QOL, the other on the components of QOL.

(A) *The venue which focuses on the determinants of QOL.* It includes different possibilities. The first consists in identifying those determinants which lower QOL in general or in a specific case and changing them. This can be done by weakening their impact, by replacing them through other factors, or by activating other factors that negate them. For example, if the identified reason for lower QOL is lack of social support, or difficulty in mobility or pain, the options for improving QOL would be to find sources for providing social support (e.g., volunteers), devising means for improving the patient's possibilities for mobility (e.g., instruments or drivers), and organizing a proper treatment for the patient's pain. These examples demonstrate a head-on attack on the factors depressing the patients' QOL. Another way of improving QOL consists in strengthening those determinants that are relatively accessible to change in general or in specific cases. The list of determinants shows several possibilities. The major ones are different alternatives or complementary interventions that are often offered to cancer patients (Determinants no. 3); applying adequate psychosocial interventions (Determinants no. 4); treating symptoms that are often side effects of treatments (Determinants no. 6; e.g., fatigue, lack of appetite, dyspnea, nausea) which are mostly addressed in oncological clinics or wards; improving the patient's functional status, for example, by addressing nutritional difficulties; training in performing different daily chores (Determinants no. 7); teaching the patient new, adaptive, and useful coping mechanisms (Determinants No. 9; see also Chap. 9); improving conditions of care in the clinic or hospital as well as communication with the doctors and healthcare personnel in general (Determinants no.10); applying interventions for developing the patient's meaningfulness of life (see Chap. 9), hope, and resilience (Determinants no. 11); improving support of family members and communication in the family (Determinants no. 12; see also Chap. 11); improving contact and support of friends, acquaintances, colleagues; and mobilizing other social community resources as is being done in many countries (Determinants no. 13).

(B) *The venue which focuses on the components of QOL.* The key to applying this venue for improving QOL is the findings which show that the overall summative evaluation an individual has of one's overall QOL is not related under all circumstances to the scores of the evaluations in all specific domains of QOL [95]. Under regular conditions, the summative score of QOL is correlated only with three major subscales of QOL: state of one's major occupation (work or studies), state of one's health, and state of one's family relations (nuclear family or one's partner). The scores of the other subscales of QOL are important but usually are not correlated with the overall score of QOL, i.e., they do not contribute significantly to the summative overall impression one has of one's QOL. However, when one of the mentioned major subscales is impaired, the overall level of QOL gets lower and stays that way as long as the impairment is considered as temporary. But when the impairment in occupation, health or family is grasped as chronic, then the overall score of QOL becomes correlated with an increasing number of the different subscales, in line with the patient's preferences or situational options. This change in correlations is attended by a reinstitution of the original level of QOL.

The practical implication of the described study is that in order to reconstruct the habitual overall level of QOL in cancer patients who consider their disease as chronic, it is advisable to help them improve their situation in as many of the subscales that are possible. For example, the patients can be helped to improve their living conditions, increase their use of entertainment options, expand their manifestations of creativity, invest in their personal development, improve their body image, develop their cognitive abilities, improve their family relations and social contacts, or deepen their occupation with spiritual issues. The mentioned examples represent different scales of the QOL inventory [16] which have been applied for raising the level of QOL. It is evident that not all domains of QOL can or should be expanded by every patient in order to raise one's QOL. Sometimes the improvement in a certain domain takes place by positive additions, sometimes by removal or reduction of disturbing components, for example, solving a disrupting issue of old standing in the family.

However, in some cases patients say that their QOL after the disease has become better than prior to it. This statement, which is barely credible to many outsiders, may reflect the improvement in QOL due to the efforts invested by these patients in improving many or most of the domains in their life, beyond the number that is necessary for maintaining one's previous level of QOL.

Assessment of Quality of Life

The assessment of QOL is an important issue mainly because of the ubiquity of the assessments and the important role they fulfill in oncological practice. QOL assessments have become required information for introducing a new drug or treatment. Further, QOL assessments are used for important decisions concerning treatments in general and in regard to specific patients.

One major issue concerns the manner of assessment. Assessment of QOL is done by means of questionnaires. Questionnaires are the preferred tool because of their proven reliability and validity. Nevertheless there are clinics and health professionals who still use for assessment general questions about satisfaction or QOL which provide less adequate assessment.

However, even if questionnaires are applied, it needs to be kept in mind that not all questionnaires are equal. Some questionnaires emphasize health issues either in the content of many items or in the basic paradigm which asks about the impact of health concerning each QOL item. These health-related questionnaires (e.g., [15, 17]) are limited in scope and in addition require answers about the degree to which health issues have affected domains in one's life (e.g., to what degree has your health problem affected your social life?). Answers to questions of this kind are difficult to give and difficult to interpret because they refer to two intermingled issues: the state of the domain and the effect of health on it. However, on the other hand, the health-related questionnaires are very commonly used so that they provide easily available platforms for comparison of results in different cancer diseases and oncology wards all over the world.

When checking results of QOL assessment, it is necessary to examine whether the QOL questionnaire is a generic one, i.e., whether it refers to QOL in general or to the whole range of cancer diseases or whether it addresses only a specific cancer disease.

Further, with regard to a generic cancer questionnaire, it is advisable to check the domains to which the questionnaire refers so as to make sure that a sufficient number of the basic ones are addressed. However, since two different QOL questionnaires were found to provide different scores for the same domain [22], in order to evaluate adequately the result of QOL assessment, it seems to be necessary sometimes to check also the specific items that represent a domain, as noted above (see The Multidimensionality of QOL). For example, an item about having at least one best friend does not necessarily provide the same information about social relations as an item about spending a lot of time with acquaintances.

An adequate evaluation of the results could also consider the form of responding to the questionnaire. The easiest way is when the form of response stays identical all through the items. When the form changes, difficulty of responding may increase while reliability of responses may be reduced.

It seems however that the most important issue in regard to QOL assessment is the identity of the responder. Since QOL is a subjective construct, it is most appropriate that the responder should be the person whose QOL is assessed. In recent years the issue about the identity of the responder arises mainly or only in the case of individuals whose age (i.e., young children) or state of mind (e.g., specific psychiatric cases or persons who are mentally challenged or suffer from dementia) raises doubts about their ability to respond. Studies showed that getting QOL assessments from others (e.g., parents or nurses or family relatives or caregivers) does not provide the adequate information. Comparing assessments given by proxy and those given by the persons themselves reveal significant differences (e.g., [109, 110]). Further, studies showed that when the questions are formulated clearly and simply, most of those who were considered unable to respond do so in a satisfactory manner [21]. Findings of this kind have led to the conclusion that whenever at all possible QOL assessments should be obtained from the persons themselves who possess the ability and the full right to report about their state of well-being [111, 112].

References

1. Theofilou, P. (2013). Quality of life: Definition and measurement. *Europe's Journal of Psychology, 9*(1), 150–162.
2. Fayers, P. M., & Machin, D. (2013). *Quality of life: The assessment, analysis and interpretation of patient-reported outcomes*. Chichester: Wiley.
3. Diener, E., Suh, E. M., Lucas, R. E., & Smith, H. L. (1999). Subjective well-being: Three decades of progress. *Psychological Bulletin, 125*(2), 276–302.

4. World Health Organization. (1947). *Constitution of the World Health Organization. Chronicle of the World Health Organization, Annex 1*. Geneva: World Health Organization.
5. Horsman, J., Furlong, W., Feeny, D., & Torrance, G. (2003). The Health Utilities Index (HUI®): Concepts, measurement properties and applications. *Health and Quality of Life Outcomes, 1*(1), 54.
6. OECD Health Statistics. Definitions, Sources and Methods. (2017). Retrieved from URL http://www.oecd.org/els/health-systems/Table-of-Content-Metadata-OECD-Health-Statistics-2017.pdf
7. Willson, I. B., & Cleary, P. D. (1995). Linking clinical variables with health related quality of life. *JAMA, 273*(1), 59–65.
8. Ware, J. E., Jr. (1995). The status of health assessment 1994. *Annual Review of Public Health, 16*(1), 327–354.
9. Aaronson, N. K., Ahmedzai, S., Bergman, B., Bullinger, M., Cull, A., Duez, N. J., & Kaasa, S. (1993). The European Organization for Research and Treatment of Cancer QLQ-C30: A quality-of-life instrument for use in international clinical trials in oncology. *JNCI: Journal of the National Cancer Institute, 85*(5), 365–376.
10. Leidy, N. K. (1994). Using functional status to assess treatment outcomes. *Chest, 106*(6), 1645–1646.
11. Karnofsky, D. A., Abelmann, W. H., Craver, L. F., & Burchenal, J. H. (1948). The use of the nitrogen mustards in the palliative treatment of carcinoma with particular reference to bronchogenic rcinoma. *Cancer, 1*(4), 634–656.
12. Oken, M. M., Creech, R. H., Tormey, D. C., Horton, J., Davis, T. E., Mcfadden, E. T., & Carbone, P. P. (1982). Toxicity and response criteria of the Eastern Cooperative Oncology Group. *American Journal of Clinical Oncology, 5*(6), 649–656.
13. Niv, D., & Kreitler, S. (2001). Pain and quality of life. *Pain Practice, 1*(2), 150–161.
14. Sprangers, M. A. G., Cull, A., Bjordal, K., Groenvold, M., & Aaronson, N. K. (1993). The European Organization for Research and Treatment of Cancer approach to quality of life assessment: Guidelines for developing questionnaire modules. *Quality of Life Research, 2*(4), 287–295.
15. WHOQoL Group. (1995). The World Health Organization quality of life assessment (WHOQOL): Position paper from the World Health Organization. *Social Science & Medicine, 41*(10), 1403–1409.
16. Kreitler, S., & Kreitler, M. M. (2006). Multidimensional quality of life: A new measure of quality of life in adults. *Social Indicators Research, 76*(1), 5–33.
17. WHOQoL Group. (1998). Development of the World Health Organization WHOQOL-BREF quality of life assessment. *Psychological Medicine, 28*(3), 551–558.
18. Burckhardt, C. S., & Anderson, K. L. (2003). The quality of life scale (QOLS): Reliability, validity and utilization. *Health and Quality of Life Outcomes, 1*(1), 60.
19. Ware, J. E. (1993). *SF-36 health survey: manual and interpretation guide*. Boston: New England Medical Center, The Health Institute.
20. Cella, D. F., Tulsky, D. S., Gray, G., Sarafian, B., Linn, E., Bonomi, A., & Brannon, J. (1993). The functional assessment of cancer therapy scale: Development and validation of the general measure. *Journal of Clinical Oncology, 11*(3), 570–579.
21. Kreitler, S., Kreitler, M. M., & Alkalay, Y. (2015). The children's quality of life questionnaire: A multidimensional measure for the assessment of quality of life in children and adolescents. *Journal of Psychological Sciences, 1*(2), 62–81.
22. Kemmler, G., Holzner, B., Kopp, M., Dünser, M., Margreiter, R., Greil, R., & Sperner-Unterweger, B. (1999). Comparison of two quality-of-life instruments for cancer patients: The functional assessment of cancer therapy-general and the European Organization for Research and Treatment of Cancer Quality of Life Questionnaire C30. *Journal of Clinical Oncology, 17*(9), 2932–2932.
23. Jacobsen, P. B., Davis, K., & Cella, D. (2002). Assessing quality of life in research and clinical practice. *Oncology (Williston Park, NY), 16*(9 Suppl. 10), 133–139.
24. Higginson, I. J., Daveson, B. A., Morrison, R. S., Yi, D., Meier, D., Smith, M., & Normand, C. (2017). Social and clinical determinants of preferences and their achievement at the end of

life: Prospective cohort study of older adults receiving palliative care in three countries. *BMC Geriatrics, 17*(1), G271.
25. Dapueto, J. J., Servente, L., Francolino, C., & Hahn, E. A. (2005). Determinants of quality of life in patients with cancer. *Cancer, 103*(5), 1072–1081.
26. Wan, G. J., Counte, M. A., Cella, D. F., Hernandez, L., Deasy, S., & Shiomoto, G. (1999). An analysis of the impact of demographic, clinical, and social factors on health-related quality of life. *Value in Health, 2*(4), 308–318.
27. Ringdal, G. I., Ringdal, K., Kvinnsland, S., & Götestam, K. G. (1994). Quality of life of cancer patients with different prognoses. *Quality of Life Research, 3*(2), 143–154.
28. Deng, Y., Tu, H., Pierzynski, J. A., Miller, E. D., Gu, X., Huang, M., Chang, D. W., Ye, Y., Hildebrandt, M. A. T., Klein, A. P., Zhao, R., Lippman, S. M., & Wu, X. (2018). Determinants and prognostic value of quality of life in patients with pancreatic ductal adenocarcinoma. *European Journal of Cancer, 92*, 20–32.
29. Ravasco, P., Monteiro-Grillo, I., Vidal, P. M., & Camilo, M. E. (2004). Cancer: Disease and nutrition are key determinants of patients' quality of life. *Supportive Care in Cancer, 12*(4), 246–252.
30. Yucel, B., Akkaş, E. A., Okur, Y., Eren, A. A., Eren, M. F., Karapınar, H., Babacan, N. A., & Kılıçkap, S. (2014). The impact of radiotherapy on quality of life for cancer patients: A longitudinal study. *Supportive Care in Cancer, 22*(9), 2479–2487.
31. Chu, W. O., Dialla, P. O., Roignot, P., Bone-Lepinoy, M. C., Poillot, M. L., Coutant, C., Arveux, P., & Dabakuyo-Yonli, T. S. (2016). Determinants of quality of life among long-term breast cancer survivors. *Quality of Life Research, 25*(8), 1981–1990.
32. Siddiqi, A., Give, C. W., Give, B., & Sikorski, A. (2009). Quality of life among patients with primary, metastatic and recurrent cancer. *European Journal of Cancer Care, 18*(1), 84–96.
33. Grey, J., & Winter, K. (2018). Patient quality of life and prognosis in multiple endocrine neoplasia type 2. *Endocrine-Related Cancer, 25*(2), T69–T77.
34. Chabowski, M., Polański, J., Jankowska-Polanska, B., Lomper, K., Janczak, D., & Rosinczuk, J. (2017). The acceptance of illness, the intensity of pain and the quality of life in patients with lung cancer. *Journal of Thoracic Disease, 9*(9), 2952–2958.
35. Chagani, P., Parpio, Y., Gul, R., & Jabbar, A. A. (2017). Quality of life and its determinants in adult cancer patients undergoing chemotherapy treatment in Pakistan. *Asia-Pacific Journal of Oncology Nursing, 4*(2), 140–146.
36. Ganz, P. A., Desmond, K. A., Leedham, B., Rowland, J. H., Meyerowitz, B. E., & Belin, T. R. (2002). Quality of life in long-term, disease-free survivors of breast cancer: A follow-up study. *Journal of the National Cancer Institute, 94*(1), 39–49.
37. Stein, K. D., Syrjala, K. L., & Andrykowski, M. A. (2008). Physical and psychological long-term and late effects of cancer. *Cancer, 112*(S11), 2577–2592.
38. Kreitler, S., Kovner, F., Inbar, M., Wigler, N., Lelchuk, S., Chaitchik, S., & Kreitler, H. (1993). Quality of life in breast cancer patients with mastectomy and lumpectomy. In J. C. Holland, M. J. Massie, W. S. Breitbart, P. B. Jacobsen, & S. D. Passik (Eds.), *Psycho-oncology V: Psychosocial factors in cancer risk and survival* (p. 219). New York: Memorial Sloan-Kettering Cancer Center.
39. Kovner, F., & Kreitler, S. (1996). Effect of palliative radiation therapy on quality of life in cancer patients. *Radiology, 201*, 566.
40. Kreitler, S., Krivoy, E., & Toren, A. (2012). Psychosocial aspects of radiotherapy in pediatric cancer patients. In S. Kreitler, M. W. Ben-Arush, & A. Martin (Eds.), *Pediatric psycho-oncology: Psychosocial aspects and clinical interventions* (2nd ed., pp. 62–70). Oxford: Wiley-Blackwell.
41. Kreitler, S., Ben-Arush, M. W., Kriboy, E., Golan, H., Yalon, M., & Toren, A. (2016). Psychosocial aspects of radiotherapy for the child and family with cancer. In L. S. Constine, N. J. Tarbell, & E. C. Halperin (Eds.), *Pediatric radiation oncology* (pp. 1–12). Alphen aan den Rijn: Wolters Kluwen Health.
42. Ness, K. K., Armenian, S. H., Kadan-Lottick, N., & Gurney, J. G. (2011). Adverse effects of treatment in childhood acute lymphoblastic leukemia: General overview and implications for long-term cardiac health. *Expert Review of Hematology, 4*(2), 185–197.

43. Su, X., Zhen, L., Zhu, M., Kuang, Y., Qin, F., Ye, X., Yin, X., & Wang, H. (2017). Determinants of self-efficacy and quality of life in patients with temporary enterostomy: A cross-sectional survey. *Journal of Clinical Nursing, 26*(3–4), 477–484.
44. Liu, Z., Zhang, L., Shi, S., & Xia, W. (2017). Objectively assessed exercise behavior in Chinese patients with early-stage cancer: A predictor of perceived benefits, communication with doctors, medical coping modes, depression and quality of life. *PLoS One, 12*(1), e0169375.
45. McNeely, M. L., Campbell, K. L., Rowe, B. H., Klassen, T. P., Mackey, J. R., & Courneya, K. S. (2006). Effects of exercise on breast cancer patients and survivors: a systematic review and meta-analysis. *Canadian Medical Association Journal, 175*(1), 34–41.
46. Parás-Bravo, P., Salvadores-Fuentes, P., Alonso-Blanco, C., Paz-Zulueta, M., Santibañez-Margüello, M., Palacios-Ceña, D., Boixadera-Planas, E., & Fernández-de-las-Peñas, C. (2017). The impact of muscle relaxation techniques on the quality of life of cancer patients, as measured by the FACT-G questionnaire. *PLoS One, 12*(10), e0184147.
47. Oh, B., Butow, P. N., Mullan, B. A., Clarke, S. J., Beale, P. J., Pavlakis, N., Lee, M. S., Rosenthal, D. S., Larkey, L., & Vardy, J. (2012). Effect of medical Qigong on cognitive function, quality of life, and a biomarker of inflammation in cancer patients: A randomized controlled trial. *Supportive Care in Cancer, 20*(6), 1235–1242.
48. Geue, K., Goetze, H., Buttstaedt, M., Kleinert, E., Richter, D., & Singer, S. (2010). An overview of art therapy interventions for cancer patients and the results of research. *Complementary Therapies in Medicine, 18*(3–4), 160–170.
49. Bradt, J., Dileo, C., Grocke, D., & Magill, L. (2011). Music interventions for improving psychological and physical outcomes in cancer patients. *Cochrane Database Systematic Reviews, 8*(8), CD006911.
50. Zimmermann, F. F., Burrell, B., & Jordan, J. (2018). The acceptability and potential benefits of mindfulness-based interventions in improving psychological well-being for adults with advanced cancer: A systematic review. *Complementary Therapies in Clinical Practice, 30*, 68–78.
51. Yan, B., Yang, L. M., Hao, L. P., Yang, C., Quan, L., Wang, L. H., Wu, Z., Li, X. P., Gao, Y. T., Sun, Q., & Yuan, J. M. (2016). Determinants of quality of life for breast cancer patients in Shanghai, China. *PLoS One, 11*(4), e0153714.
52. Richardson, A. E., Tennant, G., Morton, R. P., & Broadbent, E. (2017). A self-regulatory intervention for patients with head and neck cancer: Pilot randomized trial. *Annals of Behavioral Medicine, 51*(5), 629–641.
53. Wu, P. H., Chen, S. W., Huang, W. T., Chang, S. C., & Hsu, M. C. (2018). Effects of a psychoeducational intervention in patients with breast cancer undergoing chemotherapy. *The Journal of Nursing Research*. https://doi.org/10.1097/jnr.0000000000000252. [Epub ahead of print].
54. Luckett, T., Britton, B., Clover, K., & Rankin, N. M. (2011). Evidence for interventions to improve psychological outcomes in people with head and neck cancer: A systematic review of the literature. *Supportive Care in Cancer, 19*(7), 871–881.
55. D'Egidio, V., Sestili, C., Mancino, M., Sciarra, I., Cocchiara, R., Backhaus, I., Mannocci, A., De Luca, A., Frusone, F., Monti, M., & La Torre, G. (2017). Counseling interventions delivered in women with breast cancer to improve health-related quality of life: a systematic review. *Quality of Life Research, 26*(10), 2573–2592.
56. Lu, Q., Wong, C. C. Y., Gallagher, M. W., Tou, R. Y., Young, L., & Loh, A. (2017). Expressive writing among Chinese American breast cancer survivors: A randomized controlled trial. *Health Psychology, 36*(4), 370–379.
57. Krebber, A. M. H., van Uden-Kraan, C. F., Melissant, H. C., Cuijpers, P., van Straten, A., Becker-Commissaris, A., Leemans, C. R., & Verdonck-de Leeuw, I. M. (2017). A guided self-help intervention targeting psychological distress among head and neck cancer and lung cancer patients: Motivation to start, experiences and perceived outcomes. *Supportive Care in Cancer, 25*(1), 127–135.

58. Beatty, L., Kemp, E., Butow, P., Girgis, A., Schofield, P., Turner, J., Hulbert-Williams, N. J., Levesque, J. V., & Koczwara, B. (2017). A systematic review of psychotherapeutic interventions for women with metastatic breast cancer: Context matters. *Psycho-Oncology, 27*(1), 34–42.
59. Tabrizi, F. M., Radfar, M., & Taei, Z. (2016). Effects of supportive-expressive discussion groups on loneliness, hope and quality of life in breast cancer survivors: A randomized control trial. *Psycho-Oncology, 25*(9), 1057–1063.
60. Grégoire, C., Bragard, I., Jerusalem, G., Etienne, A. M., Coucke, P., Dupuis, G., Lanctôt, D., & Faymonville, M. E. (2017). Group interventions to reduce emotional distress and fatigue in breast cancer patients: A 9-month follow-up pragmatic trial. *British Journal of Cancer, 117*(10), 1442–1449.
61. Scheier, M. F., Helgeson, V. S., Schulz, R., Colvin, S., Berga, S. L., Knapp, J., & Gerszten, K. (2007). Moderators of interventions designed to enhance physical and psychological functioning among younger women with early-stage breast cancer. *Journal of Clinical Oncology, 25*(36), 5710–5714.
62. Andersen, B. L. (1992). Psychological interventions for cancer patients to enhance the quality of life. *Journal of Consulting and Clinical Psychology, 60*(4), 552–568.
63. Hedman, C., Djärv, T., Strang, P., & Lundgren, C. I. (2016). Determinants of long-term quality of life in patients with differentiated thyroid carcinoma–a population-based cohort study in Sweden. *Acta Oncologica, 55*(3), 365–369.
64. Huang, I. C., Hudson, M. M., Robison, L. L., & Krull, K. R. (2017). Differential impact of symptom prevalence and chronic conditions on quality of life in cancer survivors and non-cancer individuals: A population study. *Cancer Epidemiology and Prevention Biomarkers, 26*(7), 1124–1132.
65. Kreitler, S., Barak, F., Alkalay, Y., & Ostrovsky, A. (2014). *Nutrition and quality of life in advanced cancer patients*. Poster presented at the 21st annual conference of the International Society for Quality-of-Life Studies (ISQOLS), Berlin, Germany.
66. Kreitler, S., & Barak, F. (2012). Nutrition and quality of life in cancer patients with advanced disease. *Supportive Care in Cancer, 20*(Supp. 1), S132–S133.
67. Barak, F., Kreitler, S., Isimov, V., Segal, S., Shlanger, S., & Kinchin, I. (2001). Nutritional habits of patients with advanced cancer. *European Journal of Palliative Care, 85.*
68. Galindo, D. E. B., Vidal-Casariego, A., Calleja-Fernández, A., Hernández-Moreno, A., de la Maza, B. P., Pedraza-Lorenzo, M., Rodríguez-García, M. A., Ávila-Turcios, D. M., Alejo-Ramos, M., Villar-Taibo, R., & Urioste-Fondo, A. (2017). Appetite disorders in cancer patients: Impact on nutritional status and quality of life. *Appetite, 114*, 23–27.
69. Wu, Z., Wu, M., Wang, Q., Zhan, T., Wang, L., Pan, S., & Chen, G. (2018). Home enteral nutrition after minimally invasive esophagectomy can improve quality of life and reduce the risk of malnutrition. *Asia Pacific Journal of Clinical Nutrition, 27*(1), 129.
70. Teng, F. F., Kalloger, S. E., Brotto, L., & McAlpine, J. N. (2014). Determinants of quality of life in ovarian cancer survivors: A pilot study. *Journal of Obstetrics and Gynaecology Canada, 36*(8), 708–715.
71. Chabowski, M., Polański, J., Mazur, G., Janczak, D., & Rosińczuk, J. (2017). Sociodemographic and clinical determinants of quality of life of patients with non-small cell lung cancer. In *Clinical management of pulmonary disorders and diseases* (pp. 1–10). Cham: Springer.
72. Dai, Y. L., Yang, C. T., Chen, K. H., & Tang, S. T. (2017). Changes in and determinants of quality of life in patients with advanced non-small-cell lung cancer undergoing initial chemotherapy. *Journal of Nursing Research, 25*(3), 203–215.
73. Penson, D. F. (2001). The effect of erectile dysfunction on quality of life following treatment for localized prostate cancer. *Reviews in Urology, 3*(3), 113–119.
74. Vitale, S. G., La Rosa, V. L., Rapisarda, A. M. C., & Laganà, A. S. (2018). Fertility preservation in women with gynaecologic cancer: The impact on quality of life and psychological well-being. *Human Fertility, 21*(1), 35–38.

75. Wittmann, V., Látos, M., Horváth, Z., Simonka, Z., Paszt, A., Lázár, G., & Csabai, M. (2017). What contributes to long-term quality of life in breast cancer patients who are undergoing surgery? Results of a multidimensional study. *Quality of Life Research, 26*(8), 2189–2199.
76. DeRouen, M. C., Smith, A. W., Tao, L., Bellizzi, K. M., Lynch, C. F., Parsons, H. M., & Keegan, T. H. (2015). Cancer-related information needs and cancer's impact on control over life influence health-related quality of life among adolescents and young adults with cancer. *Psycho-Oncology, 24*(9), 1104–1115.
77. Ghodraty, V. J., Alibhai, S. M. H., Fitch, M., Tourangeau, A. E., Ayala, A. P., & Puts, M. T. E. (2017). Antecedents and outcomes of uncertainty in older adults with cancer: A scoping review of the literature. *Oncology Nursing Forum, 44*(4), E152–E167.
78. Chapple, A., Ziebland, S., & McPherson, A. (2004). Stigma, shame, and blame experienced by patients with lung cancer: Qualitative study. *British Medical Journal, 328*(7454), 1470.
79. Arraras, J. I., Illarramendi, J. J., Viudez, A., Ibáñez, B., Lecumberri, M. J., Cruz, S., Hernandez, B., Zarandona, U., Cambra, K., Martinez, M., & Salgado, E. (2013). Determinants of patient satisfaction with care in a Spanish oncology Day Hospital and its relationship with quality of life. *Psycho-Oncology, 22*(11), 2454–2461.
80. Barinková, K., & Mesároová, M. (2013). Anger, coping, and quality of life in female cancer patients. *Social Behavior and Personality, 41*(1), 135–142.
81. Czerw, A. I., Religioni, U., Deptała, A., & Fronczak, A. (2017). Pain, acceptance of illness, adjustment to life with cancer and coping strategies in prostate cancer patients. *Archives of Medical Science, 13*(6), 1459.
82. Nipp, R. D., Greer, J. A., El-Jawahri, A., Moran, S. M., Traeger, L., Jacobs, J. M., Jacobsen, J. C., Gallagher, E. R., Park, E. R., Ryan, D. P., Jackson, V. A., Pirl, W. F., & Temel, J. S. (2017). Coping and prognostic awareness in patients with advanced cancer. *Journal of Clinical Oncology, 35*(22), 2551–2557.
83. Greer, J. A., Jacobs, J. M., El-Jawahri, A., Nipp, R. D., Gallagher, E. R., Pirl, W. F., & Temel, J. S. (2017). Role of patient coping strategies in understanding the effects of early palliative care on quality of life and mood. *Journal of Clinical Oncology, 36*(1), 53–60.
84. Chaturvedi, S. K., Shenoy, A., Prasad, K. M. R., Senthilnathan, S. M., & Premlatha, B. S. (1996). Concerns, coping and quality of life in head and neck cancer patients. *Supportive Care in Cancer, 4*(3), 186–190.
85. Wiggers, J. H., Donovan, K. O., Redman, S., & Sanson-Fisher, R. W. (1990). Cancer patient satisfaction with care. *Cancer, 66*(3), 610–616.
86. Nguyen, T. V. F., Anota, A., Brédart, A., Monnier, A., Bosset, J. F., & Mercier, M. (2014). A longitudinal analysis of patient satisfaction with care and quality of life in ambulatory oncology based on the OUT-PATSAT35 questionnaire. *BMC Cancer, 14*(1), 42.
87. Aboshaiqah, A., Al-Saedi, T. S. B., Abu-Al-Ruyhaylah, M. M. M., Aloufi, A. A., Alharbi, M. O., Alharbi, S. S. R., Al-Saedi, A. S., & Al-Erwi, A. F. (2016). Quality of life and satisfaction with care among palliative cancer patients in Saudi Arabia. *Palliative and Supportive Care, 14*(6), 621–627.
88. Kreitler, S., & Kreitler, H. (1991). Cognitive orientation and physical disease or health. *European Journal of Personality, 5*(2), 109–129.
89. Kreitler, S., Chaitchik, S., Rapaport, Y., & Algor, R. (1991, October). *Cognitive-motivational determinants of quality of life in cancer patients.* Lecture presented at the 6th European conference on clinical oncology and cancer nursing (ECCO 6), Florence.
90. Kreitler, S., Chaitchik, S., Kreitler, H., & Rapoport, Y. (1991). Psychosocial effects of information in head and neck cancer patients. In J. C. Holland, L. M. Lesko, & M. J. Massie (Eds.), *Current concepts in psycho-oncology IV* (p. 207). New York: Memorial Sloan-Kettering Cancer Center.
91. Mazanec, S. R., Daly, B. J., Douglas, S. L., & Lipson, A. R. (2010). The relationship between optimism and quality of life in newly diagnosed cancer patients. *Cancer Nursing, 33*(3), 235.
92. Herzberg, P. Y., Lee, S. J., Heussner, P., Mumm, F. H., Hilgendorf, I., von Harsdorf, S., Hemmati, P., Rieger, K., Greinix, H. T., Freund, M., Holler, E., & Wolff, D. (2013). Personality

influences quality-of-life assessments in adult patients after allogeneic hematopoietic SCT: Results from a joint evaluation of the prospective German Multicenter Validation Trial and the Fred Hutchinson Cancer Research Center. *Bone Marrow Transplantation, 48*(1), 129.
93. Lattie, E. G., Asvat, Y., Shivpuri, S., Gerhart, J., O'Mahony, S., Duberstein, P., & Hoerger, M. (2016). Associations between personality and end-of-life care preferences among men with prostate cancer: A clustering approach. *Journal of Pain and Symptom Management, 51*(1), 52–59.
94. Rousseau, P. (2000). Topics in review: Hope in the terminally ill. *Western Journal of Medicine, 173*(2), 117–118.
95. Kreitler, S., Chaitchik, S., Rapoport, Y., Kreitler, H., & Algor, R. (1993). Life satisfaction and health in cancer patients, orthopedic patients and healthy individuals. *Social Science and Medicine, 36*(4), 547–556.
96. Kreitler, S. (2016). Meaningfulness of life and its impact on quality of life. In C. Pracana & M. Wang (Eds.), *International psychological applications and trends (InPact)* (pp. 392–394). Lisbon: W.I. R. S.
97. Lee, M. K., & Yun, Y. H. (2018). Family functioning predicts end-of-life care quality in patients with cancer: Multicenter prospective cohort study. *Cancer Nursing*, 41(3), E1–E10.
98. Lim, J. W., & Ashing-Giwa, K. T. (2013). Is family functioning and communication associated with health-related quality of life for Chinese-and Korean-American breast cancer survivors? *Quality of Life Research, 22*(6), 1319–1329.
99. Colloca, G., & Colloca, P. (2016). The effects of social support on health-related quality of life of patients with metastatic prostate cancer. *Journal of Cancer Education, 31*(2), 244–252.
100. Costa, A. L. S., Heitkemper, M. M., Alencar, G. P., Damiani, L. P., Da Silva, R. M., & Jarrett, M. E. (2017). Social support is a predictor of lower stress and higher quality of life and resilience in Brazilian patients with colorectal cancer. *Cancer Nursing, 40*(5), 352–360.
101. White, M., & Dorman, S. M. (2001). Receiving social support online: Implications for health education. *Health Education Research, 16*(6), 693–707.
102. Rogers, S. N., Harvey-Woodworth, C. N., Hare, J., Leong, P., & Lowe, D. (2012). Patients' perception of the financial impact of head and neck cancer and the relationship to health related quality of life. *British Journal of Oral and Maxillofacial Surgery, 50*(5), 410–416.
103. Gangane, N., Khairkar, P., Hurtig, A. K., & San Sebastián, M. (2017). Quality of life determinants in breast cancer patients in Central Rural India. *Asian Pacific Journal of Cancer Prevention: APJCP, 18*(12), 3325–3332.
104. Ringdal, K., & Ringdal, G. I. (2017). Quality of life and living with cancer: findings from the European social survey (2014) special module on the social determinants of health. *The European Journal of Public Health, 27*(suppl_1), 115–119.
105. Goździewicz, B., Strugała, M., Talarska, D., Stanisławska, J., & Bączyk, G. (2017). Functioning of people with colorectal cancer during chemotherapy: Demographic and clinical determinants of quality of life of patients with colorectal cancer receiving chemotherapy. Pilot study. *European Journal of Cancer, 26*(3), e12616.
106. Kreitler, S., Peleg, D., & Ehrenfeld, M. (2007). Stress, self-efficacy and quality of life in cancer patients. *Psycho-Oncology, 16*(4), 329–341.
107. Kypriotakis, G., Vidrine, D. J., Francis, L. E., & Rose, J. H. (2016). The longitudinal relationship between quality of life and survival in advanced stage cancer. *Psycho-Oncology, 25*(2), 225–231.
108. Kim, G. M., Kim, S. J., Song, S. K., Kim, H. R., Kang, B. D., Noh, S. H., Chung, H. C., Kim, K. R., & Rha, S. Y. (2017). Prevalence and prognostic implications of psychological distress in patients with gastric cancer. *BMC Cancer, 17*(1), 283.
109. Challinor, J. M., Miaskowski, C. A., Franck, L. S., Slaughter, R. E., Matthay, K. K., Kramer, R. F., Veatch, J. J., Paul, S. M., Amylon, M. D., & Moore, I. M. (1999). Somatization, anxiety and depression as measures of health-related quality of life of children/adolescents with cancer. *International Journal of Cancer, 83*(S12), 52–57.

110. Eiser, C., & Morse, R. (2001). Can parents rate their child's health-related quality of life? Results of a systematic review. *Quality of life Research, 10*(4), 347–357.
111. Kreitler, S., & Kreitler, M. M. (2012). Quality of life in children with cancer. In S. Kreitler, M. W. Ben-Arush, & A. Martin (Eds.), *Pediatric psycho-oncology* (2nd ed., pp. 18–31). Oxford, UK: Wiley-Blackwell.
112. Logsdon, R. G., Gibbons, L. E., McCurry, S. M., & Teri, L. (2002). Assessing quality of life in older adults with cognitive impairment. *Psychosomatic Medicine, 64*(3), 510–519.

Chapter 11
The Family in Cancer

The Involvement of Family in the Cancer Disease

When an individual becomes sick, many more people than the individual himself or herself become involved. This may concern friends, acquaintances, colleagues at work, and many others but primarily one's family. The family is always involved, for better or worse, regardless of how close or distant one's relationship with the family has been and regardless of the socioeconomic or psychological state of the family. The approach which expects the family to be involved in the situation rests on four major anchors: the patient, who may be in need of support; members of the family, who may want or feel obliged to contribute as much as possible to the patient's welfare and health; the healthcare team including the physician who may expect to rely at least partly on the family's help; and the state system, including the ministry of health, which would like to use some of the nursing family resources for helping the patient.

Although it has become a commonplace assumption that the family is involved when a person becomes a cancer patient, it is still legitimate to ask why and how it is involved. The question may seem superfluous or even surprising in regard to a "normative" family in a so-called regular environment, in which there have been good relations between the patient and one's family. In families of this kind, it is expected and it is the rule that the family is a major and necessary participant in the cancer situation and trajectory.

The Family as the Solution

A normative well-functioning family can be an important component in the patient's coping with the disease. First, the family as a whole as well as in terms of specific members of the family provides the patient support. The support is

S. Kreitler, *Psycho-Oncology for the Clinician*,
https://doi.org/10.1007/978-3-030-06126-5_11

usually of different kinds. The family provides emotional support in that the patient is actually never required to deal on one's fears and problems. There is mostly someone who listens, advises, and can alleviate the anxiety. Family members can help the patient realize at least emotionally that what seems to be very scary or even catastrophic may turn out to be tolerable. one's depression, distress, and different kinds of misery are held at bay in the context of a supportive family. The family support can also be of the cognitive kind in that the family members help the patient to get information from the health professionals, the Internet, or even other patients and may also help in understanding the information or exploring modes of dealing with it, such as treatment options. In cases when the patient tends to deny the information, the family is of great importance in getting the information or helping the patient get it at a rate acceptable to him or her. In addition, there is the social support which implies that the patient needs never to be alone or at least not for long. In the family context, there is mostly someone available to keep the patient company, and there may be occasions prompting attendance in different social events concerning the family or extended family. The family members often provide also instrumental support, which may range from accompaniment to the hospital for getting treatment to purchasing medication. Instrumental support includes mostly also taking care of daily needs, such as getting food, washing, and grooming.

Help in coping and decision-making concerning medical issues may be one of the most important contributions of the family. There is a lot of uncertainty involved in these decisions because of lack of complete information and difficulty of assuming responsibility for crucial issues concerning sometimes the risk of serious health outcomes (see Chap. 7; see also Chap. 13). Some patients though possibly not all derive confidence from sharing with family members the discussion, the information, and sometimes the decision itself.

There is a lot of evidence that families can be a great help for cancer patients in coping with the disease and treatments in the different phases of the disease (see Chap. 3). In the stage of diagnosis, family members can help in getting the relevant information, coordinating it, finding out about treatment options, helping in decisions, and supporting the patient emotionally in the waiting period. In the treatment period, family members provide instrumental support and may help the patient to function despite the treatment difficulties. In the survivorship phase, the family may be a great help in constructing and adjusting to the changes in lifestyle necessitated by the disease. In the phase of disease recurrence, the family may help in guiding the patient in decisions about tests and treatments. In the palliative stage, the family may contribute by providing directly and indirectly all the necessary nursing and emotional support.

Notably, studies show that family care and support have not only direct beneficial effects for the patient but also indirect ones. For example, patients who had a family caregiver reported better coping with challenges, more positive changes in life, adopting healthier habits [1], and participating more in computer-mediated support groups [2].

Difficulties of Families in the Cancer Situation

It has become evident that in view of the shift to outpatient and home-based care, the family is slowly becoming the primary caretaker especially in regard to non-hospitalized patients [3–5]. Hence, it is important to examine the difficulties of families and alleviate their burden as much as possible so as to keep this resource of patient support in an optimal state.

Any family whose member has become a cancer patient has difficulties. The difficulties dealt within the present context may characterize any family, without dwelling on any particular circumstances. Studies show an increase in stress and reduction in the quality of life in families with a cancer patient [6–9]. A major reason has to do with the necessity to perform a load of new requirements, duties, and obligations related to the patient's needs in addition to one's regular tasks. The obligations related to the patient include, for example, contacting with one or more doctors and other health professionals; getting the required medications; obtaining the right kind and amount of information about the patient's diagnosis, state, and treatment [10, 11]; accompanying the patient when he or she cannot go alone; providing food and other necessities; etc. These requirements are diverse; invovle different people; are time-consuming; concern contact with several institutions, such as clinics, hospitals, and insurance agencies; may be urgent; should be done on time without delay; are subject to changes sometimes from 1 day to the next and certainly over time; and are mostly unfamiliar to the family members. These duties have to be performed while the family member is engaged in one's regular responsibilities at home and at work. Further, the tasks – both new ones and the regular ones – are performed under the pressure of anxiety, worry, and concern for the patient's state and perhaps even survival. Sometimes financial worries are added to the burden [12].

Carrying out the load of new and regular tasks requires planning, changes in one's behavior, effective strategies, flexibility, and energy – all of which make for effective coping. This, however, needs to be complemented by a more or less radical change in the functioning of the whole family which may include a redistribution and redefinition of the roles in the family [13, 14]. For example, grown-up children who have devoted all their time to studies and entertainment are called upon to participate in household chores; a grandmother may be mobilized for attending to the patient several hours per day; and an uncle may be asked to travel to a pharmacy to get some medication. However, not rarely, the perspectives of the family caretaker and of the patient about the challenges of the situation do not match and may generate further tension [15].

The changes do not skip the patient himself or herself. A family member who has become a patient is automatically placed on the accepting end, rather than the giving one. The patient becomes the needy person; the one who should be getting help, attention, and care; and the one who evokes concern and worries and increases the workload and possibly also the burden of financial expenses of the family involved in getting medical help, nursing support, and other requirements [16, 17]. Needless to mention, the patient may feel uncomfortable, responsible for the extra troubles, and even guilty.

Changes of this kind in the family functioning do not represent merely temporary changes in functions but culminate sooner or later in a change of roles in the family. However, roles are not defined merely by a set of tasks assigned to or performed regularly by a certain family member. Roles carry the connotation of psychological function in the family system and often imply also one's status. Investigators of the family system have identified basic roles that characterize family members. Some of the most typical roles are that of "the hero," "the problem-solver," the enabler" "the clown," "the scapegoat," "the lost child," "the just one," "the responsible adult," or "the sufferer" [18]. While these roles are defined in terms of the so-called general skills or approaches, there may be also other roles defined in terms of domains, such as the expert for health issues, the expert for entertainment and hospitality, and the expert for resolving family conflicts, or the decision-maker role [19].

The roles in the family are determined both by the personality tendencies of the individual and the requirements of the family system. They are mostly fixed and contribute to maintaining the stability of the family functioning. However, a crisis such as a major health issue may disrupt the role structure of a family and hence promote disorientation and anxiety which affect negatively the quality of life and especially the emotional well-being of the family members. A reinstatement of the role structure of the family involves changes in the functioning and the status of the different family members. Often some tension remains in the system since the load of tasks assigned to at least some members is increased, both because of the need to take care of the patient and because the patient is not always capable of performing all his or her previously performed tasks in the family. Increasing the burden of one or more family members is likely to evoke at least some anger on their part. They often consider it as both difficult and unjust that the extra load of obligations falls on them.

In order to better understand the functioning of the family in the case of a cancer patient, it is necessary to consider also the contribution of the culture to which the family and the patient belong [20, 21]. It is the culture which shapes to some extent the responsibilities of the family in regard to a sick family member. In some cultures the responsibilities of the family toward the individual member include providing far-reaching care in all stages and accompanying the patient in all phases so as to help physically and psychologically as much as possible. On the other end, there are cultures which barely consider the responsibilities of the family toward the individual member, regardless of whether he or she is sick or healthy. The former are more likely to be found in the so-called collectivistic cultures and the latter rather in individualistic cultures [22–24]. In collectivistic cultures, family members are more aware of their obligations toward the individual members because the family system is considered as consisting mainly of relations, bonds, interactions, and interdependencies rather than of independent individuals, as is more characteristic of the individualistic cultures. It is likely that the difficulties of caring for a sick family member are relatively smaller in families that function in the context of a collectivistic approach.

However, beyond the cultural background, there is the contribution of the specific family to defining its responsibilities toward the individual member who has become a patient. Some families have a tradition of taking care of their members, for example, because of their values or experience in the past or profession of their members. Some families may devote more resources to taking care of their members because they possess the resources, for example, in the form of members who are unemployed or retired, space at home, and finances they can spare. Again, it is likely that the burden of caring for a cancer patient is relatively easier for families which have the tradition of caring for their members or dispose over a wider range of resources. Further, the role transitions in a family depend also on the specific needs of the patient, in line with the kind of cancer and disease stage, e.g., in the end stage, it is different than in the course of initial chemotherapy (e.g., [12]); when the patient has brain cancer, the load and stress of the caretaker are larger than in the case of other cancers [25].

Difficulties of Spouses

Spouses of cancer patients are exposed to a lot of suffering. Some of the reasons are related to the particular kind of cancer the partner got. For example, the female partners of prostate cancer patients often suffer from reduced or changed sexual intimacy because their partner's sexual functioning has been impaired through the treatments [26, 27]. Similarly, the male partners of women who had gynecological malignancies or even breast cancer may suffer from sexual difficulties because of the changes in the sexual organs or hormonal state of their partners [28].

Regardless of the site of the partner's cancer, it is likely that the partners of cancer patients tend to suffer from anxiety, a gradually increasing sadness or even depression in view of the deterioration in their partner's state [29]. The sick patient seems to slowly lose his or her abilities and sinks into another kind of existence. The patient may be unable physically or emotionally to share his/her state with the spouse, possibly trying to spare the spouse the pain of parting. The spouse feels increasingly alone and suffers from the reduced communication with the patient. In addition, the spouse may also experience empathically the sadness of the partner. The spouse becomes increasingly aware that his or her beloved partner and friend of many years is approaching death and that there is nothing that can stop the inevitable end. It is not surprising that some studies showed that spouses had similar levels of anxiety and distress as the patients themselves [30, 31].

In addition to the emotional burden of anxiety and sadness, spouse caretakers often suffer also from physical exhaustion brought about by the continuous caretaking of a sick partner. Studies show that spouse caretakers have fewer hours of sleep, take less care of themselves, have weight problems, neglect self-care in general, withdraw from their lifestyle, and often disengage from different social activities [32–36]. Sometimes the spouse caregivers have death fears [37] or become confused in regard to their self-identity [35]. The physical difficulty and exhaustion over time added to the emotional burden may amount to what may be called caretaker burnout, which is a common phenomenon in health professionals [38]. In this state the spouse caretaker could have thoughts which may express wishes for the death of the patient, such as "it would be better for him/her if death released him/her from all this suffering" or "I am not sure I can bear this any longer." Thoughts of this kind may be scaring and often evoke guilt feelings and emotional confusion for the partner [39–42]. There is evidence that the increased emotional and physical stress of spouse caretakers may lead to impairment in their physical health in the course of taking care of the patient and mainly later [43, 44].

The spouse of the patient has been often identified as the family member who is most affected by the patient's disease. This may reflect the reality or the implicit assumption of investigators who identified the spouse as the major anchor for maintaining the functioning of the family and preserving its well-being. Notably, there is a difference between men and women as caretakers. Gender seems to play an important role in regard to the caretakers' distress and overall impact on one's life and quality of life. Women are often more involved in taking care of the patient's medical symptoms, devote more time to caretaking, and often report more stress and distress [45–48].

Be it as it may, the majority of studies have focused on the spouse and his or her needs. Reviews of studies that focused on the needs of spouse caregivers in regard to different kinds of cancer patients have led to identifying five basic issues. One important issue concerns getting sufficient and correct medical information about how to help the patient most adequately and comprehensively [49]. This need gains in importance in view of the fact that an increasing number of medical services for the patient is assigned to the spouse who is mostly medically completely uneducated. Part of the assistance consists in instructing the spouse how to continue getting information as needed. Further needs of spouses are maintaining good and continuous communication with their sick partner [50], applying effective coping strategies that are based on active handling of the problems as they turn up [51], getting sufficient emotional and instrumental support from others [52, 53], and taking care of themselves [54].

In addition to the information from health professionals and external agents such as the insurance companies, hospitals, and sometimes assisting volunteers, the spouse caretaker needs to face also the issue of getting information from the patient himself or herself. There are several barriers to proper communication between family partners. The patient may be reluctant to share one's physical and emotional state with the partner possibly in order to avoid full confrontation with one's state and probably also in order to spare one's partner the pain and suffering. Additionally, studies show that patients tend not to fully trust their partners that they provide all the information they have [11]. Similarly, the partners tend not to fully rely on the information they get from the patients themselves [55].

It should however be mentioned that there is also evidence about the positive impact of caring for a cancer patient in the family. Following the caretaking, the spouse caretaker may undergo more screening for cancer [56] and may also change one's health-caring habits in general [1]. Some spouses may undergo posttraumatic growth [53]. There is also evidence for increased cohesion and closeness of relations in at least some families [57, 58].

A different situation characterizes a family in which the patient is a child (see Chap. 15).

Difficulties of Children in the Family of a Cancer Patient

A separate set of problems harasses children in families in which one member is a cancer patient. The present section focuses on the impact of a sick parent or grandparent (for the impact of sick siblings, see Chap. 15). When one parent is sick, the children may get less support both from the sick parent and from the healthy parent who takes care of the sick parent. In families of this kind, children are in distress both because they worry about the sick parent and his or her future and about their own fate [59–62]. The range of effects may be broad, including stress, lower grades in school, emotional suffering, anxiety, depression, fears, and behavioral disorder symptoms such as alcohol and drugs [63, 64]. There is some evidence that children are more affected when the father is ill [65] and that adolescent girls are more affected than the boys [66].

The amount and kind of effect depend both on the atmosphere and functioning of the family and the age and state of the child. In families with more open communication venues and sharing of difficulties and strategies of coping, the functioning of the children is better [67, 68]. Special problems arise when the parents feel guilty about the impact their disease may have on the children or the children assume that they may have something to do with the occurrence of the parent's disease or they may experience anger at the illness that threatens to separate them from the parent [69]. The situation is so much more serious when the parent is about to die (see Chap. 13).

The situation of the children and the impact on them depend to a great deal on their age. Young children are affected to a greater extent and need more physical and educational support than teenagers and adolescents. Older children may sometimes be less impacted only because they may be busy helping with different chores at home [70]. There are usually formal and informal intervention programs designed to help the children and their parents to cope with the difficulties [71–76].

Experience with families in which a parent is sick shows that children often have a realistic comprehension of the situation. Even children as young as 6 years may confront the situation by addressing the available adults with questions such as "who will take care of me when dad/mom is not with us?" or "who will prepare the food?" or "where will I sleep?" The worries of children may extend even beyond the boundaries of life, as in the case of the following 7-year-old boy who asked right after his father's death from colorectal cancer whether the dead return after they die. He further explained that although he loved his father very much, he did not want him to return in the state he was in because it would mean the family would have no fun in daily life.

Special Difficulties in Families of Cancer Patients

Some kinds of families may pose special difficulties for patients and healthcare professionals. There are different kinds of such families. Some families are not helpful for the patient because of psychological morbidity. Thus, families with one or more members with clinical levels of anxiety and depression were found to be at risk for promoting a poor psychological outcome in the cancer patients of those families [77]. Notably, families in which a third of the spouses and about half of the children were identified as suffering from depression, also about a half of the patients were depressed [69].

However, all these families seem to share the feature of being nonfunctional from the point of view of the patient. According to one commonly applied approach, the following dimensions are relevant for characterizing the functionality of families with a cancer patient: cohesiveness, conflict, and expressiveness of emotions. These dimensions are used for characterizing four kinds of families: supportive families (high in cohesiveness and in resolving conflicts), conflictual families (with medium levels of conflicts), uninvolved families (moderate in conflict and cohesion and low in expressiveness), and ordinary families (intermediate in cohesiveness, conflict, and expressiveness) [78]. In supportive families, there are the lowest levels of anxiety and depression, whereas in the conflictual and uninvolved ones, there are the highest levels. Further, families able to act openly, express feelings directly, and solve problems effectively had lower depression levels. Direct communication of information in the family was related with lower anxiety levels [69, 79] (Table 11.1, family taxonomy table which may be used by clinicians and health professionals).

The three identified dimensions may be used for defining further kinds of common kinds of families. Families that are high in cohesion and low in conflicts and expressiveness may provide the patient help but in a cool and distant manner without emotional support. Again, families that are high in expressiveness and conflicts

Table 11.1 Family taxonomy

Functionality of family	Type of family	Cohesiveness[a]	Expressiveness[b]	Conflicts[c]
Functional	Supportive	High	High	Low
Functional	Conflict resolving	Medium	High	Low
Nonfunctional	Conflictual	High	Medium	Medium
Nonfunctional	Uninvolved	High	Low	Low
Nonfunctional	Low communicators	Medium	Medium	Medium

Based on Schuler et al. [78] and reproduced with automatic permission from Elsevier through the STM permissions guidelines

For getting an assessment, one may assign to each of the three listed questions an evaluation in terms of a lot (=high), medium (=medium), or low (low), based on overall acquaintance with the family

[a]Degree to which the family members are united around one central goal and function together

[b]Degree to which the family members communicate and express openly their feelings and each member knows what the others feel and want

[c]Degree to which there are in the family disputes, conflicts, and unresolved problems

but low in cohesiveness may have the desire to help the patient but due to the conflicts and high emotional level find it difficult to decide on a course of action helpful to the patient and themselves.

There are different levels of nonfunctional families from the perspective of the cancer patient. The lowest level of functionality characterizes families that fall apart because one partner withdraws temporarily or divorces. Sometimes the grown-up children or teenagers escape from the home. It may happen that the patient who may be married and living with his/her family is withdrawn from one's family by his/her mother who takes control of the patient not trusting the partner. Other difficulties may arise when a family member breaks down mentally and requires extra attention and resources that are withdrawn from the cancer patient. Further manifestations of nonfunctionality occur when the family resists accepting the fact about the seriousness of the patient's disease and denies it. The denial may lead to concealing or throwing away the medications prescribed for the patient.

The functionality of families is disrupted at least to a medium degree when the family behaves in an over-defensive manner in regard to the patient, shielding him or her against getting treatments or even medical tests so that he/she will supposedly suffer no harm. Sometimes the shielding leads also to social isolation of the patient so that he/she can supposedly rest without being disturbed. Defensive families behave so as to keep the patient to themselves as much as possible. Sometimes the defensiveness is rooted in denial of the patient's medical situation; at other times, it may be enhanced by the family's general attitude of keeping closed, focused on itself, with minimal contacts with others.

In other cases one or more family members try to take advantage of the contact they have with hospitals and healthcare professionals in order to take care of themselves physically and psychologically. For example, when they meet the doctor, they present their own symptoms and not those of the patient. Sometimes they may even justify or rationalize their behavior by the claim that in order to help the patient, it is necessary for them to be healthy.

Some families may be too preoccupied by other issues and tensions to be able to free themselves for addressing the patient's needs. For example, there may be in the family conflicts and disagreements between the partners or between them and the children which render difficult or even impossible for the family members to take care of the patient. Other cases arise when the family is in a bad financial situation [12] or is in bereavement over another family member who has recently died.

Interventions and Help for the Family

In recent years there has been a growing tendency to provide the families of cancer patients attention, support, and help in different forms. "Thinking family" and "family-centered" cancer therapy have become commonplace approaches in cancer treatment. Basically there are four kinds of interventions: those that focus on the family as a whole system, those that focus on the caretaking spouse, those that focus on the relationship between partners, and those that focus on the care of children in the family of a parent with cancer. The participants in the intervention sessions may be all family members with or without the patient, all family members and other family relatives such as the grandparent, the spouse alone or with the patient, and the spouse with the children. It may be safely assumed that the boundaries between the different foci tend to get blurred. An intervention that targeted the family as a whole may easily turn into an intervention that deals with the relationship between the partners or between one of them and the children. All different interventions seem to share the same set of goals which is to improve or maintain the quality of life of the family members, help the family system to function properly, and maintain its stability despite the crisis. Attaining these goals is assumed to help the patient undergo the difficulties of the disease and the treatments and regain one's health and quality of life. The assumption is probably correct, although the theoretical relations between these goals and the patient's state are not always spelled out (e.g., [3, 80]).

The major tools of intervention are offering general and specific support; providing educational information; teaching the caregiver spouse how to deal with the patient's symptoms, how to deal with one's own stress, or how to cope in general with life situations; and improving the skills of couples for communication or resolving family conflicts by means of common psychotherapeutic means. Some of the teaching programs are systematized (e.g., Australian CanCope program).

The results of the different interventions are on the whole positive. Thus, supportive and educational interventions most commonly result in better quality of life of patients and partner [81–83], better coping by partner and better satisfaction with his/her caretaking [81, 84, 85], better physical health of caregiver [82, 86], and better information about helpful community resources [84]. In particular, symptom management interventions resulted in helping the caregiver to become more knowledgeable in dealing with symptoms, more confident and better informed about community resources [84, 87], and less depressed [88]. Focusing on coping skills of the partners and/or patients has resulted in better skills and confidence of caregiver and their lower distress [89, 90]. Focusing on relationships has resulted in improved relations between the partners facing the need for changes [91], but intervention only with the wives of prostate cancer helped the wives' distress but not communication with the husbands [85], which implies that the intervention needs to be targeted specifically.

An exceptional program for helping adult patients who are parents to children up to 18 years is the parents' guidance model called PACT (Parenting at a Challenging Time) [76]. It is not a traditional psychotherapy for family or couples or parents or children but a supportive intervention that deals with identifying and using the skills that parents have, assuming that parents are the best supporters of their children and can best help them when they get the proper guidance from experts. The major guiding principles are open, honest, and child-centered communication in the family; minimizing disruption; protecting family time; maximizing the support system; and legacy leaving. The practical approach is defined in terms of the following six steps of learning: about the parents, about the children and their specific concerns, about how the family has faced previous challenges, about the parents' support system, about what is expected of the children, and about specific strategies that may facilitate the family's optimal adjustment to the parent's illness. PACT is an example of a program exceptional in its simplicity and easy applicability in any context or community and in its focusing on the target directly and evoking minimal resistance or anxiety on the part of the family members.

Conclusions: The Family as the Solution and as the Problem

The different facts, approaches, and considerations presented about the family show that insofar as the cancer patient is considered, the family may indeed be the solution, but not less than that also the problem. It is the solution for some of the issues concerning the patient, mainly the provision of basic care, supplying support and help in various respects, in the different phases of the disease, and mainly in the end-of-life phase. However, getting all these benefits from one's family may require adjustments, concessions, and special considerations on the part of the patient. Yet, it may be worthwhile and operable. However, some families may be difficult to get along with. These families that are identified as nonfunctional may be conflicted, tension-laden, anxious, stressed, preoccupied, not trained in expressing emotions, in offering empathy, in communicating freely, and mainly in changing as required by the unpredictability of the disease and patient situation. In cases of this kind, the family may require the special attention of the health professionals so as to minimize the burden on the patient and maximize the support for the patient.

Yet, studies show that even in the functional families, characterized by good communication, cohesion, expressiveness of emotions, and ability to solve problems, it is necessary to provide help, support, and instruction to the caregivers so as to alleviate their burden and increase their contribution to the patient's well-being.

However it may be, special care should be taken not to get swept away in the interventions focused on the caregiving family so that the psychological treatment does not turn into a family-centered treatment, but regardless of whoever benefits or is considered, it remains always primarily patient-centered.

References

1. Litzelman, K., Blanch-Hartigan, D., Lin, C. C., & Han, X. (2017). Correlates of the positive psychological byproducts of cancer: Role of family caregivers and informational support. *Palliative & Supportive Care, 15*, 1–11.
2. Yoo, W., Shah, D. V., Shaw, B. R., Kim, E., Smaglik, P., Roberts, L. J., Hawkins, R. P., Pingree, S., McDowell, H., & Gustafson, D. H. (2014). The role of the family environment and computer-mediated social support on breast cancer patients' coping strategies. *Journal of Health Communication, 19*(9), 981–998.

3. Ferrell, B., & Wittenberg, E. (2017). A review of family caregiving intervention trials in oncology. *CA: A Cancer Journal for Clinicians, 67*(4), 318–325.
4. Teschendorf, B., Schwartz, C., Ferrans, C. E., O'Mara, A., Novotny, P., & Sloan, J. (2007). Caregiver role stress: When families become providers. *Cancer Control, 14*, 183–189.
5. Williams, A. L., & McCorkle, R. (2011). Cancer family caregivers during the palliative, hospice, and bereavement phases: A review of the descriptive psychosocial literature. *Palliative & Supportive Care, 9*(3), 315–325.
6. Schumacher, K. L., Dodd, M. J., & Paul, S. M. (1993). The stress process in family caregivers of persons receiving chemotherapy. *Research in Nursing & Health, 16*, 395–404.
7. Caruso, R., Nanni, M. G., Riba, M. B., Sabato, S., & Grassi, L. (2017). The burden of psychosocial morbidity related to cancer: Patient and family issues. *International Review of Psychiatry, 29*(5), 389–402.
8. Sales, E. (1991). Psychosocial impact of the phase of cancer on the family: An updated review. *Journal of Psychosocial Oncology, 9*, 1–18.
9. Schulz, K. H., Schulz, H., Schulz, O., et al. (1996). Family structure and psychosocial stress in families of cancer patients. In L. Baider, C. L. Cooper, & A. De-Nour Kaplan (Eds.), *Cancer and the family* (pp. 225–256). New York: Wiley.
10. Datta, S. S., Tripathi, L., Varghese, R., Logan, J., Gessler, S., Chatterjee, S., Bhaumik, J., & Menon, U. (2017). Pivotal role of families in doctor-patient communication in oncology: A qualitative study of patients, their relatives and cancer clinicians. *European Journal of Cancer Care, 26*(5), e12543.
11. Costantini, A., Grassi, L., Picardi, A., Brunetti, S., Caruso, R., Nanni, M. G., Bonetti, L., de Feudis, R., Barni, S., & Marchetti, P. (2015). Awareness of cancer, satisfaction with care, emotional distress, and adjustment to illness: An Italian multicenter study. *Psycho-Oncology, 24*(9), 1088–1096.
12. Bradley, C. J. (2017). Cancer, financial burden, and medicare beneficiaries. *Journal of Clinical Oncology, 35*(22), 2461–2462.
13. Vess, J. D., Jr., Moreland, J. R., & Schwebel, A. L. (1985). A follow-up study of role functioning and the psychological environment of families of cancer patients. *Journal of Psychosocial Oncology, 3*, 1–14.
14. Lewis, F. M. (1996). The impact of breast cancer on the family: Lessons learned from the children and adolescents. In L. Baider, C. L. Cooper, & A. Kaplan De-Nour (Eds.), *Cancer and the family* (pp. 271–288). New York: Willey.
15. Mosher, C. E., Adams, R. N., Helft, P. R., O'Neil, B. H., Shahda, S., Rattray, N. A., & Champion, V. L. (2016). Family caregiving challenges in advanced colorectal cancer: Patient and caregiver perspectives. *Support Care Cancer, 24*(5), 2017–2024.
16. Barbaret, C., Brosse, C., Rhondali, W., Ruer, M., Monsarrat, L., Michaud, P., Schott, A. M., Delgado-Guay, M., Bruera, E., Sanchez, S., & Filbet, M. (2017). Financial distress in patients with advanced cancer. *Plos One, 12*(5), e0176470.
17. Gordon, L. G., Beesley, V. L., Mihala, G., Koczwara, B., & Lynch, B. M. (2017). Reduced employment and financial hardship among middle-aged individuals with colorectal cancer. *European Journal of Cancer Care, 26*(5), e12744.
18. Marks, J., Bun, L. C., & McHale, S. M. (2009). Family patterns of gender role attitudes. *Sex Roles, 61*(3–4), 221–234.
19. Trees, A. R., Ohs, J. E., & Murray, M. C. (2017). Family communication about end-of-life decisions and the enactment of the decision-maker role. *Behavioral Science, 7*(2), 36.
20. Yeh, L. C., Kellet, U., Henderson, S., & Chen, K. H. (2015). How does culture shape roles and relationships in Taiwanese family caregiving for an adolescent with cancer? *Cancer Nursing, 38*(3), E35–E41.
21. Githaiga, J. N. (2017). Culture, role conflict and caregiver stress: The lived experiences of family cancer caregivers in Nairobi. *Journal of Health Psychology, 22*(12), 1591–1602.
22. Hofstede, G. H. (2001). *Culture's consequences: Comparing values, behaviours, institutions, and organizations across nations*. Thousand Oaks: Sage.

23. Kim, U., Triandis, H. C., Kagitcibasi, C., Choi, S. C., & Yoon, G. (Eds.). (1994). *Individualism and collectivism: Theory, method, and applications*. Thousand Oakes: Sage.
24. Triandis, H. C. (1995). *Individualism and collectivism*. Boulder: West View Press.
25. Aoun, S. M., Deas, K., Howting, D., & Lee, G. (2015). Exploring the support needs of family caregivers of patients with brain cancer using the CSNAT: A comparative study with other cancer groups. *Plos One, 10*(12), e0145106.
26. Regan, T. W., Lambert, S. D., Kelly, B., McElduff, P., Girgis, A., Kayser, K., & Turner, J. (2014). Cross-sectional relationships between dyadic coping and anxiety, depression, and relationship satisfaction for patients with prostate cancer and their spouses. *Patient Education and Counseling, 96*(1), 120–127.
27. Traa, M. J., De Vries, J., Bodenmann, G., & Den Oudsten, B. L. (2015). Dyadic coping and relationship functioning in couples coping with cancer: A systematic review. *British Journal of Health Psychology, 20*(1), 85–114.
28. Lopes, V. B., Lobo, A. P. A., Da Silva, G. B., Jr., Melo, A. K., Lamboglia, C. G., & Silva, C. A. B. D. (2017). The experience of male spouses in the context of breast cancer: A systematic review of the literature. *Psychology, Health & Medicine*, *22*, 1–10.
29. Popek, V., & Hönig, K. (2015). Cancer and family: Tasks and stress of relatives. Krebs und Familie: Aufgaben und Belastungen Angehöriger. *Der Nervenarzt, 86*(3), 266, 268–70, 272–273.
30. Northouse, L. L., Mood, D. W., Montie, J. E., Sandler, H. M., Forman, J. D., Hussain, M., Pienta, K. J., Smith, D. C., Sanda, M. G., & Kershaw, T. (2007). Living with prostate cancer: Patients' and spouses' psychosocial status and quality of life. *Journal of Clinical Oncology, 25*(27), 4171–4177.
31. Song, L., Northouse, L. L., Braun, T. M., Zhang, L., Cimprich, B., Ronis, D. L., & Mood, D. W. (2010). Assessing longitudinal quality of life in prostate cancer patients and their spouses: A multilevel modeling approach. *Quality of Life Research, 20*(3), 371–381.
32. Mosher, C. E., Champion, V. L., Azzoli, C. G., Hanna, N., Jalal, S. I., Fakiris, A. J., Birdas, T. J., Okereke, I. C., Kesler, K. A., Einhorn, L. H., Monahan, P. O., & Ostroff, J. S. (2013). Economic and social changes among distressed family caregivers of lung cancer patients. *Support Care Cancer, 21*(3), 819–826.
33. Mosher, C. E., Bakas, T., & Champion, V. L. (2013). Physical health, mental health, and life changes among family caregivers of patients with lung cancer. *Oncology Nursing Forum, 40*(1), 53–61.
34. Northouse, L., Williams, A. L., Given, B., & McCorkle, R. (2012). Psychosocial care for family caregivers of patients with cancer. *Journal of Clinical Oncology, 30*(11), 1227–1234.
35. Ugalde, A., Krishnasamy, M., & Schofield, P. (2012). Role recognition and changes to self-identity in family caregivers of people with advanced cancer: A qualitative study. *Support Care Cancer, 20*(6), 1175–1181.
36. Fujinami, R., Sun, V., Zachariah, F., Uman, G., Grant, M., & Ferrell, B. (2015). Family caregivers' distress levels related to quality of life, burden, and preparedness. *Psycho-Oncology, 24*(1), 54–62.
37. Bachner, Y. G., O'Rourke, N., & Carmel, S. (2011). Fear of death, mortality communication, and psychological distress among secular and religiously observant family caregivers of terminal cancer patients. *Death Studies, 35*(2), 163–187.
38. Bloniaz, E. R. (2011). Caring for the caretaker: A nursing process approach. *Creative Nursing, 17*, 12–15.
39. Kreitler, S., Barak, F., & Siegelmann-Danieli, N. (2009). Survivor's guilt: The case of cancer. In D. Cooley, L. Steffen, & R. Fisher (Eds.), *Death and dying*. Oxford: Inter-Disciplinary Press.
40. Kreitler, S., Barak, F., Alkalay, Y., & Siegelman-Danieli, N. (2012). Survivor's guilt in the caretakers of cancer. In A. Kasher & A. Glahn (Eds.), *The presence of the dead in our lives, A.* Interface/Probing the Boundaries Series. Amsterdam: Rodopi.

41. Kreitler, S., Barak, F., Alkalay, Y., & Siegelman-Danieli, N. (2012). Survivor's guilt in the caretakers of cancer. In N. Hinerman & J. A. Glahn (Eds.), *The presence of the dead in our lives, B* (pp. 77–98). Amsterdam: Rodopi.
42. Kreitler, S., Barak, F., & Siegelman-Danieli, N. (2012). The guilt of the survivors. In S. Kreitler & H. Shanun-Klein (Eds.), *Studies of grief and bereavement*. Book 2 in the Series Death Education. Hauppauge: Nova Publishers.
43. Jianguang, J., Zöller, B., Sundquist, K., & Sundquist, J. (2012). Increased risks of coronary heart disease and stroke among spousal caregivers of cancer patients. *Circulation, 125*, 1742–1747.
44. Girgis, A., Lambert, S., Johnson, C. D., Waller, A., & Currow, D. (2013). Physical, psychosocial, relationship, and economic burden of caring for people with cancer: A review. *Journal of Oncology Practice, 9*(4), 197–202.
45. Kim, Y., Loscalzo, M. J., Wellisch, D. K., & Spiller, R. L. (2006). Gender differences in caregiving stress among caregivers of cancer survivors. *Psychooncology, 15*(12), 1086–1092.
46. Kim, Y., & Carver, C. S. (2007). Frequency and difficulty in caregiving among spouses of individuals with cancer: Effects of adult attachment and gender. *Psycho-Oncology, 16*(8), 714–723.
47. Bakas, T., Lewis, R. R., & Parsons, J. E. (2001). Caregiving tasks among family caregivers of patients with lung cancer. *Oncology Nursing Forum, 28*(5), 847–854.
48. Given, B., Given, C. W., Sikorskii, A., Jeon, S., Sherwood, P., & Rahbar, M. (2006). The impact of providing symptom management assistance on caregiver reaction: Results of a randomized trial. *Journal of Pain and Symptom Management, 32*(5), 433–443.
49. Kim, Y., Kashy, D. A., Spillers, R. L., & Evans, T. V. (2010). Needs assessment of family caregivers of cancer survivors: Three cohorts comparison. *Psychooncology, 19*(6), 573–582.
50. Porter, L. S., Keefe, F. J., Hurwitz, H., & Faber, M. (2005). Disclosure between patients with gastrointestinal cancer and their spouses. *Psychooncology, 14*(12), 1030–1042.
51. Kershaw, T. S., Mood, D. W., Newth, G., Ronis, D. L., Sanda, G., Vaishampayan, U., & Northouse, L. L. (2008). Longitudinal analysis of a model to predict quality of life in prostate cancer patients and their spouses. *Annals of Behavioral Medicine, 36*(2), 117–128.
52. Mellon, S., Northouse, L. L., & Weiss, L. K. (2006). A population-based study of the quality of life of cancer survivors and their family caregivers. *Cancer Nursing, 29*(2), 120–131.
53. Weiss, Z. (2004). Correlates of posttraumatic growth in married breast cancer survivors. *Journal of Social and Clinical Psychology, 23*(5), 733–746.
54. McCorkle, R., Ercolano, E., Lazenby, M., Schulman-Green, D., Schilling, L. S., Lorig, K., & Wagne, E. H. (2011). Self-management: Enabling and empowering patients living with cancer as a chronic illness. *CA: A Cancer Journal for Clinicians, 61*(1), 50–62.
55. Kreitler, S., Chaitchik, S., Rapoport, Y., & Algo, R. (1995). Psychosocial effects of information and disease severity in head-and-neck cancer patients. *Journal of Cancer Education, 10*, 144–154.
56. Koca, D., Oztop, I., & Yilmaz, U. (2013). Evaluation of changes in the attitudes and behaviors of relatives of lung cancer patients toward cancer prevention and screening. *Indian Journal of Cancer, 50*(3), 233–238.
57. Kissil, K., Niño, A., Jacobs, S., Davey, M., & Tubbs, C. Y. (2010). "It has been a good growing experience for me": Growth experiences among African American youth coping with parental cancer. *Families, Systems & Health, 28*(3), 274–289.
58. Phillips, F. (2015). The experience of adolescents who have a parent with advanced cancer: A phenomenological inquiry. *Palliative & Supportive Care, 13*(04), 1057–1069.
59. Sieh, D. S., Oort, F. J., Visser-Meily, J. M. A., & Meijer, A. M. (2014). Mediators for internalizing problems in adolescents of parents with chronic medical condition. *Journal of Developmental and Physical Disabilities, 26*(1), 67–82.
60. Krattenmacher, T., Kühne, F., Ernst, J., Bergelt, C., Romer, G., & Möller, B. (2012). Parental cancer: Factors associated with children's psychosocial adjustment – A systematic review. *Journal of Psychosomatic Research, 72*(5), 344–356.

61. Lindqvist, B., Schmitt, F., Santalahti, P., Romer, G., & Piha, J. (2007). Factors associated with the mental health of adolescents when a parent has cancer. *Scandinavian Journal of Psychology, 48*(4), 345–351.
62. McDonald, F. E., Patterson, P., White, K. J., Butow, P. N., Costa, D. S., & Kerridge, I. (2016). Correlates of unmet needs and psychological distress in adolescent and young adults who have a parent diagnosed with cancer. *Psycho-Oncology, 25*(4), 447–454.
63. Morris, J. N., Martini, A., & Preen, D. (2016). The well-being of children impacted by a parent with cancer: An integrative review. *Support Care Cancer, 24*, 3235–3251.
64. Visser, A., Huizinga, G. A., van der Graaf, W. T., Hoekstra, H. J., & Hoekstra-Weebers, J. E. (2004). The impact of parental cancer on children and the family: A review of the literature. *Cancer Treatment Reviews, 30*(8), 683–694.
65. Visser, A., Huizinga, G. A., Hoekstra, H. J., van der Graaf, W. T., Klip, E. C., Pras, E., & Hoekstra-Weebers, J. E. (2005). Emotional and behavioural functioning of children of a parent diagnosed with cancer: A cross-informant perspective. *Psychooncology, 14*(9), 746–758.
66. Osborn, T. (2007). The psychosocial impact of parental cancer on children and adolescents: A systematic review. *Psychooncology, 16*(2), 101–126.
67. Chen, Y.-C., & Fish, M. C. (2013). Parental involvement of mothers with chronic illness and children's academic achievement. *Journal of Family Issues, 34*(5), 583–606.
68. Thastum, M., Johansen, B. M., Gubba, L., Olesen, L. B., & Romer, G. (2008). Coping, social relations, and communication: A qualitative exploratory study of children of parents with cancer. *Clinical Child Psychology and Psychiatry, 13*(1), 123–138.
69. Kissane, D. W., Bloch, S., Burns, W. I., McKenzie, D., & Posterino, M. (1994). Psychological morbidity in the families of patients with cancer. *Psycho-Oncology, 3*(1), 47–56.
70. Visser, A., Huizinga, G. A., Hoekstra, H. J., van den Graaf, W. T. A., & Hoekstra-Weebers, J. E. H. M. (2006). Parental cancer: Characteristics of parents as for child functioning. *Cancer, 106*(5), 1178–1187.
71. Inhestern, L., Haller, A.-C., Wlodarczyk, O., & Bergelt, C. (2016). Psychosocial interventions for families with parental cancer and barriers and facilitators to implementation and use – A systematic review. *Plos One, 11*(6), e0156967.
72. Niemela, M., Vaisanen, L., Marshall, C., Hakko, H., & Rasanen, S. (2010). The experiences of mental health professionals using structured family-centered interventions to support children of cancer patients. *Cancer Nursing, 33*(6), E18–E27.
73. Ernst, J. C., Beierlein, V., Romer, G., Moller, B., Koch, U., & Bergelt, C. (2012). Parents with cancer and their minor children—A nationwide survey of outpatient psychosocial cancer counselling service regarding needs and its utilisation. *Gesundheitswesen, 74*, 742–746.
74. Lewis, F. M., Brandt, P. A., Cochrane, B. B., Griffith, K. A., Grant, M., Haase, J. E., et al. (2015). The enhancing connections program: A six-state randomized clinical trial of a cancer parenting program. *Journal of Consulting and Clinical Psychology, 83*(1), 12–23.
75. Ernst, J. C., Beierlein, V., Romer, G., Moller, B., Koch, U., & Bergelt, C. (2013). Use and need for psychosocial support in cancer patients: A population-based sample of patients with minor children. *Cancer, 119*(12), 2333–2341.
76. Swick, S. D., Martin, A. S., & Rauch, P. (2012). When a parent has cancer: Supporting healthy child development during challenging times. In S. Kreitler, M. Weyl Ben-Arush, & A. Martin (Eds.), *Pediatric psycho-oncology: Psychosocial aspects and clinical interventions* (2nd ed., pp. 246–259). Oxford: Wiley Blackwell.
77. Edwards, B., & Clarke, V. (2005). The validity of the family relationships index as a screening tool for psychological risk in families of cancer patients. *Psycho-Oncology, 14*(7), 546–554.
78. Schuler, T. A., Zaider, T. I., Li, Y., Hichenberg, S., Masterson, M., & Kissane, D. W. (2014). Typology of perceived family functioning in an American sample of advanced cancer patients. *Journal of Pain and Symptom Management, 48*(2), 281–288.
79. Edwards, B., & Clarke, V. (2005). The psychological impact of a cancer diagnosis on families: The influence of family functioning and patients' illness characteristics on depression and anxiety. *Psycho-Oncology, 13*(8), 562–576.

80. Northouse, L. L., Katapodi, M. C., Song, L., Zhang, L., & Mood, D. W. (2010). Interventions with family caregivers of cancer patients: Meta-analysis of randomized trials. *CA: A Cancer Journal for Clinicians, 60*(5), 317–339.
81. Northouse, L. L., Mood, D. W., Schafenacker, A., Kalemkerian, G., Zalupski, M., Lorusso, P., Hayes, D. F., Hussain, M., Ruckdeschel, J., Fendrick, A. M., Trask, P. C., Ronis, D. L., & Kershaw, T. (2013). Randomized clinical trial of a brief and extensive dyadic intervention for advanced cancer patients and their family caregivers. *Psycho-Oncology, 22*(3), 555–563.
82. Budin, W. C., Hoskins, C. N., Haber, J., Sherman, D. W., Maislin, G., Cater, J. R., Cartwright-Alcarese, F., Kowalski, M. O., McSherry, C. B., Fuerbach, R., & Shukla, S. (2008). Breast cancer: Education, counseling, and adjustment among patients and partners: A randomized clinical trial. *Nursing Research, 57*(3), 199–213.
83. Northouse, L. L., Mood, D. W., Schafenacker, A., Montie, J. E., Sandler, H. M., Forma, J. D., Hussain, M., Pienta, K. J., Smith, D. C., & Kershaw, T. (2007). Randomized clinical trial of a family intervention for prostate cancer patients and their spouses. *Cancer, 110*(12), 2809–2818.
84. Robinson, K. D., Angeletti, K. A., Barg, F. K., Pasacreta, J. V., McCorkle, R., & Yasko, J. M. (1998). The development of a family caregiver cancer education program. *Journal of Cancer Education, 13*(2), 116–121.
85. Manne, S., Babb, J., Pinover, W., Horwitz, E., & Ebbert, J. (2004). Psychoeducational group intervention for wives of men with prostate cancer. *Psychooncology, 13*(1), 37–46.
86. Pasacreta, J. V., Barg, F., Nuamah, I., & McCorkle, R. (2000). Participant characteristics before and 4 months after attendance at a family caregiver cancer education program. *Cancer Nursing, 23*(4), 295–303.
87. Giarelli, E., McCorkle, R., & Monturo, C. (2003). Caring for a spouse after prostate surgery: The preparedness needs of wives. *Journal of Family Nursing, 9*(4), 453–485.
88. Kozachik, S. L., Given, C. W., Given, B. A., Pierce, S. J., Azzouz, F., Rawl, S. M., & Champion, V. L. (2001). Improving depressive symptoms among caregivers of patients with cancer: Results of a randomized clinical trial. *Oncology Nursing Forum, 28*(7), 1149–1157.
89. McMillan, S. C., Small, B. J., Weitzner, M., Schonwetter, R., Tittle, M., Moody, L., & Haley, W. E. (2006). Impact of coping skills intervention with family caregivers of hospice patients with cancer: A randomized clinical trial. *Cancer, 106*(1), 214–222.
90. Scott, J. L., Halford, W. K., & Ward, B. G. (2004). United we stand? The effects of a couple-coping intervention on adjustment to early stage breast or gynecological cancer. *Journal of Consulting and Clinical Psychology, 72*(6), 1122–1135.
91. Kuijer, R. G., Buunk, B. P., de Jong, G. M., Ybema, J. F., & Sanderman, R. (2004). Effects of a brief intervention program for patients with cancer and their partners on feelings of inequity, relationship quality and psychological distress. *Psycho-Oncology, 13*(5), 321–334.

Chapter 12
Relations with the Physicians and Medical Institutions

Introduction

When a person becomes a cancer patient, one finds oneself in a new environment, physically and psychologically, interacting with people whose identity and profession are new, doing things one has not done before, and struggling with problems and situations that until now have stayed outside one's regular action zone. It is a stressful environment because of its unfamiliarity, complexity, and significance for the patient.

The Medical Environment

The medical environment is the site or stage where the whole drama of diagnosis, treatments, recovery, survival, and recurrence is played. It is an environment with rules of its own. The goals, the major figures, the manner of operation, the regulations, the basic issues, and the interactions between the protagonists are different than in any other environment. Patients find themselves in the medical environment without any prior preparation. They are kind of thrown into it and are pressured to function fast and even make decisions without being quite oriented about its contents and procedures. This new environment resembles a system, and as in a system, any specific aspect depends in its operation and realization on the others in the system. It takes time, experience, patience, and openness of mind to learn about how the system functions so as to be able to promote one's goals without losing too much energy and without getting too often frustrated. The medical environment is highly complex because of the multiplicity of its components and their interrelations. Although the environment in a big hospital and in a smaller clinic may differ, the major aspects do not change. These are health professionals who go about their business with concentration and devotion, caring for a great many patients in

S. Kreitler, *Psycho-Oncology for the Clinician*,
https://doi.org/10.1007/978-3-030-06126-5_12

different states and with different needs, all of whom try to promote the state and needs of only one major component – themselves. This situation constitutes the groundwork for potential tension and stress. The reasons are that the health professionals, on the one hand, and the patients, on the other hand, are not completely aware of the needs and manner of operation of the other party, despite good intentions and readiness for cooperation on both sides. In addition, there are two major factors that enhance the tension in the situation: the seriousness of the tasks which may even escalate to issues of life and death and time pressure due to the multiplicity of tasks or extremity of danger.

The major component in the medical environment are the health professionals, even though it is often claimed that the major component are the patients. The health professionals are not a homogenous group. They include the doctors and in addition the nurses, dieticians, technicians of all kinds, psychologists, social workers, physiotherapists, secretaries, and other helpers. The whole system is hierarchical, in its overall structure as well as its internal structure. The overall structure refers to the pyramid of doctors at the top followed by nurses down to the nonmedical personnel. The internal structure refers to the stratification within each of the professions. Thus, for example, within the medical personnel there may be differences between a specialist doctor and a resident physician, or between doctors with different specializations, e.g., a surgeon versus a specialist in internal medicine, or within the nursing team where a registered nurse may have a different status than a nurse practitioner. Status differences between and within the professional groups are based on differences in education, pay, expertise, and power [1]. The different teams of health professionals and their members interact in many different ways as determined by the common goal they share of helping the patient and by the formal and informal interpersonal relations they may have.

The nature and complexity of the structure and interrelations in the medical environment are not always evident and transparent for the outside observer and may be quite difficult to decipher. Yet, the patients need to be aware of the different roles and interactions characterizing the medical environment in which they are treated in order to be able to get the help they need in the best manner. Understanding the system may help the patients to learn who is responsible for what and whom to address for whatever they may need. Patients often find out that they need to approach various health professionals beyond the doctor, especially the nurses, in order to proceed in implementing their treatment plan, and beyond that – their recovery. There are goals that are implemented best by specific health professionals, e.g., social workers and psychologists, rather than others. The task of integrating the advices, services, and help of the different teams may not always be easy. The task may be so complicated especially in the initial phases of the patient's introduction into the system that a patient navigator has been considered to be necessary for guiding the patient through the intricacies [2].

Understanding the system includes also learning the specific language used by the health professionals in the particular medical environment in which the patient is treated so as to comprehend what the various verbal and nonverbal expressions by the health professionals actually mean, e.g., "we will see," "it will be OK," "patience," etc.

Learning the system is necessary for the patient in order to avoid avoidable delays, to get responses and guidance, to circumvent the real or imaginary barriers, to find out what to expect in general and specifically, and to adjust one's expectations to what is actually necessary and possible.

The Doctor-Patient Relationship: The Components

The relations of the patient with the health professionals play a major role in the life of the cancer patient. These relations are unique, complex, dynamic, and highly important for the physical and psychological well-being of the patient. They are unique in comparison to other relations the patient may have; they are complex because of their multiple components – medical, mental, and interpersonal; they are dynamic because they change, mostly in line with the changes in the patient's medical state; and they are important because of their role in regard to the patient's state of health.

The patient-doctor relationship is often the most important of the patient's relationships in the medical context. It is a unique relationship because it is personal and very close but is bounded by strict regulations concerning its goals and manner of operation. In regard to cancer patients, it is further burdened by the seriousness of the disease which may be mortal, by the suffering of the patient, and by the chronicity of the disease which often prolongs the duration of the relationship.

The most basic, steady, and important component of the doctor-patient relationship is its functionality. In matter-of-fact terms, the patient needs to get from the doctor information about disease-relevant features (e.g., diagnosis, treatment, chances of recovery), help in getting the means for treatment and recovery (e.g., medications), and support in regard to the success of the whole project of getting treated and recovering. The doctor on his or her part expects from the patient cooperation in the sense of adherence to the regulations and requirements of the treatments. However, this description is not complete. A subtext needs to be added. On the part of the patient, it is necessary to add the patient's expectations which may sometimes be based on unrealistic conceptions about the situation and the possibilities of the doctor. Many of these expectations are unexpressed and possibly even not recognized. A patient may consider the doctor as an all-powerful magician who may expel the horrors of cancer by moving the wand in the right direction. Alternately, a patient may consider the doctor as a father or mother figure who is there mainly for him or her and especially for providing reassurance. Still other unrealistic doctor images may include the conception that the doctor is the patient's subordinate expected to serve and answer to all the patient's needs and requests or that the doctor is an intimate friend expected to spend time with the patient and share his or her problems with him or her.

There may also be a subtext on the part of the doctor. The doctor may feel pressured by the patient or overwhelmed by expectations he or she is neither ready nor supposed to fulfill. Again, the doctor may feel that his or her work may perhaps be futile because of the patient's physical or psychological state that minimizes the chances for cooperation or success. Sometimes the doctor may feel closer to the patient than one expected or wanted to feel which may cause one discomfort [3].

The subtext on both sides may be determined also to some extent by the reactions of one or another party to the personality of the other. For example, the patient may experience the doctor as tense, nervous, impatient, and distant, whereas the doctor may experience the patient as critical, uncooperative, and overdependent. On the other hand, doctor and patient may experience each other in terms of positive characteristics, such as friendliness, flexibility, and openness to which neither party can respond without reservation due to the contextual regulations of the medical environment.

Since the relationship is mostly prolonged, extending over months or years, both doctor and patient may feel mutual personal obligations toward each other. For example, the doctor may develop a kind of protective attitude toward a patient, and the patient may feel that deterioration in one's state of health may imply letting the doctor down after all the investment in the patient that the doctor has done.

The explicit and implicit characteristics of the situation constitute the boundaries of the interpersonal situation between doctor and patient. Be it as it may, it is evident that there is a gap between these two worlds – of doctor and patient – which is bridged mostly only temporarily through the goal of striving for the patient's recovery. The gap is comprehensive and large, based on differences in education, expertise, experience, knowledge, behavior, and mainly status. However it is approached, the relationship of doctor-patient is asymmetrical because there is someone who is in need of something that only the other can provide.

Communication in the Doctor-Patient Relationship

Communication is often considered as the mainstay of the doctor-patient relationship. But it is also one of the most difficult components of the relationship. Communication means different things for the doctor and the patient. Studies show that for the doctor, it means basically imparting the information concerning the diagnosis and the kinds of treatments that need to be undergone. If necessary, more detailed information concerning the treatments is often imparted by the other doctors on the ward and the nurses. The patient however is interested not only in the treatment plan at large but also in treatment options and the details of side effects, such as alopecia, fatigue, and other symptoms, and their expected severity [4]. Over and beyond, the patient is interested at least as much in different themes, mainly whether he or she will ever recover from the disease or whether the doctor believes that she or he will survive [5–7]. Yet patients do not always dare to ask these questions and may not even be sure that they want to know the answers. The communication in regard to these issues is further complicated by the beliefs held by at least some patients that they need to trust the doctor to tell them what he or she consider important for them to know. Thus, at the risk of generalizing, it often seems that for the doctor, information is mainly an issue that concerns facts, whereas for the patient, it focuses more on trust (see Chap. 7).

A study of doctor-patient relations identified the following behaviors on the part of the doctor as improving the relationship: reassuring the patients that it is OK to ask questions, showing and explaining the patients their lab results, asking patients about their treatment goals and preferences, avoiding judging the patients, and providing reassurance [8]. Notably, the majority of items in the recommended list of behaviors (see the first three) refer directly to information provision.

There are further aspects that contribute to the complexity of the issue of imparting and getting information in the medical context. One aspect is commonly called "truth telling." It often refers to the dilemma of doctors whether to impart to the patient all of the relevant information, especially when it is bad news [9, 10]. When doctors do not disclose all the information, it is mostly because they want to protect the patients from psychological distress or feel the patients' reluctance to confront the whole truth [9]. From the doctor's perspective, it may often seem that even if formally all the information was presented to the patient, it is rather doubtful that the patient could understand the information in the medical sense, which implies also that the all-important prognostic implications remain unclear. The patients on their side often suspect that they did not get all the truth about their medical situation, both because they may feel uncertain about their understanding of the medical terms and because they are not sure to what extent they can trust their doctor [11, 12]. Patients may feel so uncertain about their full understanding of the doctor's message that they may revert to considering also nonverbal indices accompanying the verbal statements, hoping to get some clarification through them. Additionally, not all patients feel secure and confident enough to express their doubts about the imparted information and to pose questions in regard to unclear items. As often noted, the majority of patients do not tell their doctors about their use of complementary and alternative medicine (see Chap. 8). Getting a second opinion may become a particularly sensitive issue because of the patient's fear that it may hurt the physician knowing that the patient does not sufficiently trust him or her. It is evident that patients try to avoid hurting their doctor also because of their dependence on the doctor for treatment and recovery.

A recent study identified four kinds of patients on the basis of their attitudes in regard to information: the "questioners," who have a general overall mistrust of their doctors and the information they provide; the "undecided" ones who need time in order to process the information they got and make up their mind; the "cross-checkers" whose mistrust of the information provided by the doctor leads them to double-checking it in other sources (e.g., the Internet, other physicians); and the "experience-oriented" who feel that their experience of the disease and situation deviates from that of the doctor, so that they seek information from others, often other patients or survivors. Notably, all four types express mistrust in the information provided by the doctor and the need to complement it in some form [13].

Be it as it may, communication is not a onetime affair. It goes on all during the patient's disease and undergoes changes in the course of the growing acquaintance between doctor and patient. It may include differences in treatment introduced by the doctor, reactions of the patient to the undergone treatments, and expressions of doubt by patients about whether the treatment is functioning. Balint [14] suggested the interesting metaphor "mutual investment company" for describing the gradual acquisition of information and experience in regard to the illness and the protagonists that the doctor and patient accumulate in the course of their protracted relationship. The accumulated "capital" is put to use for the benefit of both parties: the doctor learns how best to impart information to the patient and to draw some conclusions about signs that may portend changes in the patient's state of health, while the patient may learn about the best means for getting answers to one's questions and indications about how to understand the answers.

A special difficulty concerning the transmission of information may arise because of the use patients make of the Internet. Getting information from the Internet may provide the patients empowerment, but the patients are not always able to evaluate the relevance and validity of the presented information. Not all patients dare to discuss the Internet-based information with the doctor, and when they do, not all doctors have the time and patience to explain the mistakes and irrelevance of some of this information [15, 16].

Communication of information involves more aspects than those revolving around providing trustworthy and complete information. Another aspect concerns sharing personal information about themes that do not belong strictly to the medical domain. Patients often wonder about issues, such as how much they should disclose to the doctor about themselves and what is really relevant or not from their life in general, for example, should they tell the doctor about their stressful situation at work, about the troubled relations they may have with their grown-up children, and about their future plans. Sharing information of this kind may express the tendency for enhancing the personal contact with the doctor, which may be desired by some patients in order to mitigate to some extent the asymmetry of the doctor-patient relationship. Other patients may try to avoid the sharing of personal information because it may seem to them too private or of no interest for the doctor.

Difficulties in Doctor-Patient Relations

Difficulties may often arise in the doctor-patient relations. Some of them may have to do with the involved personalities. The doctor may exert more control and evidence of authority and power than are comfortable or acceptable by the patient [17, 18]. The patient on his or her side may evidence more attachment, dependence, and weakness than are manageable easily by the doctor [19]. Further, the patient may be over demanding or suspicious of the doctor to a degree that could be unpleasant for the doctor. The patient may be in need of expressions of support and encouragement by the doctor more than is usual or habitual for the doctor. Again, the doctor may express more empathy and concern for the patient than the patient is able to deal with; or, in contrast, the doctor may remain distant and aloof to a degree that render the patient uncomfortable [20].

Further sources of problems that could disturb the doctor-patient relations may be identified in the doctor's domain and in the patient's arena. The doctor may be overburdened, may suffer from burnout, and may have personal problems in the family or at work that prevent his or her complete devotion to the patients. In the arena of the patient, difficulties may arise from the involvement of family members who may contact the doctor directly or through the patient pressuring him or her for more information, attention, and care for the patient and sometimes even for themselves. It is not rare that family members try to use the patient's meeting with the doctor in order to get medical information for themselves or present their own knowledge or other good qualities. These occasions may be frustrating for both doctor and patient (see Chap. 11).

A review of the studies of doctor-patient communication summarized the major problems in communication on the patient's side as due to patients' anxiety and fears, nondisclosure of information to the doctors, resistance to being ordered around and excluded from the decision-making process, and unrealistic expectations. The barriers on the doctors' side have been found to be deterioration of communication skills, burden of work, fear of litigation, discouragement of cooperation, fear of abuse by patients, and withdrawal from contact [18].

Some of the presented examples affect the interpersonal distance between doctor and patient. The distance is an integral part of the relationship and one of the more complicated parts. The distance defines this kind of relationship, and it is in a constant state of change. It may become too large in which case it may be disturbing for one or both parties, or it may become too narrow, in which case it may be even too intimate and may even glide onto the sexual domain [21]. The later situation is not as rare as may be mostly expected, especially in the form that is limited only to romantic approaches. The motives for it, which may be largely unintentional and unconscious, are likely to include the patient's desire to obliterate maximally the asymmetry of the doctor-patient relation or provide the doctor an incentive or a present for success in the treatment. Both parties are aware of the interpersonal distance between them and are concerned about maintaining it in the form and dimensions that conform to the needs of both parties. Attaining this goal requires often adjusting the distance to changing realities.

An important factor that may affect the relations and the interpersonal distance between doctor and patient is the frustration and anger of the patient. It is almost unavoidable for the patient not to feel occasionally frustrated. The frustration is nourished by the disease itself, the pain and suffering involved in the symptoms and the treatments, the fear of death, the withdrawal from roles at work and in the family, the delays in getting treatments, and other difficulties. When the sense of helplessness in view of the situation overpowers the patient, it may happen that he or she revert to expressing hostility and even aggression, mostly limited to verbal manifestations [22]. Physically aggressive behaviors are of course prohibited and may be legally punishable. They are also detrimental for the doctor-patient relations in the specific cases when they occur and radiate over to the doctor-patient relations in general. Fear of patient aggression and litigation are sometimes expressed by doctors [18].

The Benefits of Good Doctor-Patient Communication

In the past good doctor-patient communication was often identified as "bedside manners" which a doctor may or may not have; at present it is increasingly considered as a central requirement of efficient medical treatment. Patients tend to evaluate it as a major component of the doctor's professional competence.

Studies showed that when there is good patient-doctor communication, the patients suffer less pain and are better able to tolerate pain [23]. Further, they have a higher sense of control, are more satisfied with the medical care they get, provide the doctor more relevant information about themselves; they understand better the medical information and situation and their adherence to the treatment is better [24–26]. The doctors on their side get more information that enables a more precise diagnosis and better targeted treatment plan, are better able to identify the patients' needs and expectations and to regulate the patients' emotional reactions, and are more satisfied with the medical care they provide [25]. These circumstances were found to be associated with the patients' recovery as manifested in decreased tumor growth, improved daily functioning, shorter hospital stay, fewer visits to the doctor, better psychological adjustment, lower anxiety and depression, less frustration and less tendency to complain about the doctor, and in general better recovery from illness [18, 27–29].

Satisfaction with Care

Satisfaction with care is an increasingly used construct in order to evaluate the functioning of the medical setting and of the healthcare environment in general. The evaluation by patients of their satisfaction with the medical care is becoming an important component of this construct. There is evidence that shows the benefits of patient satisfaction. For example, patients who are satisfied with the medical care they got have a better quality of life [30–32], pressure less their physicians and complain less about them and to them, have better adherence, and on the whole have better treatment outcomes [32]. Notably, at least one study showed that the evaluation of satisfaction with care provided by patients and physicians (in radiation oncology) is fairly similar [33].

On the whole, reports of satisfaction with medical care by cancer patients are rather high, mostly above medium degree of satisfaction. Concerning the determinants of patient satisfaction with care, a review of studies showed that the major determinants of patient satisfaction are the information provided by the medical staff about the disease and treatment and the interpersonal contact with the physician. Additional factors mentioned less often are duration of waiting time for an appointment, continuity of care, contribution of the nursing staff, and empathy manifested by the staff [34]. Further specification of these factors shows that satisfaction with care is affected positively by the physician's ability to give explanation to patients, helping attitude of the staff and the staff's concern for patient safety [33], as well as improvement in the patient's overall health [35]. The following are factors that were found to reduce satisfaction rating; inconvenience during scheduling of appointments, billing and registration process; status of the changing rooms and interdepartment coordination [33]; nonattendance to the patients' spiritual needs [36]; being a smoker (in the case of lung cancer patients); lack of college education, not living in a rural location, refusing to report income; not knowing/not being sure of one's disease stage [37]; financial burden during treatments [32]; too few supportive relatives, comorbidity, self-reported health, and region of treatment [38]; older age, extent of disease, too short time dedicated by the specialist, and the type of center [39]. Some specific studies highlight factors that do not affect satisfaction with care by cancer patients, for example, applying patient navigation, especially [40], or awareness that one's family is hiding bad information about one's state of health [41].

In sum, it appears that satisfaction with care is a complex and unclear construct because it is affected by many factors most of which have little to do with the actual medical treatment that the patient gets. Moreover, it is unclear which aspect of the total context is manifested in a specific evaluation by the patient of satisfaction with care, e.g., waiting time, pain, or extent of provided information. Possibly it is necessary to consider that in view of the patients' total dependence on the doctor for treatment and care, patients may hesitate to express more openly their criticism and dissatisfaction. Be it as it may, the patients' evaluation of satisfaction with care should definitely be assessed, but it should be interpreted with caution.

References

1. Salvage, J., & Smith, R. (2000). Doctors and nurses: Doing it differently: The time is ripe for a major reconstruction. *BMJ: British Medical Journal, 320*(7241), 1019.
2. Braun, K. L., Kagawa-Singer, M., Holden, A. E., Burhansstipanov, L., Tran, J. H., Seals, B. F., Corbie-Smith, G., Tsark, J. U., Harjo, L., Foo, M. A., & Ramirez, A. G. (2012). Cancer patient navigator tasks across the cancer care continuum. *Journal of Health Care for the Poor and Underserved, 23*(1), 398.
3. Mariscotti, J. (2008). A delicate dance: Negotiating the doctor-patient relationship during cancer treatment. *The Oncologist, 13*(11), 1205–1206.
4. Oskay-Özcelik, G., Alavi, S., Richter, R., Keller, M., Cecere, S. C., Cormio, G., Joly, F., Kurtz, J. E., du Bois, A., Maciejewski, M., Jedryka, M., Vergote, I., Van Nieuwenhuysen, E., Casado, A., Mendiola, C., Achimas-Cadariu, P., Vlad, C., Reimer, D., Zeimet, A. G., Friedlander, M., & Sehouli, J. (2018). EXPRESSION III: Patient's expectations and preferences regarding physician-patient relationship and clinical management. Results of the international NOGGO/ENGOT-ov4-GCIG study in 1,830 ovarian cancer patients from European countries. *Annals of Oncology, 29*, 910–916.
5. Kreitler, S., Chaitchik, S., Rapoport, Y., & Algor, R. (1995). Psychosocial effects of level of information and severity of disease on head-and-neck cancer patients. *Journal of Cancer Education, 10*(3), 144–154.
6. Chaitchik, S., Kreitler, S., Shared, S., Schwartz, I., & Rosin, R. (1992). Doctor-patient communication in a cancer ward. *Journal of Cancer Education, 7*(1), 41–54.

7. Kreitler, S., Chaitchik, S., Kovner, F., & Kreitler, H. (1992). Information in breast cancer patients: The good and the bad news. *Journal of Cancer Education, 7*(Supplement 1), 25.
8. Dang, B. N., Westbrook, R. A., Njue, S. M., & Giordano, T. P. (2017). Building trust and rapport early in the new doctor-patient relationship: A longitudinal qualitative study. *BMC Medical Education, 17*(1), 32.
9. Grassi, L., Giraldi, T., Messina, E. G., Magnani, K., Valle, E., & Cartei, G. (2000). Physicians' attitudes to and problems with truth-telling to cancer patients. *Supportive Care in Cancer, 8*(1), 40–45.
10. Shahidi, J. (2010). Not telling the truth: Circumstances leading to concealment of diagnosis and prognosis from cancer patients. *European Journal of Cancer Care, 19*(5), 589–593.
11. Seetharamu, N., Iqbal, U., & Weiner, J. S. (2007). Determinants of trust in the patient–oncologist relationship. *Palliative & Supportive Care, 5*(4), 405–409.
12. Hillen, M. A., Koning, C. C. E., Wilmink, J. W., Klinkenbijl, J. H. G., Eddes, E. H., Kallimanis-King, B. L., de Haes, J. C. J. M., & Smets, E. M. A. (2012). Assessing cancer patients' trust in their oncologist: Development and validation of the Trust in Oncologist Scale (TiOS). *Supportive Care in Cancer, 20*(8), 1787–1795.
13. Adamson, M., Choi, K., Notaro, S., & Cotoc, C. (2018). The doctor–patient relationship and information-seeking behavior: Four orientations to cancer communication. *Journal of Palliative Care*. https://doi.org/10.1177/0825859718759881.
14. Holmes, J., & Elder, A. (2016). Bowlby, Balint, and the doctor–patient relationship: Towards a theory of human relationships in medical practice. *British Journal of General Practice, 66*(648), 384–385.
15. Welch Cline, R. J., Penner, L. A., Harper, F. W., Foster, T. S., Ruckdeschel, J. C., & Albrecht, T. L. (2007). The roles of patients' internet use for cancer information and socioeconomic status in oncologist-patient communication. *Journal of Oncology Practice, 3*(3), 167–171.
16. Harvey, S., Memon, A., Khan, R., & Yasin, F. (2017). Parent's use of the internet in the search for healthcare information and subsequent impact on the doctor–patient relationship. *Irish Journal of Medical Science, 186*(4), 821–826.
17. Porcerelli, J. H., Bornstein, R. F., Porcerelli, D., & Arterbery, V. E. (2015). The complex role of personality in cancer treatment: Impact of dependency-detachment on health status, distress, and physician-patient relationship. *The Journal of Nervous and Mental Disease, 203*(4), 264.
18. Ha, J. F., & Longnecker, N. (2010). Doctor-patient communication: A review. *The Ochsner Journal, 10*(1), 38–43.
19. Brédart, A., Kop, J. L., Fiszer, C., Sigal-Zafrani, B., & Dolbeault, S. (2015). Breast cancer survivors' perceived medical communication competence and satisfaction with care at the end of treatment. *Psycho-Oncology, 24*(12), 1670–1678.
20. Ong, L. M., Visser, V. R. M., Van Zuuren, F. J., Rietbroek, R. C., Lammes, F. B., & De Haes, J. C. J. M. (1999). Cancer patients' coping styles and doctor-patient communication. *Psycho-Oncology, 8*(2), 155.
21. Collier, R. (2016). When the doctor–patient relationship turns sexual. *Canadian Medical Association Journal, 188*(4), 247–248.
22. Grube, M. (2012). Violent behavior in cancer patients—A rarely addressed phenomenon in oncological treatment. *Journal of Interpersonal Violence, 27*(11), 2163–2182.
23. Náfrádi, L., Kostova, Z., Nakamoto, K., & Schulz, P. J. (2017). The doctor–patient relationship and patient resilience in chronic pain: A qualitative approach to patients' perspectives. *Chronic Illness*. https://doi.org/10.1177/1742395317739961.
24. Arora, N. K. (2003). Interacting with cancer patients: The significance of physicians' communication behavior. *Social Science & Medicine, 57*(5), 791–806.
25. Bredart, A., Bouleuc, C., & Dolbeault, S. (2005). Doctor-patient communication and satisfaction with care in oncology. *Current Opinion in Oncology, 17*(4), 351–354.
26. Kaplan, S. H., Greenfield, S., & Ware, J. E., Jr. (1989). Assessing the effects of physician-patient interactions on the outcomes of chronic disease. *Medical Care, 27*, S110–S127.
27. Rutter, D. R., Iconomou, G., & Quine, L. (1996). Doctor-patient communication and outcome in cancer patients: An intervention. *Psychology and Health, 12*(1), 57–71.

28. Stewart, M., Brown, J. B., Boon, H., Galajda, J., Meredith, L., & Sangster, M. (1999). Evidence on patient-doctor communication. *Cancer, 25*(1999), 30.
29. Zachariae, R., Pedersen, C. G., Jensen, A. B., Ehrnrooth, E., Rossen, P. B., & von der Maase, H. (2003). Association of perceived physician communication style with patient satisfaction, distress, cancer-related self-efficacy, and perceived control over the disease. *British Journal of Cancer, 88*(5), 658.
30. Ong, L. M., Visser, M. R., Lammes, F. B., & De Haes, J. C. (2000). Doctor–patient communication and cancer patients' quality of life and satisfaction. *Patient Education and Counseling, 41*(2), 145–156.
31. Chen, J. Y., Tao, M. L., Tisnado, D., Malin, J., Ko, C., Timmer, M., Adams, J. L., Ganz, P. A., & Kahn, K. L. (2008). Impact of physician–patient discussions on patient satisfaction. *Medical Care, 46*(11), 1157.
32. Chino, F., Peppercorn, J., Taylor, D. H., Lu, Y., Samsa, G., Abernethy, A. P., & Zafar, S. Y. (2014). Self-reported financial burden and satisfaction with care among patients with cancer. *The Oncologist, 19*(4), 414–420.
33. Kataria, T., Sharma, K., Pareek, P., Goyal, S., Gupta, D., & Abhishek, A. (2006). Perception of quality in a Radiation Oncology Department: Is it different for patients and health care providers. *Indian Journal of Cancer, 53*, 152.
34. Lis, C. G., Rodeghier, M., & Gupta, D. (2009). Distribution and determinants of patient satisfaction in oncology: A review of the literature. *Patient Preference and Adherence, 3*, 287–304.
35. Nguyen, T. V. F., Anota, A., Brédart, A., Monnier, A., Bosset, J. F., & Mercier, M. (2014). A longitudinal analysis of patient satisfaction with care and quality of life in ambulatory oncology based on the OUT-PATSAT35 questionnaire. *BMC Cancer, 14*(1), 42.
36. Astrow, A. B., Wexler, A., Texeira, K., He, M. K., & Sulmasy, D. P. (2007). Is failure to meet spiritual needs associated with cancer patients' perceptions of quality of care and their satisfaction with care? *Journal of Clinical Oncology, 25*(36), 5753–5757.
37. Weiss, J., Yang, H., Weiss, S., Rigney, M., Copeland, A., King, J. C., & Deal, A. M. (2017). Stigma, self-blame, and satisfaction with care among patients with lung cancer. *Journal of Psychosocial Oncology, 35*(2), 166–179.
38. Heerdegen, A. C. S., Petersen, G. S., & Jervelund, S. S. (2017). Determinants of patient satisfaction with cancer care delivered by the Danish healthcare system. *Cancer, 123*(15), 2918–2926.
39. Miñana-López, B., Cánovas-Tomás, M. A., & Cantalapiedra-Escolar, A. (2016). Perception and satisfaction with the information received during the medical care process in patients with prostate cancer. *Actas Urológicas Españolas (English Edition), 40*(2), 88–95.
40. Wells, K. J., Winters, P. C., Jean-Pierre, P., Warren-Mears, V., Post, D., Van Duyn, M. A. S., Fiscella, K., Darnell, J., & Freund, K. M. (2016). Effect of patient navigation on satisfaction with cancer-related care. *Supportive Care in Cancer, 24*(4), 1729–1753.
41. Costantini, A., Grassi, L., Picardi, A., Brunetti, S., Caruso, R., Nanni, M. G., Bonetti, L., de Feudis, R., Barni, S., & Marchetti, P. (2015). Awareness of cancer, satisfaction with care, emotional distress, and adjustment to illness: an Italian multicenter study. *Psycho-Oncology, 24*(9), 1088–1096.

Chapter 13
Confronting Dying and Death

Introduction

Dying is an event, a process, a journey, an experience, and a concept, which gradually comes to dominate the life of the cancer patient. In the course of this development, it acquires new meanings, gets involved with a variety of evoked emotions, and is transformed in terms of the individual's narrative of life and dying.

Individuals who get the diagnosis of cancer approach it with a preceding conception of death. In the Western world, it is likely that their conception is the product of a deep-rooted fear of death, supported by existential anxieties, religious concepts, and possibly some prior exposure to death observed in friends or family members. Hence, confronting death requires from the individual to overcome the previous biased conceptions and construct an approach that would support adjustment, coping, and hopefully survival. There is a lot of learning to do in regard to dying from cancer because death has many faces, and the death from each kind of disease is unique, not only for each individual person but for each kind of context or set of circumstances in which this event occurs [1].

Death Considered from Different Perspectives

Each perspective represents a set of issues that highlight some of the involved problems in regard to dying. One type of perspective focuses on analyzing death from the different professional approaches that deal with death, namely, the medical, the physical, and the psychological. The medical approach consists in specifying in diagnostic and medical terms the different stages representing the formal aspects, such as being tested for cancer, getting the diagnosis, or entering the palliative stage. The physical approach focuses on the changes that occur in the body – in its functioning, its structure, its movement capacities, and its sensations, including pain, fatigue, restlessness,

S. Kreitler, *Psycho-Oncology for the Clinician*,
https://doi.org/10.1007/978-3-030-06126-5_13

and tension. The psychological approach refers to the changes that occur in the domains of cognition, feelings, and behaviors as the individual proceeds through the different hardships, treatments, stresses, and transformations marking the changes toward increasing disability and the slow often painful adaptation to the deterioration.

Another perspective focuses on analyzing death from the point of view of the different major individuals involved in the process and in coping with its difficulties. These are the dying patient, family members, and the healthcare professionals including the physician and the nursing personnel.

A third perspective focuses on major choices and decisions evoked by dying or referring to it. The most salient issues concern the site of death and assisting or assisted dying, for example, by suicide, euthanasia, or no-resuscitation.

The three different perspectives represent a sample of the multiple approaches or issues involved. Each provides a unique approach to death and enables the revelation of a particular aspect of death for those involved. The delineated perspectives are kinds of frameworks in which the patient is gradually exposed to different aspects of death, learns to identify them, and practices different coping means in regard to them. Thus, the perspectives complement each other and constitute the contexts through which the narrative of dying is woven.

The three mentioned perspectives of death evidently differ in their comprehensiveness. The most comprehensive one is the triad of the professional approaches, while the relatively limited one is the perspective of decisions. Moreover, the perspectives are not completely independent and interact in different multiple ways. For example, the different active or passive forms of hastening death are based on interactions between the patient, the physician, and mostly also family members. Likewise, the psychological approach is often an outcome of the physical situation of the patient in the different medically defined stages of the disease.

The Triad of Professional Approaches: The Medical, Physical, and Psychological

The triad of the professional approaches reveals dying as a multi-track set of processes, each defined in terms of its specific constituents, particular rhythm, and contents, and proceeds according to its own dynamics, all culminating in the final endpoint of death itself. Each of the three tracks exposes a particular aspect of death and brings the patient closer to considering the possibility of death [2].

The Diagnostic-Medical Approach

This approach is best reflected in the stages of the disease, which are usually the product of the impacts of the disease, the health services, and the overall context of the patient's life. *Stage 1* consists in getting tested for the disease. It is in this stage that the individual or future patient is exposed for the first time to the eventuality of death, without any particular physical or psychological preparation. Even the mere fact of being referred to tests of cancer may already be interpreted by patients as a kind of death sentence because they tend to read it as "I have cancer" and having cancer is tantamount in the naive patient's mind to "I am going to die." In this phase, which could last for weeks or even months, the patient does not have yet any help or support and is facing alone the potentiality of death. Thus, the patient's reaction to death in this phase is pure and deep anxiety, which may turn into panic. Some patients react with symptoms of acute stress disorder (e.g., avoidance of stimuli reminding cancer, hypervigilance, motor unrest), sometimes mitigated to some extent by efforts at denial. It is at this point that the process of dying starts for many cancer patients. In this interim period, the patient lives in a kind of limbo in which nothing is certain, not knowing what will follow the results of the tests. The fog of uncertainty is dispelled when the diagnosis is firmly established, but not the major question of one's survival. Not surprisingly, most cases of suicide in cancer patients have been registered in the period following diagnosis [3–5].

If the diagnosis is cancer, in *Stage 2*, patients deal mainly with undergoing the treatments, which involves managing their different side effects and surviving them without giving up one's daily routine. During this phase which may last 10–12 months, the anxiety of dying is often repressed or subsides, both because the treatments constitute a kind of weapon against the disease and death and because death anxiety may be absorbed or overshadowed by the other dominant anxieties at that time concerning life after the treatments.

In *Stage 3* the patient is in remission, freed of treatments, and expected to reconstruct one's life. Into this void the potentiality of death bursts in again. This time it is modified by the new meaning of being considered in conjunction with the issue of meaningfulness of life which often becomes pressing in view of the undergone hardships. Not surprisingly, the search for meaning in life is intimately bound to fear of death [6, 7] and even to the serious consideration of suicide. Actually, the sense of meaninglessness of life may trigger both the fear of death and the tendency for suicide, as a kind of solution for both the meaninglessness of life and fear of death [8–11]. In some cases, enhanced religiosity may provide an answer to the meaningfulness of life as well as help in overcoming the fear of death [12].

Disease recurrence which characterizes *Stage 4* ushers in the fear of death with enhanced intensity. The information about the recurrence of disease turns death into a real event with a full threatening impact that lurks in the immediate future. At this phase, undergoing a renewed series of treatments does not mitigate the fear of death because the patient's trust in the ability of the treatments to cure the disease has been shaken by previous failures. The conviction that death is unavoidable dominates this phase medically and psychologically [13]. Thus, the issue of death that has been lurking behind the scenes is pushed into the center of consciousness. The patient has done another step toward approaching death, namely, familiarizing oneself with it, interiorizing it, and preparing for it. What is given up is probably not the battle for life but rather the resistance to dying. There may be evidence for initial preparations for death, which may be manifested in taking internally leave of one's beloved ones, giving up in fantasy the ownership of some of one's personal objects (e.g., clothes, jewelry), and sometimes constructing imaginary snapshots of one's envisaged funeral. Themes of this kind are rarely shared openly with others.

Stage 5 is focused on palliative care and confronting death. Regardless of whether the patient is at home, in a hospital, or in a nursing home [14], the medical treatment is limited to medicines controlling pain or other sources of discomfort [15, 16]. The theme of death can hardly be handled by denial any more. Confronting death means that the patients find themselves thinking increasingly about death. Various surrounding stimuli sometimes help to promote this process, for example, the patients' location, the visitors and the themes or news they discuss, and sometimes the distributed information pamphlets. Different emotions may attend the process, including anger, irritability, anxiety, tension, fear, and frustration, often intermingled with memories or associations. Sometimes patients are occupied with different kinds of preparations (e.g., financial arrangements, confessions, providing information about documents or valuables, taking leave of others, transferring roles to others) which may be expected to enable the patients to have more freedom and fewer worries but often cause other worries due to misunderstandings in the family and with friends and acquaintances.

The common antedating signs of approaching death are loss of appetite, loss of weight, irregular breathing, general slowness in movement, and overall apathy. Some of the physical symptoms that actually precede the approach of death are lower blood pressure, irregular pulse, lower body temperature, increased perspiration, skin changes to pale and bluish, and difficulties in breathing, attended sometimes by congestion causing a rattling sound and cough. Hands and feet may become blotchy and purplish and then the rest of the body. The person stops responding; the eyes are open or semi-open but probably do not see. Death comes when breathing and then the heart stop. The moment of death itself varies across patients. Medically speaking, the "passage" between life and death is a transitional state called *coma*. Coma may last hours or days, and modern literature describes two aspects of coma in those dying of chronic illness:

1. The low road is characterized by an increasing silence, somnolence until natural sedation occurs, and dying. This is known as "peaceful dying."
2. The high road may be rather traumatic and occurs when the process of dying is not well controlled and is accompanied by organic brain syndromes of terminal delirium: restlessness, confusion, agitation, hallucinations, myoclonic jerks, and seizures.

The whole process is designed in terms of cardiac death or brain death, denoting complete arrest of these organs [17, 18].

The Physical Approach

The attitudes and conceptions about death are elaborated by patients in line with their physical state and changes in it, as determined by the diagnosis, the treatments, and the patient's overall state of health. The patients' evaluation of their physical state serves as basis for their conclusion how close they are to dying. In judging their physical state, patients often rely on specific kinds of information [19].

Symptoms constitute one major source of information for patients about their physical state. The symptoms most often considered by patients in this context include pain, fatigue or weakness, lack of appetite, diarrhea, bleeding, insomnia, and nausea. When patients get one or more of these symptoms recurrently or for longer periods of time, they tend to conclude that their physical state is deteriorating, often [116] without considering the cause for these symptoms. However, on the other hand, the amount of symptoms that appear as side effects of chemotherapeutic treatments may be interpreted by the patient as an optimistic sign indicating one's body is reacting well to the treatment.

The medical treatments suggested by the doctor often serve as another source of information that patients use as indicators of their physical state. When the doctor states directly or indirectly that there are no specific medical treatments that are adequate for the patient at his or her given medical state or, even worse, that no medical treatments may be of help any more, the patient interprets this communication as indicating the approach of death. Similarly, when the doctor brings up the issue of transfer to palliative care at home, in a hospice, or in a hospital, the patient concludes that the doctor gave up any hope to prevent or delay death. Even the mere amount of medication that the patient gets may serve for the patient as an indicator for the progression of the disease. Getting a lot of medication is likely to be interpreted as a sign that the doctors still believe in one's potential to recover.

The formal staging of cancer diseases from I to IV is also used by patients in evaluating their physical state, concluding that the more advanced the stage they hear from the physician or read in their file, the worse is their physical state.

Sometimes the mere name of the disease provides the patients an indication of the expected course of events. Diseases have a reputation concerning their degree of malignancy and responsiveness to treatments. Some diseases have earned the reputation of being "friendly" and others of being "dangerous." A patient who happens to identify his or her disease as highly malignant may start preparing for death earlier in the process than otherwise.

Patients may evaluate the prospects of their disease manifestations and course of disease on the basis of what they learn from or through other patients whom they meet in the hospital or clinics or self-help groups. By observing the developments in other patients, they tend to conclude – rightfully or not – that a similar fate awaits them too.

Memories of the death of other patients with whom patients have been in close contact or memories of the death of family members who had cancer may also play a role in shaping one's attitude to death in view of the physical phenomena characterizing one's disease.

The Internet is an important source of information for many patients who may use it in order to answer the questions "how am I doing?" The Internet presents information from varied sources – for example, other patients, personal opinions, anonymous doctors, cancer societies, medical journals, or other data sources.

Patients may select the information they like or which they expect or which they evaluate as most reliable or helpful.

The physician is another important source of information about one's physical state. The physician often communicates to the patients and their families what the state of the disease is. The physician may present in this context the results of medical tests or rely on statistical or scientific evidence, such as "studies show that patients who use this medication survive for 12 months" or "patients diagnosed with this kind of cancer survive a maximum of 2 years." Communications of this kind may be highly disconcerting when patients live longer than the limits established in this manner.

Some patients extract information about their physical state from the nonverbal expressions accompanying the physicians' verbal communications. Nonverbal indicators may be used for concluding rightly or erroneously whether the doctor believes in their chances to survive, regardless of the verbally stated message they get. In the doctor's facial expressions, bodily posture, or voice melody, patients may read doubt, skepticism, or disbelief in the chances of their survival which may or may not correspond to the contents of the verbal communication. Sometimes patients read optimistic hints into the nonverbal communication of the physician [20, 21].

Patients reach a kind of conclusion about the imminence of death by integrating the different sources of information, following various principles, such as addition or selection of a salient or repetitive point [21–23], whereby the sources of the information are often forgotten or deleted. The conclusion represents a kind of overall evaluation which is however susceptible to changes in view of new information or new estimates of previously available information.

Physical symptoms are used by at least some patients to assess whether they are in the process of dying. This probably characterizes mainly those patients who may somehow experience subjectively that they are approaching death. This experience is difficult to account for, but patients often refer to it. It may be manifested in internal sensations or evoke them. Sometimes these sensations are in accord with the other informations patients may have about their physical state; sometimes they precede them [24–26].

A systematic review of studies about the prevalence of symptoms reported by patients in the last days prior to dying showed that the major ones and the most bothersome are pain and shortness of breath. Mostly no distressing symptoms are present, and only for some patients expert care is necessary [17, 18].

The Psychological Approach

Withrdrawal From Life

From the psychological perspective, the most characteristic feature of dying is the progressive withdrawal from life which is manifested in minimizing gradually one's activities in different domains of life. A most common phenomenon is the withdrawal from people, friends, and acquaintances. The patient does increasingly less in order to meet one's friends and does not evidence interest in maintaining the relationships. Initially the patient may react positively to active attempts on the part of one's friends to keep up the contacts but does nothing active on one's own part. In later phases even the reaction to the active attempts from others dies down. This phenomenon may be called "social death" [27]. Similarly, the patient loses gradually interest in what happens in one's closest environment and in one's family.

Similar phenomena take place in regard to one's work or occupation. Slowly the person loses interest in one's work environment, in one's colleagues, and in what takes place in one's former working place.

The same processes characterize the patient's attitude in regard to the external environment, including the news, politics, entertainment, and celebrity figures, actually, in regard to anything that has evoked one's interest and motivation in the past but comes to be gradually replaced by a growing indifference.

A similar fate occurs in regard to activities concerning one's health, body, and appearance. For example, the person is less interested in taking care of one's external appearance, of one's clothes, and even of one's basic hygiene. One starts to forget ingesting medications or attending doctor appointments. Lowered concern with food and eating contribute slowly to growing cachexia, attended by weakness and changes in the way one looks and moves [28–30]. Processes of this kind enhance the patient's sense of helplessness and incompetence that engender demoralization [31, 32]. In more advanced stages, the process of dissociation is manifested in losing track of time of day and losing clarity about where one is and perhaps also who one is. The slow withdrawal from the outside world and into oneself may seem as a "fading away" or "gliding away." This may evoke in family members and friends the reaction "he/she is somehow no longer with us" [33].

Loss of the meaningfulness of life

Loss of the meaningfulness of life is a phenomenon that occurs often in the palliative phase, possibly as one result of the patient's withdrawal from life and activity. Many studies showed that cancer patients score lower than healthy individuals on questionnaires assessing meaningfulness of life [e.g., 1, 32, 34–36]. Meaningfulness is a construct that is grounded in meaning, i.e., it depends on meaning, uses the tools of meaning, and results in the construction of meaning. Meaning is a system of contents and processes which is being applied continuously by humans in order to make sense of their external and internal environment and to enable behaviors of all kinds [37, 38]. Meaninglessness of life is mostly assessed by scales that provide overall estimates of meaningfulness. In contrast, the meaning-based scale of the meaningfulness of life [39–41] provides in addition information about the specific aspects of life and behavior that contribute to meaningfulness of life. These aspects may be grouped into four clusters: (a) those focused on dynamic-actional contents (e.g., actions, manner of operation, functions); (b) those focused on sensory-perceptual aspects (e.g., external appearance, colors, shapes, time, location); (c) those focused on experiential inner-world aspects (e.g., emotions, experiences, cognitions, memories, attitudes, evaluations, values, judgments); and (d) those focused on contextual aspects (e.g., possessions, causes, results). Studies showed that each person tends to base one's meaningfulness of life on one preferred group of categories, assisted by addressing also the other groups to some extent. Notably, the meaning-based assessment of the meaningfulness of life refers to life in general and not to aspects representing the concerns of cancer patients, such as resentment of the illness [34]. In cancer patients the highest scores of meaningfulness of life are in the impersonal contextual-situational cluster and the lowest in the personal experiential-cognitive cluster. On the whole, cancer patients have lower scores on meaningfulness of life because they mention fewer domains as contributing to their meaningfulness of life. Notably, lower scores on the actional-dynamic aspects reflect low levels of activity, possibly due to difficulties of mobility and limited options. Lower scores of the perceptual-sensory and contextual aspects reflect loss of interest in the environment, including interpersonal relations. Finally, lower scores on the experiential-cognitive aspects reflect dissociation from one's inner world, including one's emotions, evaluations, and cognitions in general. The result of lowered meaningfulness of life is a sense of internal void, emptiness and loneliness. It is often identified as depression or more specifically as existential distress.

Existential Distress

Existential distress is often diagnosed in cancer patients in the palliative stage [32, 36]. It describes a range of phenomena, including deterioration in health, the sense of impending death, helplessness, and loss of autonomy and hope for improvement. Some investigators consider meaningfulness of life and existential distress as components of the same construct [42]. Some regard low meaningfulness of life as a constituent of existential distress [43] or as its determinant [10]. However, empirical data show that the two constructs are indeed correlated but distinct [44]. The self and free choice are two major issues that affect existential concerns [45]. The self is affected in that a patient starts feeling worthless, alone, alienated, dysfunctional, and doing nothing for one's family. Self-esteem becomes lower and the sense of identity becomes impaired. Hence, existential distress is often affiliated with questions such as "Who am I?", "Am I still the same person I have been before the cancer?", "Why has all this befallen me?", and "Is this suffering part of my life?" [46, 47]. In addition, patients may feel that they are dependent on others in many respects; are in need of assistance; have lost their freedom of choice; have reduced control over themselves and their life – physical control, cognitive control, and control over the future [48] – and have difficulty in making up their mind about different issues, in understanding what goes on, and in adhering to basic rules of routine [49]. Loss of the meaningfulness of life and existential distress are major components in shaping the patients' emotional life.

The Stage Theory

The emotional sphere plays a most prominent role in the life of cancer patients in the palliative stage. Indeed, the psychological approach to dying has become known through the five stages of dying described by Kübler-Ross [50], which is largely based on emotional responses: (1) *denial and isolation*, expressing the patient's shock reaction upon the first encounter with dying; (2) *anger*, which may be directed at different targets, e.g., the health professionals who have not prevented the outcome of death, at others who are not dying, or at God for not having selected other victims; (3) *bargaining*, which may be used by offering the higher-power "deals" for mitigating the sentence of death; (4) *depression*, expressing one's sorrow about the losses one experiences or expects as a result of death; and (5) *acceptance*, expressing the attitude of giving up and surrendering to the unavoidable.

This stage theory has evoked a lot of criticism, mainly because it assumes a linear sequential progression from one stage to the next, whereas in reality, patients undergo a variety of stages even repetitive ones, without necessarily following a regular sequence [51]. Additionally, the stage-bound emotions are not the only ones that have been described in dying patients and which may include also hope, guilt, fear, anxiety, irritability, guilt, euphoria, gratitude, longing, panic, surprise, shame, regret, curiosity, excitement, peaceful harmony, and indifference [52, 53], often dotted with stretches of denial [54]. Moreover, the five-stage model was not designed initially to describe the situation in regard to cancer patients, who may have a particular approach to death. It seems that a two-phase approach, defined by the recurrent aspects of denial and acceptance, is often more adequate [55].

Depression

Depression is undoubtedly the emotion that has been most often observed and studied in patients in the palliative stage. Some of the reasons may be its commonness, and the dangers of suicide and the tendency of opting for hastened death that depression may enhance. Since depression has earned many different names (e.g., despair, existential despair, demoralization, grief, dysphoria, hopelessness, and anhedonia) and has been assessed in different ways, there are widely varying estimates of its prevalence in the palliative stage, ranging from 2% to 49% [56] or 33% to 58% [57]. The observed symptoms include lack of sleep, loss of interest in life, irritation, loss of concentration, sometimes even suicidal thoughts, and anxiety that is often observed in conjunction with depression. The risk factors for depression are female gender, younger age, prior history of depression, lack of social support, functional disability, pain, and other serious symptoms [56]. To these one may add the more general risk factors, mainly a sense of responsibility even in the absence of control, guilt evoked by failure, and giving up one's wishes for the sake of adherence to norms and obligations [58].

Although the differences between the various terms describing depression are not always clear, the distinction between depression and demoralization has been supported by several studies [32, 59]. Demoralization is a distinctive psychological state characterized by helplessness, hopelessness, giving up and subjective incompetence, sense of failure, inability to cope [60], and the potential to give up on life and desire death [59].

Death Anxiety

Patients with terminal cancer often experience anxiety concerning issues such as the disease progression, treatment process, uncontrolled pain, dying, and uncertainty after dying. Anxiety in cancer patients has been assessed under different names, including generalized anxiety disorder, panic, phobia, fear, adjustment disorder, as well as mixed phenotype of depression and anxiety. Hence the reports about rates of prevalence vary from 2% for generalized anxiety disorder to 48% [61]. In the present context the focus is on death anxiety.

Death anxiety is an issue of concern for most cancer patients, not in the least because of the ubiquitous connotations of cancer as causing death. It is shared by many human beings and has been widely researched. The following kinds of fear of death recur in many studies: (a) fear of afterlife, e.g., fear of boredom, loneliness, of longing to come back to life, of punishment, torture in hell, suffering for one's deeds in life, rejection by the "authorities" in the hereafter, alienation from God, and even facing the dead whom one may fear; (b) fear of dying, e.g., fear of pain, suffering, suffocation, losing one's body parts, and immobility; (c) fear of extinction, i.e., of annihilation, of "ceasing to be", and of nothingness; and (d) fear of dying prematurely, e.g., before having fulfilled one's goals and duties in this life, prior to having asked for forgiveness or not having found the reason for one's existence [62].

Psychometric studies identified death anxiety as a multidimensional phenomenon including four factors: (a) the cognitive-affective component; (b) component of physical changes; (c) awareness of the unstoppable flow of time, compressing the future and expanding the past; and (d) fear of dying a painful, stressful death [63]. A study about the cognitive tendencies characterizing death anxiety showed that it consists of more components of anxiety than of fear and may be characterized better as a variant of anxiety than of fear. Individuals (cancer patients or healthy controls) scoring high on death anxiety tend to overlook the matter of fact aspects of the theme of death itself and focus rather on their emotional and cognitive reactions to it, elaborating their subjective conceptions of death which result in enhanced anxiety-evoking images [62].

A further exploratory study of attitudes that enhance death anxiety has led to the following list of core beliefs characterizing the high scorers on death anxiety: the essence of life is activity; the basic unit of existence is the individual (rather than the family, the community, the nation, etc.); a person should produce things and be productive (in the sense of producing material or specific things, rather than merely be or experience or know things); life is the highest value, beyond everything else; the most important goal is maintaining what is while avoiding any changes; the most important time is the future, followed by the present and in the last rank by the past; one's major duty in life is to enact all of one's potentialities; one is held accountable for everything one has done in life, as well as for everything one has not done in life; and responsibility lies only with the individual even though there are circumstances that may promote or hinder certain activities.

It seems likely that many of the core beliefs form part of the cultural background in which we live and function. Some of the core beliefs in that culture promote death anxiety but others may serve to mitigate it. Different cultures and religions do it in different ways, thus contributing ultimately to maintaining the delicate balance between the information that we will all die and the desire for living, keeping death anxiety at a tolerable level [62]. The findings about the cognitive and attitudinal bases of death anxiety may be applied for interventions designed to control this distressing emotion.

Pediatric oncology patients also suffer from death anxiety. Terminally ill children are aware of the potentiality of their death, even when not told, but they often conceal this knowledge from their own parents and the medical staff [64]. The awareness of death is a slowly developing process, fed, on the one hand, by the child's personal experiences of disease and treatments and, on the other hand, by information obtained from the adults directly and indirectly through eavesdropping and observing their behaviors toward oneself or among themselves. Their fears increase especially after they have been through the relapse-remission cycle. The fears are manifested in playing less, moving less around, being less interested in things, planning for only very short periods, grieving over the things that they will probably not do, decreased communication with adults, and lowered cooperation with the medical procedures [65, 66].

Anger

Anger is a common emotional reaction in terminal cancer patients [67, 68]. It is a negative emotion that is difficult to control. The reasons are mainly that patients feel the unfairness of the illness [68] and their helplessness in handling it. In prostate cancer patients, it was found to support pessimism in regard to one's prognosis [69]. When uncontrolled or inhibited, it is related to lower partner support [70]. Quite often the anger is directed against God, who has "allowed" the illness [71], or against the doctors who are often blamed for their inability to heal the patient or to communicate with sufficient compassion and understanding [72].

Hope

Hope is a completely different emotion that may appear in terminally sick patients and is very important for cancer patients. In general it is related negatively with the symptom burden and with depression [73]. Patients' hope was found to be beneficial for patients because basically it turns out to be life affirming, enhancing the value of their lives and the connections with others [74]. There are different kinds of hope, e.g., for complete cure, for improvement in health, for comfort, for peace, for continued relations with relatives [75], or simply for good moments. Sometimes the hope of patients is for miraculous instantaneous cure, which they try to maintain despite its apparent irrationality and lack of support from the environment [76], not rarely with a lot of mental labor and self-convictions [77]. Hope may be unsteady and often change with despair prior to being revived by the patients [76]. Notably, hope does not disappear even when patients have a realistic conception of the inevitable progression of their disease [78]. However, the patients' hope may seem problematic to health professionals when it appears to be unrealistic and does not conform to medical facts [79].

Dying or the Moment of Death

From the psychological perspective, there are specific phenomena characterizing death. The most frequently mentioned ones are confusion, disorientation, hallucinations including talking to non-present people or even dead ones, as well as extreme mood changes, such as fear from imagined threats or hidden enemies followed by elation and bursts of energy [17]. Some patients report that the experience of dying is sometimes enacted in preparatory phases which do not reach completion, prior to death itself. Others described the slow progression of the process of death when it takes over the body and its organs [1, 19]. Most remarkable are recollections of so-called out-of-body experiences (OBEs) or near-death experiences (NDEs), reported by many people who have been close to death. Experiences of this kind are often considered to be hallucinatory or illusory, but they should also be studied as possible manifestations of the cognitive changes the brain undergoes in the course of dying [80].

Death from the Points of View of the Major Involved Individuals

The major issues dealt with in this section concern problems and difficulties with which the major protagonists of the great drama of death need to cope with. Some of these problems are unique to each of the three protagonists, but other difficulties are shared by them or their efforts at resolution may converge.

Coping with Dying from the Point of View of the Patient

The cancer patient who enters the phase of advanced disease is confronted with medical as well as psychological issues, although it is likely that the two kinds of issues may not be quite distinct. The issues about which patients complain in this phase are mostly pain [81], sleeplessness, breathlessness, low mood [82], nutritional problems (i.e., loss of appetite, constipation, vomiting or nausea, dry mouth or thirst) [29], helplessness and powerlessness [83], need for help in activities of daily living [81], and insufficient information [84]. By information patients usually mean not only the bare medical facts but mainly a kind of communication that would be comprehensible, truthful and honest, and would express respect for them as human beings [85].

Dealing with Resolving Different Tasks

Awareness of the closeness of death may involve for many patients concern with resolving specific tasks. Some of these tasks may have to do with in the individuals' religion or family tradition. others may be invented by the person himself/herself [86, 87]. The commonly mentioned tasks are reviewing, confessing, taking care of interpersonal relations, closure, and leaving a will. Reviewing implies evaluating one's achievements and failures in different domains. In contrast, confessing includes exposing to the relevant persons one's deeds that one considers evil or harmful and disclosing secrets from the past. Further, taking care of interpersonal relations involves expressing one's attitude and mainly positive emotions, such as gratefulness, and forgiveness to the significant others in one's life or environment. Similarly, closure indicates finishing duties, obligations, or things one has wanted to do in one's life, e.g., leaving notes about different unfinished business, writing a final or preliminary chapter for one's book, and making a decision about something that has bothered one for a long time. Finally, preparing a will refers to financial, practical, and spiritual things one would like to bequeath to others.

The mentioned tasks are only examples of obligations which dying people impose on themselves or others expect them to perform. They are assumed to ease the psychological burden or distress of the dying person by enabling freedom of the so-called duties of life. Yet, in some cases, tasks of the mentioned kind may bring about an increase in the burden or distress of dying, because of time pressure, limited mobility, fatigue, and other difficulties attending attempts to solve problems that may not be easy and which one has been unable to solve earlier in life. Furthermore, the tasks of closure may enhance the realization of unfilled aspirations in the past and the futility or impossibility of further efforts [88] which may evoke despair when one starts grieving over oneself and one's lost life.

The Role of Spirituality

In recent years the importance and benefit of meeting the patients' spiritual needs have become increasingly clear. Studies show that the majority of cancer patients in advanced stages express the need for spirituality, regardless of their medical diagnosis and treatment or their religious background [89]. A review of several studies showed that spiritual needs are understood by most patients as referring to the following major themes: finding the meaning and purpose of life; finding the meaning in experiencing the disease; being connected to other people, God, and nature; having access to religious/spiritual practices; physical, psychological, social, and spiritual well-being; talking about death and the experience of dying; making the best out of their time; and being independent and being treated like a normal person [90]. The major recurrent meanings of spirituality are peace, hope, and relationships [85, 91]. Patients consider spiritual care as part of the overall care they expect. Spirituality seems to be a real need rather than an option [92]. Meeting the patients' spiritual needs decreases symptom severity, the level of hopelessness, and the desire for hastened death by enhancing their sense of dignity [92] and increasing their quality of life [91] [see also Spirituality and Religion, Chap. 8).

Psychosocial Interventions in the Palliative Phase

The psychosocial interventions in the palliative phase focus on providing the patients relief, enhancing a sense of peace and harmony, enabling freedom from duties and obligations, and creating an atmosphere in which the patients may consider at will issues that bother them. These issues are often though not always of an existential nature, concerning for example the nature of the self, their interpersonal relationships, and the meaning of their life.

One kind of interventions deals directly or indirectly with meaning. The best known is the meaning-centered therapy, which is based on promoting the patients' freedom of choice in regard to shaping their views and decisions about who they are and what they want to do in their remaining time [93]. Another approach to meaning making is exemplified by the psychodynamic life narrative which focuses on the meanings of one's life narrative, elaborating one's self-identity through the life review [94]. A different approach consists in developing the components of the meaningfulness of life, e.g., actional or emotional, which the patients can then apply at will in order to expand the range of their meaningfulness of life. There is evidence that increasing the level of the meaningfulness of life decreases the scores on existential despair [44].

Another kind of interventions focuses on upholding dignity by addressing more directly concrete concerns of everyday life rather than existential issues. The dignity-conserving repertoire includes both dignity-conserving perspectives, such as maintenance of pride, role preservation, and resilience or fighting spirit, and dignity-conserving practices, such as living in the moment and maintaining normalcy. Dignity therapy provides patients also the possibility of preparing a document about their legacy [95]. A third kind of interventions focuses on helping the patients find peace and respite from stress and anxieties by means of different approaches using mostly fantasy and relaxation practices. The best known are mindfulness interventions [96], relaxation [97], guided imagery [98], and meditation [99]. Notably, practices of this kind work also for pediatric cancer patients, who may apply fantasy, for example, in order to construct in imagination fulfillments of wishes and projects that would never be realized [65, 66] (see also Meaning-Based Interventions, Chap. 8).

The "Good" Death.

In recent years some studies were devoted to exploring patients' views about what would constitute for them a "good death." In most cases the good death inventory designed for the bereaved was used with the patients (see next section). The descriptions of good death are similar though not quite identical in different studies. In one study patients answered that it was associated with living with the prospect of imminent death, preparing for death, and dying comfortably, e.g., quickly, independently, without suffering, and without harming in any way their social relations [100]. Patients in a nursing home gave the following descriptions: pain relief, religious services, giving care to others, and appreciation of respectful and prompt care [101]. The following themes were mentioned in a third study: physical and cognitive control, unawareness of death, good relationship with family, maintaining hope, and physical and psychological comfort [102]. In Taiwan patients referred to respect for autonomy, decision-making participation, and getting verbal support [103]. In another study, the following themes were salient: not being a burden to the family, presence of family, resolving unfinished business, freedom from pain, feeling that life was meaningful, and being at peace with God [104]. The following themes recurred in still another study: controlled pain, not being a burden on one's family, and having sorted out one's personal affairs [105]. Further descriptions included clear consciousness, short stay in the hospital, good physical care, high physician-assessed autonomy, good emotional support, good communication, and good continuity of life [106]. Finally, a review of 36 studies in this domain showed that there were 3 descriptions that recurred: preferences for a particular dying process (mentioned in 94% of reports), followed by freedom from pain and emotional well-being [107]. The most interesting one is the first which indicates that patients seem to have a personal vision of death which is their own personal conception which reflects their needs. Addressing this conception is probably an important constituent of providing adequate help to dying cancer patients.

Coping with Dying from the Point of View of the Family

Coping with a seriously sick cancer patient is one of the most difficult tasks facing family members. It is particularly difficult when the dying patient is a close family member, such as one's children, parents, or partner, or a relative who is especially loved. The stress is so much larger when the family member is also the caretaker of the patient, who may be residing at home or outside home, e.g., hospital or nursing home.

Knowing that someone in your family is dying from cancer constitutes a serious source for worry. The family member worries about the patient, about the other relatives who may be affected by the patient's state, and even about themselves. They may feel distressed by the patient's suffering, by their own limited ability to help him or her, by the possible genetic bonds between themselves and the patient, and often even by mundane issues, such as wills and other financial arrangements [108].

For the family members, the period of the patient's palliative care denotes a time of parting, taking leave, and separating. Yet, this connotation generates pressure to use the remaining time optimally by staying with the patient as close as possible. Not spending enough time with the patient or not doing enough for him or her may generate in the family member a feeling of dissatisfaction with oneself or even guilt [109].

A further source of guilt that is common in family members of dying patients is the wish that they may have for the patient to be already dead. This wish may reflect not only one's desire to be free from all the worries and obligations related to the patient's state but also reflect the desire to see the patient already liberated from suffering. Sometimes the sense of guilt is grounded in the anticipatory grief that family members may experience [110].

Particularly complicated is the case of family members who take care of the dying patient. They suffer from the stress of daily contact with their beloved family member whom they watch in the process of deterioration, as well as from a deep sense of powerlessness and inability to stop the process or even merely to alleviate the suffering. Their situation is further complicated by the unclear status they have as caretakers which may cause problems with getting the adequate information and instructions from the formal health professionals about what the patient's state really is and how to deal adequately with the symptoms and with approaching death. Guilt may be more pronounced in family members who take care of the patient, more than in those who do not do so, possibly because they feel that their care is not as perfect as they would like it to be. Moreover, studies show that the family caretakers feel more guilt about things they have done than about those they have not done [111]. Sometimes the stress may cause them physical and psychological symptoms, such as muscle tension, headache, loss of appetite, anxiety, and depression evoked by feelings of guilt, anger, and loneliness [112]. In addition to the survivors' guilt [113], family members may be prone even to posttraumatic stress [114].

Studies devoted to the definition of the "good" death by bereaved family members showed that the definition included the following ten major domains: "environmental comfort," "life completion," "dying in a favorite place," "maintaining hope and pleasure," "independence," "physical and psychological comfort," "good relationship with medical staff," "not being a burden to others," "good relationship with family," and "being respected as an individual" [115]. These aspects are partly but not completely identical to those emphasized by the patients "good" death (see former section) (see also Chap. 11).

Coping with Dying from the Point of View of the Doctor and Other Health Professionals

Health professionals dealing with palliative care patients are exposed to specific and difficult problems. A dying patient confronts the doctor with one's insufficiency as a professional. Doctors are prepared, taught, and motivated for healing and promoting life. These goals are unfortunately not the dominant ones in the palliative care setting. Dealing with a dying patient requires from the doctors mobilizing their skills for a goal that is difficult to integrate within the framework of classical medicine, at least as it has been formally defined until recent decades. Hence, dealing with death functions as a reminder of the limits of one's profession and may involve helplessness and even guilt. It may even engender learned helplessness in the oncologists of palliative care. Not infrequently the medical limitations may cause anger outbursts on the part of patients and their family against the health professionals [116].

In addition, there are particular symptoms of the dying patient, including confusion, restlessness, agitation, delirium, and severe bouts of anxiety or depression that may cause the patient and the family members suffering. Studies show that the doctors' conceptions about what is needed in the situation do not always conform with the views of the patients or the family members. One particularly delicate issue concerns the continuation of active treatment against cancer in the dying patient. The doctors who consider the patients' welfare and the utility of the treatments may not always be supportive of the patients or the family's desire to continue "fighting the cancer" [117].

The need to communicate with the patient and the family about the present and expected state of the patient may constitute another kind of difficulty for the health professionals. As health professionals they are bound and motivated to present the truth. But this may be difficult if it does not conform to the expectations of the patient and the family members or when it may aggravate their suffering and suppress any hopes they may have.

The constant confrontation with impeding or occurring death may be difficult for doctors and the other health professionals. Some of them may feel discomfort in the presence of death or may experience some personal difficulty dealing with it. Sometimes a patient's dying process may remind the clinician of similar losses suffered in his or her own personal life, leading the physician to have surprisingly strong feelings toward a specific patient.

A particular task of the health professionals in the palliative setting is expressing empathy and providing emotional support to the patients and often their family members too. This task is more salient and expected in the palliative setting than in other settings of providing medical care. It is particularly difficult because its performance, constituents, time frame, extent, and degree of personal involvement are not specified. It is required of doctors, nurses, and all formal and informal health carers in the situation. Additionally, the difficulty consists also in that empathy may be a limited resource, and its repeated manifestations may bring about depletion and compassion fatigue. Special preparation, by acquiring specific tools for the adequate management of empathy manifestation, may be advisable [118].

The difficulties of dealing with dying patients are shared by all involved health professionals, who, in addition to the oncologists, include primarily also the nursing personnel, psychologists and psychooncologists, social workers, individuals who provide spiritual care and help, sometimes also religious helpers, and often also volunteers with differing degrees of preparation for the tasks. Most of these experts focus on providing human, social, emotional, and personal support to the dying, each, in his or her specialty, responding as best as they can to the different and often changing needs of the patients. The complex situation requires teamwork although the patients are not always able or ready to use all the options.

Due to the professional, personal, and circumstantial difficulties of treatment in the palliative setting, high levels of burnout are manifested by the working staff, and several programs have been devised for helping them [119]. (see also Chap. 16).

Decisions in the Palliative Care Phase

There are several major decisions that may weigh heavily on the individuals involved in the palliative phase of cancer patients. Although these decisions may be assigned to one or the other of the major protagonists – doctors and health professionals, family members, and patients – in reality all are involved and participate in reaching the decisions and in implementing them.

Decisions for Doctors/Clinicians

As is well known, the decision whether a patient is dead or not is not clear cut or easy. Relying neither on cardiorespiratory criteria nor on brain death [80, 120] provides the basis for determining unambiguously that a patient is completely dead. One reason for the unclarity is that dying is a process rather than an instantaneous event [121]. A similar issue is determining whether a certain patient is in the dying phase or not. This decision determines to a certain extent important issues, such as the kind of treatment that will be offered to the patient if at all and the recommended place of hospitalization. This decision too is quite difficult. One method is to base the decision on physical symptoms, such as breathlessness, weak pulse, or falling blood pressure. However, the validity of these and even improved indices has not been proven [122, 123]. Another method consists in focusing on estimates of likely survival of the patient. However, this method too is not foolproof. Comparing clinicians' predictions of survival with actual survival showed quite serious deviations (overestimation in 27% and underestimation in 12%) [124].

Studies showed that the decision of doctors whether the patient is approaching death is mostly reached on an intuitive basis, relying more on impression and previous experience than on clear-cut criteria. The decision may be described as "fluid" because the distinction between a treatable and a dying patient is blurred and subject to changes as new information becomes available [122]. Additionally, psychological factors affect death in addition to physiological ones. The prediction of whether a patient in ICU will die or not was less accurate on the basis of medical evaluation than by psychological factors, identified by the cognitive orientation approach, such as beliefs referring to readiness for changes, focusing on the relevant, acceptance of limits, and only weak tendencies for obsessive-compulsive behaviors [125].

The difficulties and unclarities of determining whether a patient is dying are reflected also in the affiliated decisions that doctors have to make about whether to resuscitate [126], or whether to intubate [127], and whether to withdraw or withhold treatment or not [128]. Actually, in reality, decisions of this kind are met increasingly on the basis of consultation between the doctor, the patient, and the patient's family. In these borderline situations, the role of the oncologist is to define the issues, open up the discussion, and guide gently the decision about when and how to pass to the formal palliative stage [129].

Decisions of Family Members

As mentioned above, family members are often active participants in the decisions about whether measures, such as resuscitation and intubation, should be undertaken in regard to the patient and whether medical treatments in general should be continued for prolonging the patient's life and if yes how much and for how long. The role of the family depends to some extent on the state of the patient and on the role the family has played in sustaining the patient all along.

A specific decision that family members have to undertake is the extent to which they will be involved in actively taking care of the patient. The decision depends to some extent on the state of the patient. When the medical situation is challenging and requires expert care, it is likely that the family would find it hard to undertake the task, without additional nursing help which may not be available. The decision depends also on the family member's financial situation. If it is necessary for the family member to continue working outside the home, it may be difficult if not impossible for him or her to devote the time and resources to taking care of the patient. In some cases family members stop altogether all their other duties and obligations in order to devote themselves completely to assisting the patient, regardless of the cost. In many other cases, some kind of compromise between the family member's own life and the caring for the patient is reached.

The abovementioned decisions are closely related to another important decision in the palliative phase concerning where the patient will die. Actually, the place where the patient stays during the palliative period (months, weeks, days) and where he or she dies is not necessarily the same. Many patients who stay at home or in a nursing home when they deteriorate are transferred to a hospital where they eventually die. There are multiple possibilities of where to live/die in the palliative phase, depending on the patient, the family, the country, the availability of adequate locations, and the patient's financial resources. The major places include the home, an oncology ward in a general hospital, a specialized palliative care unit in a hospital, communal establishments, a nursing home, and a hospice. The different locations differ in various respects. For example, as compared to patients who die in hospitals, those who die in specialized palliative care units show less indirectly expressed anger but more directly expressed anger and helplessness and more positive feelings and report more anxiety about death but less anxiety about isolation and general anxiety and fewer shared relationships [130].

Most patients (about 70%) in different countries would like to die at home, probably because it represents a most personal, safe, and pleasant place for many, but the percentage of those who actually die at home is closer to 25–30% [131, 132].

Predictors of preferred home death differ in different countries. For example, the predictors in Western countries are younger age, being male, born in the UK/Ireland or Italy/Greece, better physical health, poorer mental health, and fewer concerns about dying at home. In Japan decisions about dying at home are based on considerations of quality of life, of availability and the patient has ability of family caregivers, desire to minimize being a burden to others and relationships with healthcare providers [131, 132]. Different factors may play a role in determining the actual place of death. In Japan, the chances to die at home are higher when both the patient and the family share the preference for death at home [133]. In Israel, the major factors predicting the patient's death at home are having a non-Ashkenazi background, having social work care for the family, living in one's own house and not a rented one, belonging to a family whose members worked, and having immigrated to Israel a long time ago. Secondary predictors are being married and having a diagnosis other than breast cancer. Hence, the variables that proved to be predictors of site of death are partly economical (e.g., living in an owned and not rented house), partly sociological (e.g., being non-Ashkenazi, living with one's family), and partly medical (e.g., having a diagnosis other than breast cancer). A review of 58 studies [134] showed that the following 6 factors were strongly related to dying at home: the patient's low functional status, the patient's preference, the availability of home care, the intensity of home care, living with relatives, and extended family support. The environmental factors of living in nonurban locations and the availability of healthcare were the most highly predictive ones.

Decisions of the Patient

A basic issue concerning the palliative phase is the patient's minimize to live. It is unclear to what extent this desire is conscious, clear to the patient, and based on what could be described as "decision." In any case, it is a reflection of a complex set of factors. On the one hand, there are life-supporting factors. Major among these may be the so-called will to live. This drive may be related to self-preservation in the evolutionary sense and is assumed to be activated in those who survive difficult life-threatening situations, such as the holocaust or serious physical states. Studies suggest that the will to life may be affected negatively by factors, such as hopelessness, depression, low level of dignity, feeling one is a burden to one's family, dissatisfaction with the support of family and healthcare workers, as well as physical distress due to breathlessness [135, 136].

The cognitive orientation of survival [125] is likely to be a major component of the will to live or survive. The cognitive orientation of survival is a set of beliefs of four types (about oneself, about reality and others, about rules and norms, and about one's goals) referring to themes, such as readiness for changes, focusing on the relevant, acceptance of limits, and only weak tendencies for obsessive-compulsive behaviors. Its validity was proven in studies which showed that it predicted whether a patient in ICU will die or more accurately than the medical evaluation [125] as well as the duration of a positive response to the treatment of HIV [137]. It may be assumed that the cognitive orientation of survival is effective under conditions when physical survival is challenged.

A similar construct of the life evaluation questionnaire [138], designed to assess psychological aspects of the will to live, identified the following themes in high scorers: clearer perception of the meaning of life, freedom versus restriction of life, resentment of the illness, contentment with past and present life, and past and present social integration.

On the other hand, there seem to be also life-negating factors. One of them has been referred to as the death drive, which Freud conceptualized as the anti-pleasure principle and anti-sexual life-producing drive. Others viewed it as the tendency for self-destruction or self-punishment. Accordingly, life is considered as based on the balance between the life-supporting and life-negating forces. The attraction toward death is strengthened when the former become weaker, for example, through the loss of success, hope, love, or support [139].

In cancer patients in the advanced palliative phase, there may be manifestations of life-negating forces, for example, active attempts at suicide (e.g., using medication), suicidal thoughts, passive attempts at suicide (e.g., stopping eating and drinking or stopping one's medications), succumbing to lethargy and wasting, desire for hastened death, and cooperating with physician-assisted dying (i.e., euthanasia). If these and possibly other less explicit manifestations of the positive consideration of ending life are taken into account, it seems that up to 50% of patients in this phase would qualify [140]. This is not surprising when we consider the suffering of these patients, their helplessness, dependence on others, limited perspective for improvement in the future, hopelessness, pain, fatigue and other symptoms, depression, and the feeling of being a burden on others. Another contributing factor that is not negligible is the uplifting of the legal and social taboo on choosing hastened death in the final palliative phase. It seems that more patients express ideas of suicide or discuss hastened death with their health professionals or family members than those who actually undertake any concrete steps. One reason is the application of different interventions to reducing the desire for death, including the alleviation of pain [140, 141].

Another reason may be the support of family members who would like to be with the patient as long as possible. A still further reason may be the lack of energy, the difficulty to decide, or even the fear of death of the patients themselves. But it is certainly difficult to assess the number of those who commit suicide because it is not always clear what the situation actually was or perhaps not even known down to all details.

Some Afterthoughts

The different approaches to the themes of death and dying explored in the present chapter support several general conclusions. One is that dying is a process, whose beginning and whose end are difficult to determine. Another conclusion is that multiple approaches are possible and are needed, based on different professional and personal points of view. Despite the fact that in some cases the different approaches overlap, it is evident that the themes of death and dying require and profit from the multiplicity of approaches. The most important conclusion however seems to be that death and dying are a complex phenomenon – or event or construct or experience or phase – whose minimal description, not to mention, deciphering, requires considering medical, physical, physiological, psychological, social, cultural, and religious information and concepts. All of these however get integrated and fused in the dying human being.

References

1. Kreitler, S. (Ed.). *Confronting dying and death*. Hauppauge: Nova Publishers.
2. Kreitler, S. (2012). Death in cancer patients: Meanings, attitudes and feelings. In S. Kreitler (Ed.), *Confronting dying and death* (pp. 247–258). Hauppauge: Nova Publishers.
3. Crocetti, E., Arniani, S., Acciai, S., Barchielli, A., & Buiatti, E. (1998). High suicide mortality soon after diagnosis among cancer patients in central Italy. *British Journal of Cancer, 77*, 1194–1196.
4. Levi, F., Bulliard, J. L., & La-Vecchia, C. (1991). Suicide risk among incident cases of cancer in the Swiss Canton of Vaud. *Oncology, 48*, 4–47.
5. Storm, N. H., Christensen, N., & Jensen, O. M. (1992). Suicides among Danish patients with cancer: 1971 to 1986. *Cancer, 69*, 1507–1512.
6. Tang, P. L., Chiou, C. P., Lin, H. S., Wang, C., & Liand, S. L. (2011). Correlates of death anxiety among Taiwanese cancer patients. *Cancer Nursing, 34*(4), 286–292.
7. Lyke, J. (2013). Associations among aspects of meaning of life and death anxiety in young adults. *Death Studies, 37*(5), 471–482.
8. Breitbart, W., & Poppito, S. (2014). *Individual meaning centered psychotherapy treatment manual*. New York: Oxford University Press.
9. Camus, A. (1955). *The myth of Sisyphus and other essays*. New York: Alfred A. Knopf.
10. Frankl, V. (2006). *Man's search for meaning*. Boston: Beacon Press.
11. Yalom, I. D. (1980). *Existential psychotherapy*. New York: Basic Books.

12. Jong, J., Ross, R., Philip, T., Chang, S.-H., Simons, N., & Halberstadt, J. (2018). The religious correlates of death anxiety: A systematic review and meta-analysis. *Religion, Brain & Behavior, 8*(1), 4–20.
13. Barak, F., Lipshitz, S., Kaufer, H., Nathanel, R., Siegelmann, N., Alkalay, Y., & Kreitler, S. (2013). Where to die? Factors affecting the place of death. Presentation in MASCC/ISOO International Symposium on Supportive Care in Cancer, Berlin, Germany, June 27–30, 2013.
14. Kreitler, S., Barak, F., Siegelmann, N., Nathanel, R., Lifshitz, S., & Kaufer, H. (2013). Where to die? This is the question. Presentation in 15th World Congress of Psycho-Oncology and Psychosocial Academy, Rotterdam, The Netherlands, November 4–8, 2013.
15. Fauli, C., Caestecker, S., de Nicholson, A., & Black, F. (2012). *Handbook of palliative care* (3rd ed.). Essex: Wiley-Blackwell.
16. Watson, M., Lucas, C., Hoy, A., & Wells, J. (2009). *Oxford handbook of palliative care* (2nd ed.). New York: Oxford University Press.
17. Berkovic, M. (2012). The medical point of view: Is the care for the dying a part of our profession? In S. Kreitler (Ed.), *Confronting dying and death* (pp. 1–12). Hauppauge: Nova Publishers.
18. Clark, C. (2017). Care at the very end-of-life: Dying cancer patients and their chosen family's needs. *Cancers(Basel), 9*(2), 11.
19. Kreitler, S. (2012). The psychological point of view: The individual facing death and dying. In S. Kreitler (Ed.), *Confronting dying and death* (pp. 89–102). Hauppauge: Nova Publishers.
20. Mast, M. S. (2007). On the importance of nonverbal communication in the physician-patient interaction. *Patient Education and Counseling, 67*(3), 315–318.
21. Trovo de Araujo, M. M., & da Silva, M. J. (2012). Communication strategies used by health care professionals in providing palliative care to patients. *Revista da Escola de Enfermagem, 46*(3), 626–632.
22. Anderson, N. H. (2014). *Contributions to information integration theory* (Cognition) (Vol. I). New York: Psychology Press, Francis & Taylor Group.
23. Tonoti, C. (2004). An information integration theory of consciousness. *BMC Neuroscience, 5*, 42.
24. Hinton, J. M. (1963). The physical and mental distress of the dying. *Journal of Chronic Diseases, 17*, 201–205.
25. Saunders, D. C. (1994). Pain and impending death. In P. D. Wall & R. Melzack (Eds.), *Textbook of pain* (3rd ed., pp. 861–868). Edinburgh: Churchill Livingstone.
26. Witzel, L. (1971). Das Verhalten von sterbenden Patienten. Medizinische Klinik. No. 557.
27. Kreitler, S. (2018). Dying from cancer – The four tracks. In H. S. Watanabe (Ed.), *Horizons in cancer research* (Vol. 69, pp. 145–172). Hauppage: Nova Publishers.
28. Amano, K., Morita, T., Miyamoto, J., Uno, T., Katayama, H., & Tatara, R. (2018). Perception of need for nutritional support in advanced cancer patients with cachexia: A survey in palliative care settings. *Supportive Care in Cancer, 26*(8), 2793–2795.
29. Kreitler, S., Barak, F., Alkalay, Y., & Ostrovsky, A. (2014). Nutrition and quality of life in advanced cancer patients. The 21st Annual Conference of the International Society for Quality-of-Life Studies (ISQOLS), Berlin, Germany, 15–18 October, 2014.
30. Kreitler, S., & Barak, F. (2012). Nutrition and quality of life in cancer patients with advanced disease. *Supportive Care in Cancer, 20*(1), S132–S133.
31. Barbosa, M., Moutinho, S., & Gonçalves, E. (2011). Demoralization: Introducing the concept and its importance for palliative care. *Acta Medica Portuguesa, 24*(Suppl 4), 779–782.
32. Robinson, S., Kissane, D. W., Brooker, J., & Burney, S. (2016). A review of the construct of demoralization: History, definitions, and future directions for palliative care. *American Journal of Hospice and Palliative Care, 33*(1), 93–101.
33. Kreitler, S. (1999). Die Todesproblematik bei Krebspatienten [The problem of death in cancer patients]. Interdisciplinary Symposium: Der Tod: Das Grosse Tabu der Gegenwart [Death: The great taboo of the present] Vienna, Austria, September 13–14, 1999.

34. Hassankhani, H., Soheili, A., Hosseinpour, I., Ziaei, J. E., & Nahamin, M. (2017). A comparative study on the meaning in life of patients with cancer and their family members. *Journal of Caring Science, 6*(4), 325–333.
35. Hannum, S. M., & Rubinstein, R. L. (2016). The meaningfulness of time; Narratives of cancer among chronically ill older adults. *Journal of Aging Studies, 36*, 17–25.
36. Vehling, S., & Philipp, R. (2018). Existential distress and meaning-focused interventions in cancer survivorship. *Current Opinion in Supportive and Palliative Care, 12*(1), 46–51.
37. Kreitler, S. (2014). Meaning and its manifestations: The meaning system. In S. Kreitler & T. Urbanek (Eds.), *Conceptions of meaning* (pp. 3–32). Hauppauge: Nova Publishers.
38. Kreitler, S. (2013). The construction of meaning. In D. Cervone, M. Fajkowska, M. Eysenck, & T. Maruszewski (Eds.), *Personality dynamics: Embodiment, meaning construction, and the social world* (pp. 47–63). Clinton Corners: Eliot Werner Publications.
39. Kreitler, S. (2016). Meanings of meaningfulness of life. In A. Batthyany (Ed.), *Logotherapy and existential analysis* (Vol. 1, pp. 95–106). Vienna: Springer.
40. Kreitler, S. (2016). Meaningfulness of life and its impact on quality of life. In C. Pracana & M. Wang (Eds.), *International psychological applications conference and trends*. (InPact (pp. 392–394). Lisbon: W.I.A.R.S.
41. Kreitler, S. (2017). Meaning-based assessment of the meaningfulness of life. Paper presented at European Conference on Psychological Assessment ECPA 14, Lisbon, Portugal.
42. Steger, M. F., Frazier, P., Oishi, S., & Kaler, M. (2006). The meaning in life questionnaire: Assessing the presence of and search for meaning in life. *Journal of Counseling Psychology, 53*(1), 80.
43. Lo, C., Panday, T., Zeppieri, J., Rydall, A., Murphy-Kane, P., Zimmermann, C., Rodin, G. (2017). Preliminary psychometrics of the existential distress scale in patients with advanced cancer. *European Journal of Cancer Care*. 26(6).
44. Kreitler, S. (2018). Meaningfulness of life and existential distress. *Advances in Clinical and Experimental Psychology, 1*, 1–10.
45. Cassell, E. J. (1991). *The nature of suffering and the goals of medicine*. Oxford: Oxford University press.
46. Shinar, Y. R., & Marks, A. D. (2015). Distressing visions at the end of life: Case report and review of the literature. *Journal of Pastoral Care & Counseling, 69*(4), 251–253.
47. Chochinov, H. M., Kristjanson, L. J., Breitbart, W., McClement, S., Hack, T. F., Hassard, T., & Harlos, M. (2011). Effect of dignity therapy on distress and end-of-life experience in terminally ill patients: A randomised controlled trial. *The Lancet Oncology, 12*(8), 753–762.
48. Morita, T., Tsunoda, J., Inoue, S., & Chihara, S. (2000). An exploratory factor analysis of existential suffering in Japanese terminally ill cancer patients. *Psycho-Oncology, 9*(2), 164–168.
49. BolmsJo, I. (2000). Existential issues in palliative acre – Interviews with cancer patients. *Journal of Palliative Care, 16*(2), 20.
50. Kübler-Ross, E. (1981). *Living with death and dying*. New York: Macmillan.
51. Neimeyer, R. A. (Ed.). (2001). *Meaning reconstruction and the experience of loss*. Washington, DC: American Psychological Association.
52. Hafen, B. Q., & Framdsen, K. J. (1983). *Faces of death: Grief, dying, euthanasia, suicide*. Englewood Cliffs: Prentice-Hall.
53. Kalish, R. A. (1981). *Death, grief, and caring relationships*. Monterey: Brooks/Cole.
54. Kreitler, S. (1999). Denial in cancer patients. *Cancer Investigation, 17*, 514–534.
55. Weisman, A. D., & Worden, W. (1975). Psychological analysis of cancer deaths. *Omega, 6*, 61–75.
56. Wilson, K. G., Lander, M., & Chochinov, H. M. (2009). Diagnosis and management of depression in palliative care. In H. M. Chochinov & W. Breitbart (Eds.), *Handbook of psychiatry in palliative medicine* (2nd ed., pp. 39–68). New York: Oxford University Press.
57. Wasteson, E., Brenne, E., Higginson, I. J., Hotopf, M., Lloyd-Williams, M., Kaasa, S., Loge, J. H., & the European Palliative Care Research Collaorative (EPCRC). (2009). Depression

assessment and classification in palliative cancer patients: A systematic literature review. *Palliative Medicine, 23*(8), 739–753.
58. Kreitler, S. (2015). Psychopathology: The cognitive orientation approach. In C. Pracana (Ed.), *InPACT international psychological applications conference and trends* (pp. 58–63). Portugal: W.I.A.R.S. Lisbon.
59. Kissane, D. W., Clarke, D. M., & Street, A. F. (2001). Demoralization syndrom- A relevant psychiatric diagnosis for palliative care. *Journal of Palliative Care, 17*(1), 12–21.
60. Tecuta, L., Tomba, E., Grandi, S., & Fava, G. A. (2015). Demoralization: A systematic review on its clinical characterization. *Psychological Medicine, 45*(4), 673–691.
61. Kolva, E., Rossenfeld, B., Pessin, H., Breitbart, W., & Brescia, R. (2011). Anxiety in terminally ill cancer patients. *Journal of Pain and Symptom Management, 42*(5), 691–701.
62. Kreitler, S. (2005). Fear of death. In P. L. Gower (Ed.), *New research on the psychology of fear* (pp. 59–89). Hauppage: Nova Science.
63. Lonetto, R., & Templer, D. I. (1986). *Death anxiety*. New York: Hemisphere Publishing Corporation.
64. Bluebond-Langner, M. (1978). *The private worlds of dying children*. Princeton: Princeton University Press.
65. Kreitler, S., & Krivoy, E. (2004). Psychological intervention with the dying child. In S. Kreitler & M. W. Ben Arush (Eds.), *Psychological aspects of pediatric oncology* (pp. 389–414). Chichester: Wiley.
66. Kreitler, S., & Krivoy, E. (2012). Psychological intervention with the dying child. In S. Kreitler, M. W. Ben Arush, & A. Martin (Eds.), *Pediatric psycho-oncology* (2nd ed., pp. 209–222). Oxford: Wiley-Blackwell.
67. Houston, R. E. (1999). The angry dying patient. *Primary Care Companion to the Journal of Clinical Psychiatry, 1*(1), 5–8.
68. Kissane, D. W. (1994). Managing anger in palliative care. *Australian Family Physician, 23*(7), 1257–1259.
69. Gerhart, J., Schmidt, E., Lillis, T., O'Mahony, S., Duberstein, P., & Hoerger, M. (2017). Anger proneness and prognostic pessimism in men with prostate cancer. *American Journal of Hospice and Palliative Care, 34*(6), 497–504.
70. Julkunen, J., Gustavsson-Lilius, M., & Hietanen, P. (2009). Anger expression, partner support, and quality of life in cancer patients. *Journal of Psychosomatic Research, 66*(3), 235–244.
71. Exline, J. J., Park, C. L., Smyth, J. M., & Carey, M. P. (2011). Anger toward God: Social-cognitive predictors, prevalence, and links with adjustment to bereavement and cancer. *Journal of Personality and Social Psychology, 100*(1), 129–148.
72. Ha, F. J., & Longnecker, N. (2010). Doctor-patient communication. *The Ochsner Journal, 10*(1), 38–43.
73. Davis, M. P., Lagman, R., Parala, A., Patel, C., Sanford, T., Fielding, F., Brumbaugh, A., Gross, J., Rao, A., Majeed, S., Shinde, S., & Rybicki, L. A. (2017). Hope, symptoms and palliative care. *American Journal of Hospice and Palliative Care, 34*(3), 223–232.
74. Eliott, J. A., & Olver, I. N. (1982). Hope and hoping in the talk of dying cancer patients. *Social Science & Medicine, 64*(1), 138–149.
75. Duggleby, W., Holtslander, L., Steeves, M., Duggleby-Wenzel, S., & Cunningham, S. (2010). Discursive meaning of hope for older persons with advanced cancer and their caregivers. *Canadian Journal on Aging [La Revue Canadienne Du Vieillissement], 29*(3), 361–367.
76. Daneault, S., Lussier, V., Mongeau, S., Yelle, L., Côté, A., Sicotte, C., Paillé, P., Dion, D., & Coulombe, M. (2016). Ultimate journey of the terminally ill: Ways and pathways of hope. *Canadian Family Physician [Medecin De Famille Canadien], 62*(8), 648–656.
77. Nierop-van Baalen, C., Grypdonck, M., van Hecke, A., & Verhaeghe, S. (2016). Hope dies last … A qualitative study into the meaning of hope for people with cancer in the palliative phase. *European Journal of Cancer Care, 25*(4), 570–579.

78. Soylu, C., Babacan, T., Sever, A. R., & Altundag, K. (2016). Patients' understanding of treatment goals and disease course and their relationship with optimism, hope, and quality of life: A preliminary study among advanced breast cancer outpatients before receiving palliative treatment. *Supportive Care in Cancer, 24*(8), 3481–3488.
79. Nierop-van Baalen, C., Grypdonck, M., van Heck, A., & Verhaeghe, S. (2018). Health professionals' dealing with hope in palliative patients with cancer, an explorative qualitative research. *European Journal of Cancer Care, 18*, e12889.
80. Parnia, S. (2014). Death and consciousness – An overview of the mental and cognitive experience of death. *Annals of the New York Academy of Sciences, 1330*, 75–93.
81. van den Beuken-van Everdingen, M. H., Hochstenbach, L. M., Joosten, E. A., Tjan-Heijnen, V. C., & Janssen, D. J. (2016). Update on prevalence of pain in patients with cancer: Systematic review and meta-analysis. *Journal of Pain and Symptom Management, 51*(6), 1070–1090.
82. Addington-Hall, J., & McCarthy, M. (1995). Dying from cancer: Results of a national population-based investigation. *Palliative Medicine, 9*(4), 295–305.
83. Sand, L., Strang, P., & Milberg, A. (2008). Dying cancer patients' experiences of powerlessness and helplessness. *Supportive Care in Cancer, 16*(7), 853–862.
84. Sherman, A. C., Simonton-Atchley, S., Mikeal, C. W., Anderson, K. M., Arnaoutakis, K., Hutchins, L. F., Makhoul, I., Mahmoud, F., Milojkovic, N., Harrington, S. E., & Suen, J. Y. (2018). Cancer patient perspectives regarding preparedness for end-of-life care: A qualitative study. *Journal of Psychosocial Oncology, 36*(4), 454–469.
85. Kuhl, D. (2009). What dying people want. In H. M. Chochinov & W. Breitbart (Eds.), *Handbook of psychiatry in palliative medicine* (2nd ed., pp. 141–156). New York: Oxford University Press.
86. Hester, M. (2010). *End-of-life care and pragmatic decision making: A bioethical perspective*. New York: Cambridge University Press.
87. Hallenbeck, J. L. (2003). *Palliative care perspectives*. Oxford: Oxford University Press.
88. Cherny, N. I., Coyle, N., & Foley, K. M. (1996). Guidelines in the care of the dying cancer patient. *Hematology/Oncology Clinics of North America, 10*, 261–286.
89. Höcker, A., Krüll, A., Koch, U., & Mehnert, A. (2014). Exploring spiritual needs and their associated factors in an urban sample of early and advanced cancer patients. *European Journal of Cancer Care, 23*(6), 786–794.
90. Forouzi, M. A., Tirgari, B., Safarizadeh, M. H., & Jahani, Y. (2017). Spiritual needs and quality of life of patients with cancer. *Indian Journal of Palliative Care, 23*(4), 437–444.
91. Mesquita, A. C., Chaves, É. C. L., & Barros, G. A. M. (2017). Spiritual needs of patients with cancer in palliative care: An integrative review. *Current Opinion in Supportive and Palliative Care, 11*(4), 334–340.
92. Ripamonti, C. I., Giuntoli, F., Gonella, S., & Miccinesi, G. (2018). Spiritual care in cancer patients: A need or an option? *Current Opinion in Oncology, 30*(4), 212–218.
93. Breitbart, W., & Appelbaum, A. (2011). Meaning-centered group psychotherapy. In M. Watson & D. W. Kissane (Eds.), *Handbook of psychotherapy in cancer care* (pp. 137–148). Hoboken: Wiley-Blackwell.
94. Charon, R. (2004). Narrative and medicine. *New England Journal of Medicine, 350*, 862–864.
95. Chochinov, H. M., Hack, T., Hassard, T., Kristjanson, L. J., McClement, S., & Harlos, M. (2005). Dignity therapy: A novel psychotherapeutic intervention for patients near the end of life. *Journal of Clinical Oncology, 23*(24), 5520–5525.
96. Payne, D. K. (2011). Mindfulness interventions for cancer patients. In M. Watson & D. W. Kissane (Eds.), *Handbook of psychotherapy in cancer care* (pp. 39–47). Hoboken: Wiley-Blackwell.
97. Benson, H. (1975). *The relaxation response*. New York: Morow.
98. Kreitler, S. (2012). Guided imagery: A psychological tool in the service of health psychology. In K. R. Carter & G. E. Murphy (Eds.), *Alternative medicine: Practices, health benefits and controversies* (pp. 1–26). Hauppauge: Nova Publishers.

99. Kabat-Zinn, J. (2003). Mindfulness-based interventions in context: Past, present, and future. *Clinical Psychology Science and Practice, 10*(2), 144–156.
100. Kastbom, L., Milberg, A., & Karlsson, M. (2017). A good death from the perspective of palliative cancer patients. *Supportive Care in Cancer, 25*(3), 933–939.
101. Engle, V. F., Fox-Hill, E., & Graney, M. J. (1998). The experience of living-dying in a nursing home: Self-reports of black and white older adults. *Journal of the American Geriatric Society, 46*(9), 1091–1096.
102. Miyashita, M., Kawakami, S., Kato, D., Yamashita, H., Igaki, H., Nakano, K., Kuroda, Y., & Nakagawa, K. (2015). The importance of good death components among cancer patients, the general population, oncologists, and oncology nurses in Japan: Patients prefer "fighting against cancer". *Supportive Care in Cancer, 23*(1), 103–110.
103. Cheng, S. Y., Hu, W. Y., Liu, W. J., Yao, C. A., Chen, C. Y., & Chiu, T. Y. (2008). Good death study of elderly patients with terminal cancer in Taiwan. *Palliative Medicine, 22*(5), 626–632.
104. Yun, Y. H., Kim, K. N., Sim, J. A., Kang, E., Lee, J., Choo, J., Yoo, S. H., Kim, M., Kim, Y. A., Kang, B. D., Shim, H., Song, E. K., Kang, J. H., Kwon, J. H., Lee, J., Lee, S. N., Maeng, C. H., Kang, E. J., Do, Y. R., Choi, Y. S., & Jung, K. H. (2018). Priorities of a "good death" according to cancer patients, their family caregivers, physicians, and the general population: A nationwide survey. *Supportive Care in Cancer, 26*(10), 3479–3488.
105. Waghorn, M., Young, H., & Davies, A. (2011). Opinions of patients with cancer on the relative importance of place of death in the context of a 'good death'. *BMJ Supportive & Palliative Care, 1*(3), 310–314.
106. Cheng, S. Y., Lin, W. Y., Cheng, Y. H., Huang, C. H., Chen, C. Y., Hwang, S. J., Tsa, S. T., & Chiu, T. Y. (2016). Cancer patient autonomy and quality of dying-a prospective nationwide survey in Taiwan. *Psycho-Oncology, 25*(2), 179–186.
107. Meier, E. A., Gallegos, J. V., Thomas, L., Depp, C. A., Irwin, S. A., & Jeste, D. V. (2016). Defining a good death (Successful dying): Literature review and a call for research and public dialogue. *American Journal of Geriatric Psychiatry, 24*(4), 261–271.
108. Kreitler, S. (2007). Coping with death by family members. The Glickman Center for Education and Training, Eshel – The association for the planning and development of services for the aged in Israel. Tel Hashomer, Israel, May 17, 2007.
109. Kreitler, S., Barak, F., & Siegelmann-Danieli, N. (2009). Survivor's guilt: The case of cancer. In D. Cooley, L. Steffen, & R. Fisher (Eds.), *Death and dying*. Oxford: Inter-Disciplinary Press.
110. Chapman, K. J., & Pepler, C. (1998). Coping, hope, and anticipatory grief in family members in palliative home care. *Cancer Nursing, 21*(4), 226–234.
111. Kreitler, S., Barak, F., Alkalay, Y., & Siegelman-Danieli, N. (2012). Survivor's guilt in the caretakers of cancer. In A. Kasher & A. Glahn (Eds.), *The presence of the dead in our lives* (Interface/Probing the Boundaries Series) (pp. 77–98). Amsterdam: Rodopi.
112. Milberg, A., Strang, P., & Jakobsson, M. (2004). Next of kin's experience of powerlessness and helplessness in palliative home care. *Supportive Care in Cancer, 12*(2), 120–128.
113. Kreitler, S., Barak, F., & Siegelman-Danieli, N. (2008). The survivors' guilt: The case of cancer. 6th global conference, making sense of dying and death, probing the boundaries project, interdisciplinary. Salzburg, Austria, November 3–5, 2008.
114. Hirooka, K., Fukahori, H., Taku, K., Togari, T., & Ogawa, A. (2017). Quality of death, rumination, and posttraumatic growth among bereaved family members of cancer patients in home palliative care. *Psycho-Oncology, 26*(12), 2168–2174.
115. Miyashita, M., Morita, T., Sato, K., Hirai, K., Shima, Y., & Uchitomi, Y. (2008). Good death inventory: A measure for evaluating good death from the bereaved family member's perspective. *Journal of Pain and Symptom Management, 35*(5), 486–498.
116. Granek, L., Ben-David, M., Bar-Sela, G., Shapira, S., & Ariad, S. (2018). "Please do not act violently towards the staff": expressions and causes of anger, violence, and aggression in Israeli cancer patients and their families from the perspective of oncologists. *Transcultural Psychiatry*. 2018, Jul 27: 1363461518786162 [Epub ahead of print].

117. Kaur, J., & Mohandi, B. K. (2011). Transition from curative to palliative care in cancer. *Indian Journal of Palliative Care, 17*(1), 1–5.
118. Kreitler, S. (2018). Empathy: How much is right? Tools for the management of empathy in the context of healthcare. In C. Pracana & M. Wang (Eds.), *Psychology applications & developments IV*. Lisboa: Science Press.
119. Parola, V., Coelho, A., Cardoso, D., Sangren, A., & Apóstolo, J. (2017). Prevalence of burnout in health professionals working in palliative care: A systematic review. *JBI (Joanna Briggs Institute) Database of Systematic Reviews and Implementation Reports, 15*(7), 1905–1933.
120. Ganapathy, K. (2018). Brain death revisited. *Neurology India, 66*(2), 308–315.
121. Sade, R. M. (2011). Brain death, cardiac death, and the dead donor rule. *Journal of the South Carolina (JSC) Medical Association, 107*(4), 146–149.
122. Taylor, P. M., & Jonson, M. (2011). Recognizing dying in terminal illness. *British Journal of Hospital Medicine, 72*, 446–450.
123. Taylor, P., Crouch, S., Howell, D. A., Dowding, D. W., & Johnson, M. J. (2015). Change in physiological variables in the last 2 weeks of life: An observational study of hospital inpatients with cancer. *Palliative Medicine, 29*, 120–127.
124. Glare, P., Virik, K., Jones, M., Hudson, M., Eychmuller, S., Simes, J., & Christakis, N. (2003). A systematic review of physicians' survival predictions in terminally ill cancer patients. *British Medical Journal, 327*(7408), 195–198.
125. Harel, S. (2014). The relation between psychological, familial and supportive features and course of disease and quality of life in patients hospitalized in intensive care units. Thesis for Master's Degree (M.A.) in the Department of Nursing, Haifa University.
126. Eliott, J. A., & Olver, I. (2011). Dying cancer patients talk about physician and patient roles in DNR decision making. *Health Expectations, 14*(2), 147–158.
127. Kim, K., Chakravarthy, B., Anderson, C., & Liao, S. (2017). To intubate or not to intubate: Emergency medicine physicians' perspective on intubating critically ill, terminal cancer patients. *Journal of Pain and Symptom Management, 54*(5), 654–660.
128. Randén, M., Helde-Frankling, M., Runesdotter, S., & Strang, P. (2013). Treatment decisions and discontinuation of palliative chemotherapy near the end-of-life, in relation to socioeconomic variables. *Acta Oncologica, 52*(6), 1062–1066.
129. Lacey, J., & Sanderson, C. (2010). The oncologist's role in care of the dying cancer patient. *Cancer Journal, 16*(5), 532–541.
130. Viney, L. L., Walker, B. M., Robertson, T., Lilley, B., & Ewan, C. (1994). Dying in palliative care units and in hospital: A comparison of the quality of life of terminal cancer patients. *Journal of Consulting and Clinical Psychology, 62*(1), 157–164.
131. Barak, F., Livshits, S., Kaufer, H., Netanel, R., Siegelmann-Danieli, N., Alkalay, Y., & Kreitler, S. (2015). Where to die? This is the question: A study of cancer patients in Israel. *Palliative and Supportive Care, 13*, 165–170.
132. Higginson, I. J., Astin, P., & Dolan, S. (1998). Where do cancer patients die? Ten-year trends in the place of death of cancer patients in England. *Palliative Medicine, 12*(5), 353–363.
133. Ikezaki, S., & Ikegami, N. (2011). Predictors of dying at home for patients receiving nursing services in Japan: A retrospective study comparing cancer and non-cancer deaths. *BMC Palliative Care, 10*(3), 1–11.
134. Gomes, B., & Higginson, I. J. (2006). Factors influencing death at home in terminally ill patients with cancer: Systematic review. *British Medical Journal, 332*, 515–521.
135. Chochinov, H. M., Tataryn, D., Clinch, J. J., & Dudgeon, D. (1999). Will to live in the terminally ill. *The Lancet, 354*, 816–819.
136. Chochinov, H. M., Hack, T., Hassard, T., Kristjanson, L. J., McClement, S., & Harlos, M. (2005). Understanding the will to live in patients nearing death. *Psychosomatics, 46*(1), 7–10.
137. Kedem, E., Karkom, M., & Kreitler, S. (submitted). The cognitive orientation of survival as a predictor of responses to treatment in Israeli and Russian HIV patients.
138. Salmon, P., Manzi, F., & Valori, R. M. (1996). Measuring the meaning of life for patients with incurable cancer: The life evaluation questionnaire (LEQ). *European Journal of Cancer, 32A*(5), 755–760.

139. Comer, R. J. (2016). *Fundamentals of abnormal psychology* (8th ed.). New York: Worth Publishers.
140. Breitbart, W., Pessin, H., & Kolva, E. (2011). Suicide and desire for hastened death in people with cancer. In D. W. Kissane, M. Maj, & N. Sartorius (Eds.), *Depression and cancer* (pp. 125–150). Chichester: Wiley.
141. Breitbart, W. S., & Alici, Y. (2014). Suicide, assisted suicide, and desire for hastened death. In W. S. Breitbart & Y. Alici (Eds.), *Psychosocial palliative care*. (Chapter 6 (pp. 49–54). New York: Oxford University Press.

Chapter 14
Specific Cancer Diseases: The Psychological Perspective

Introduction

Cancer is not one specific disease but a family of diseases that differ greatly in almost any conceivable respect – medical, pathological, genetic, and epidemiological. Although patients refer to their disease mostly in terms of the general label "cancer," they soon find out how different the cancer diseases are. They learn about the particular characteristics of cancers from the different kinds of health professionals who take care of them but no less from the other patients whom they meet in the clinics and hospitals, self-help groups, and Internet reports and groups.

The number of different cancers runs into the hundreds. According to ASCO, there are over 100 cancer types and according to the NIH over 200 [1]. They are often named in line with the organs or tissues in which they form but sometimes also by the type of cell that created them. The five major groups of cancer are the carcinomas, leukemias, sarcomas, lymphatic system cancers, and brain and spinal cord cancers. The cancers differ in the primary symptoms, in the way they are detected, in the manner in which a diagnosis is established, in the stages, in the treatment options, in the manner and degree and sites of metastases, in the overall course of disease, in the follow-up care, and in the chances for recurrence and survival. These medical aspects include also variations in severity, stages, and the underlying anomaly in the cells. Additionally, cancer differs in prevalence, ethnic backgrounds, populations, susceptibility to different risk factors, and incidence in specific groups (e.g., gender, age), environments, and geographical regions.

Patients are mostly familiar only with the general characteristics of the kind of cancer with which they have been diagnosed, and it is only gradually that they learn to appreciate the differences between the kinds of cancer and stop generalizing the facts about cancer they find out from patients with other cancers.

There are major psychological differences in experiencing and being treated for different kinds of cancer. These depend on the kind of cancer itself, including stage and

S. Kreitler, *Psycho-Oncology for the Clinician*,
https://doi.org/10.1007/978-3-030-06126-5_14

grade, but also on the personality of the patient, the kind of treatment, and the environment, including culture, lifestyle, family factors, and the support the patient gets.

The attitude of the patient toward the disease is a major determinant of the total experience. Having cancer is in most cases an engrossing event for the patient. However, some patients let the disease invade the whole of their life and revolutionize it, believing that only a major change in themselves and their lifestyle will enable recovery. Others keep a distance between themselves and the disease, do not let the disease invade or control them, and change their lifestyle and behavior as little as possible, awaiting as it were the passage of the storm until quieter times arrive.

The present chapter focuses on the psychological aspects of cancers of different kinds. Most patients with different cancer diseases pass through the difficulties of undergoing diagnosis with its uncertainties and treatments attended by their difficult side effects and embark on the track of survivorship with the fears of recurrence. There are phases and fears likely to be shared by cancer patients with varied cancer diagnoses. Aspects of this general kind have been dealt with in other chapters (see Chaps. 3, 6, 7, 8, 9, and 10). However, living with one kind of cancer is not like living with another kind. An attempt is made in the present chapter to emphasize the specific and characteristic aspects of the different cancers rather than the general ones characterizing cancers across the board. Yet, since it is likely that heterogeneity characterizes the psychological aspects of dealing with cancer possibly more than the physiological and medical aspects, the following discussions need to be considered as general overviews.

Breast Cancer

Breast cancer is the most common and most dreaded cancer in women in the Western world. Many women have been exposed to at least some of the medical aspects and terminology of breast cancer through contact with their friends or family members who have been diagnosed with breast cancer. Some have accompanied their sick friends through several of the stages of the disease and treatments. In addition, breast cancer is discussed in the media quite often, exposing the results of new research or describing the experiences or attitudes of various celebrities diagnosed with breast cancer. It has been noted that breast cancer makes "good" headlines which is partly responsible for the tendency to present reports about breast cancer issues in a "sensationalized" way [2]. Information about breast cancer is reported in the websites in the form of facts or semi-facts, autobiographical confessions, proposals for help and support, or self-help group discussions. In addition, the widely publicized campaigns for screening and even self-testing in regard to breast cancer [3] contribute to keeping breast cancer in the forefront of awareness. All these easily accessible sources of information render breast cancer a kind of familiar disease, more than other cancer diseases. Yet they do not mitigate the emotional impact and the fears it evokes in women.

The loads of facts, semi-facts, and other references to breast cancer in the media and social networks include many myths, half-truth, and incorrect statements that may enhance the fear evoked by breast cancer. These fears may contribute to the reluctance of many women to undergo breast cancer screening and to strengthening the barriers against the screening [4, 5]. Fear of detecting cancer is a major determinant of avoiding screening for breast cancer [6–8], which has strengthened the assumption that breast cancer patients tend toward repression [9, 10].

Breast cancer is usually diagnosed in a regular screening survey or after detection of some irregularity in the breast in a regular screening survey or because the patient herself or a doctor detected a lump or some other symptom. It involves some kind of imaging (e.g., mammography) and a biopsy.

The diagnosis and treatment of breast cancer usually last for about a year. It involves medical examinations, mostly surgery, medications in the form of chemotherapy or hormonal therapy, and radiotherapy. After termination of treatment, medical follow-up is required, and in many clinics, it involves examination by an oncologist and a surgeon. But after several years, it is often reduced to a once-a-year checkup unless there are changes requiring medical attention.

A diagnosis of breast cancer brings to the surface fears and anxieties that women may harbor for years without confronting or overcoming them. Women share with the majority of people the commonly cited fears of cancer which have been identified as fears about its proximity, the absence of strategies to keep it at a distance, about the personal and social implications of succumbing, and of dying from the cancer [11]. The fears of disease progression and recurrence fulfill a great role in the lives of breast cancer patients [12]. But in addition they suffer from fears concerning specific aspects.

Body Image

One major issue focuses on concerns about negative changes in their *body image* [13]. This refers primarily to the breast. The breast is a focus of sexuality in the life of many women and couples. Women are scared of the changes in the breast because of their own reactions as well as because of the reactions of their partner. In case of mastectomy, the change in body image is evident, but even following lumpectomy, the result may not be perfect or as desired by the woman. There may be changes in the shape, the volume, and the overall appearance of the breast, as well as in the skin and hardness following radiotherapy [14]. Also the symmetry of both breasts may be impaired. Sometimes women report pain in the breast and even fear that some malignant cells may have remained in the breast following lumpectomy [15]. Following breast surgery women are faced with the major decision concerning breast reconstruction. The dilemmas are multiple: whether to undergo the reconstruction, whether to undergo full or partial reconstruction, and if yes when, during the primary surgery or later. The decisions are a function of several considerations, such as desire to avoid any further surgeries and doctor visits, degree of satisfaction with the shape of the breast as is, fear that reconstruction may render detection of recurrence more difficult, and the assumed or declared attitudes of the partner [16, 17].

Further important changes take place in regard to the body image. First is alopecia, which is still a highly common side effect of different kinds of chemotherapy [18]. Although many women use wigs or partial hair additions, these help in maintaining appearance but not always the sense of femininity and beauty. The latter are further affected negatively by frequent changes in the skin, following radiotherapy, and by weight gain, due to the different maintenance drugs prescribed following termination of chemotherapy (e.g., tamoxifen) [19]. Weight gain may be a part of a more encompassing cluster of symptoms, such as hot flashes, hair thinning, fatigue, and mood swings, related to the effect of drugs such as tamoxifen creating a state of menopause [20]. This too implies for women aging coupled with loss of beauty and femininity.

Sexuality

Body image is closely associated with the feeling of being a woman and with *sexuality*. Since the breast is often treated as a symbol of femininity – including sexual attractiveness and motherhood – it is not surprising that changes in the appearance of the breast may affect the sense of womanliness and also the sexuality of women [21]. These changes may lower the woman's self-esteem and confidence, even after and despite breast reconstruction. Lumpectomy and breast reconstruction help in supporting the body image but to a lower extent sexuality [22].

Fertility

Fertility and childbearing constitute another major issue for at least the younger women affected by breast cancer. Premenopausal women worry about whether they can still bear children despite the treatments for breast cancer they have undergone. They also worry if they should have children in view of the risk of dying before the children are grown up. In case they are genetically implicated, they also worry about passing on the genes to their children [23].

Specific side effects that concern women diagnosed with breast cancer are fatigue, pain, and depression [24, 25]. In addition, breast cancer patients mention often cognitive difficulties of different kinds [26, 27]. Cognitive impairment may be due not only to chemotherapy but also to other treatments and may persist for a long time after termination of the treatments [28]. The lowering of cognitive performance is particularly worrisome for the women and may interact with depression in a cause-and-effect loop.

Analyzing the responses of a great number of women with breast cancer has led to the identification of four trajectories of psychological distress and functioning: the chronic, delayed, recovered, and resilient [29]. Notably, women who reacted with distress in the first year were still in distress 6 years later, while those who adjusted better in the first year continued so also later [30].

The psychological effects of breast cancer and the patients' responses to the disease and treatments are affected at least to some extent by the psychological characteristics of the patients. In particular, it is likely that the following tendencies identified in studies of the cognitive orientation tendencies of breast cancer patients may render it particularly difficult for them to cope with the disease and its symptoms: concern with the positive evaluation of others, perfectionism and insistence on fulfilling one's duties, not sharing with others, and need for unrestricted freedom. Tendencies of these kinds may affect especially dealing with changes in body image, giving to others, getting support from others, and adjusting one's activities to one's physical and emotional resources [31, 32].

It seems that women diagnosed with breast cancer use websites of self-help and information on the Internet to a large extent in the different phases of the disease. They also report using different psychosocial treatments, CAM, and support of different kinds in their attempts to cope with the disease. It appears that breast cancer often affects their life and lifestyle to a salient degree.

Gastrointestinal Cancers

Colorectal cancer is the most common of the gastrointestinal cancers. The diagnosis starts mostly after detection of some symptom by the patient or in a regular screening or on the basis of information about genetic family background. It is mostly experienced as an unpleasant process [33]. The treatment consists of surgery, followed often by chemotherapy and sometimes radiotherapy. Pain, and difficulties or anomalies with bowel movements, may follow, depending on the extent of the surgery and the stage of the disease. These symptoms usually weaken with time but may also persist and require more attention on the part of the patient and prolonged rehabilitation. A review showed that patients with colorectal cancer continue to suffer from depression, distress, and bowel-related problems such as constipation and diarrhea which affect their quality of life [34]. Yet, there is also evidence that the quality of life of the patients after some time does not differ from that in the general population [35].

Under certain conditions, the surgery results in a permanent ostomy, which may affect quite seriously the patients' quality of life, even when they remain disease-free. The patients reported depression, anxiety [36], social isolation, interference with work and entertainment, difficulties with sexuality, low self-esteem and impaired body image, and problems with appearance and clothing as well as with managing the colostomy (e.g., issues of odor, leakage, and noise) [37–39].

Gastrointestinal cancers include further diagnoses which may often have more serious psychological effects. These are hepatocellular carcinoma, cancer of the pancreas, and cancer of the esophagus and stomach. These types of cancer are assumed by patients to be high in malignancy. Treatments are often prolonged and are attended by different complications which may necessitate recurrent surgeries. The diseases are also often related to severe symptoms including dysphagia (e.g., esophagus cancer), pain and difficulty in digestion (e.g., pancreas), or ascites (e.g., hepatocellular carcinoma). Hence, on the whole, patients with these types of cancer often suffer physically and psychologically, are frequently preoccupied with the disease and the symptoms, and report quite a lot of distress, anxiety, and depression [40–42].

Specific psychological tendencies were found to characterize individuals diagnosed with gastrointestinal cancers [43, 44]. These include compulsiveness, pleasing others, control of oneself, self-assertion, distancing oneself from others, adhering to the rules, and performing to perfection all ones obligations. It is plausible that these tendencies may enhance the difficulty of coping with the symptoms of the disease [43, 44]. Thus, individuals characterized by compulsiveness and self-control suffer especially when they cannot adequately control their toilet behavior, while the lower ability to function as required may hurt particularly those who insist on performing all ones' obligations to perfection.

Lung Cancer

Lung cancer is a complicated disease. A study which compared distress evaluations of 9000 cancer patients of different diagnoses found that the highest rates of anxiety and depression were reported by patients with lung cancer (43.4%, as compared with the average which was 35. 1%) [45]. Also other studies found higher rates of emotional distress in lung cancer patients than in other cancer diagnoses [46, 47]. Certain characteristics, mainly younger age, being a female, current smoking, current employment, advanced disease, and undergoing treatment are related in lung cancer patients with greater risk for emotional problems, which are associated with a reduced quality of life and greater symptom burden [47]. In another study the predictors for severe emotional problems were similar and included younger age, fatigue, pain, anxiety, and depression [48]. Depression was reported even after beginning of treatment in 50% of the patients [48]. A study in China [49] showed that gender, younger age, surgical history, employment status, and medical insurance significantly predicted the severity of psychological problems in lung cancer patients. Functional impairment was found to be highly distressing [49]. The treatments may be difficult and bring about a reduction in quality of life [50].

The high rate of distress noted by patients reflects both the way they feel and the way they expect to feel in the future. Lung cancer has the reputation of a disease generating suffering. The quality of life in lung cancer patients is lower than in the healthy population and in patients suffering from other malignancies. It is affected by the severity and the number of symptoms these patients have, such as fatigue, loss of appetite, dyspnea, cough, pain, and blood in sputum, which are specific for lung tumors. Difficulties in breathing that seem to be related to lung cancer are considered by many people to be especially distressing and difficult to bear [51]. Fatigue and respiratory problems reduce the psychological dimension of quality of life, while sleep problems reduce cognitive functioning. The physical dimension of activity, related to growing disability, is reduced in most of the patients. As a result, many of these patients are unable to play their family and social roles [52]. The major symptoms in those undergoing treatment (chemotherapy 75.8%, radiotherapy 54.7%, and surgery 54.4%) are neurocognitive symptoms (e.g., fatigue, cognitive changes) especially among those receiving chemotherapy, followed by musculoskeletal/dermatologic symptoms and thoracic symptoms (13.5%) [53].

Treatment, even surgery, does not necessarily reduce distress in lung cancer patients. Postoperative psychological distress and, in particular, depression increased after surgical treatment for lung cancer. Postoperative anxiety and depression were found to be enhanced by residual symptoms after surgery [51]. Gender and family history of cancer were found as criteria for identifying patients at risk for higher levels of physical symptoms and lower self-efficacy after cancer surgery [54]. Notably, acceptance of disease, which is related to lower stress and higher self-esteem, plays an important role in the adaptive process. However, it is lower after surgery [55]. The fear of suffering may evoke the desire to avoid it at all costs, even by means of shortening one's survival period by consenting to the "do-not-resuscitate" request [56]. Not surprisingly, different psychiatric symptoms occur in these patients [57].

Depression is a particularly salient problem in lung cancer patient. Depression is higher in lung cancer patients than in other groups of patients. Thoracotomy, post-operative dyspnea, severe pain, and diabetes mellitus were identified as risk factors for postoperative depression after adjusting for preoperative depression [51]. Younger age, being female, and undergoing surgery were identified as risk factors for depression [58]. Patients with depression have higher rates of visits and admissions to emergency rooms than those without depression [58]. In patients with early-stage disease, depression was related to increased mortality [59]. In recent years new biologically based therapies causing fewer serious side effects have been developed for lung cancer [60]. Hence, it may be hoped that suffering will be reduced for at least some patients.

Personal Responsibility for The Disease

A particularly salient source of stress and distress in lung cancer patients is the fact that they are often assigned personal responsibility for the disease [61, 62]. Since smoking tobacco has been identified as a risk factor for lung cancer (e.g., by the Surgeon General's 1964 report), social attitudes toward lung cancer patients have become negative. Hence, lung cancer patients are often blamed for their disease, especially if they had been smokers. Sometimes it is even claimed that there seems to be no justification for spending public money for their treatment. Personal responsibility was found to be common – as high as in 80% of respondents – in patients who had ever smoked, whereas regret and feelings of stigmatization were less frequent, but when present they were associated with negative psychological outcomes, such as treatment nonadherence, feelings of isolation, avoidance of healthcare providers, and poor quality of life, in past smokers as well as in those who had never smoked [60]. Notably, lung cancer patients tend to assume responsibility for their disease even when they have never smoked but have been in the presence of other people who have smoked (i.e., passive smoking) or have not checked their apartment for radon gas [63].

Following diagnosis and surgery, lung cancer patients who have been smokers tend to consider quitting smoking. Many do, but they also feel the difficulty of quitting and still consider the benefits of smoking, e.g., pleasure, health benefits in relieving stress, and help in coping. Therefore, many express the wish to quit and need to get support for quitting smoking [64]. Notably, having quit smoking apparently empowers the patients because posttraumatic growth was found to function as a buffer against the negative effects of stigma on psychological distress only among those who after diagnosis quit smoking [65].

The tendency of lung cancer patients to assume responsibility for their disease is in accord with their personality characteristics, as defined by the cognitive orientation methodology which showed that they tend to be rational, realistic, and honest, try to perform what is required and right, and maintain control of the situation [66].

Due to the psychological distress of lung cancer patients, it is commonly suggested that these patients should get support and help in coping with the disease.

The major coping strategies applied by lung cancer patients were found to be reflections about the cause of the disease, the experience of inequity, repression, so-called positive attitude, focusing on the present, and adjusting of life terms [67]. There are many resources and foundations offering help and education to lung cancer patients [68]. More specifically, mindfulness training [69] and spiritual support have proven to be particularly helpful [70].

Prostate Cancer

This is one of the more common cancers. It affects an increasing number of males especially with advancing age. Early detection is possible, mainly by PSA screening, which has been noted to evoke anxiety in at least some individuals [71]. Due to improved screening and available treatments, the life span of prostate cancer patients has become longer. The primary treatment options are deferred treatments which include "watchful waiting" and "active surveillance"; surgery, i.e., prostatectomy, radical (open) operation, laparoscopic or robotic; radiation therapy, i.e., external beam, intensity modulated, proton therapy, and brachytherapy (seed implants); and focal therapies (e.g., through heat or cryotherapy). The major systemic treatments are androgen deprivation therapy (ADT) and chemotherapy.

The choice depends primarily on the grade and spread of the cancer itself, as well as on further factors, such as the patient's age, general health and comorbidities, psychological state, and attitude toward the different side effects of the treatments (e.g., on erection, incontinence).

The large choice of treatments even in the first stage of the disease produces a great difficulty for the patient. The need to make a choice and decide requires getting a lot of information, at least partly medical, to make sure that it is correct and complete and to decide in view of different considerations. The situation is stressful also because of the prolonged period of uncertainty that the decision time involves.

The different treatments are likely to cause different side effects that affect the patient's psychological state. The lowest degree of effect on quality of life is the treatment that consists in surveillance, although it is also attended by anxiety and fear concerning the time when it will be given up for more active types of treatment [72]. Prostatectomy may affect adversely erectile function if the responsible nerves are impaired. This causes the patients a lot of anxiety prior to the surgery and depression following it. In some cases there is also pain. Radiotherapy may affect adversely bladder and bowel functioning. Urinary incontinence may be distressing because of leaking and smells. Side effects of the hormonal treatments include erectile dysfunction, hot flashes, loss of sexual desire, gynecomastia, loss of bodily hair, difficulties in concentration and memory, weakness, irritability, and anxiety [73]. Beyond the side effects, there is often the accompanying anxiety about the recurrence of the disease, which increases around the periods of screening [74].

The impairment of sexual functioning, which may result from different treatments of prostate cancer, is particularly distressing because of its likely effects on couples and intimate relationships. Studies showed that partners may suffer more distress than the patients themselves [75]. Treatment by ADT may cause not only sexual dysfunction but may be also followed by diabetes, cardiovascular disorders, bone density reduction, impotence, and depression [76–78].

The personality tendencies of prostate cancer patients [79] may enhance their distress caused by different phenomena of the disease and the treatments. Thus, their tendencies as revealed by the cognitive orientation approach, to rely mainly on themselves, be independent, and do things their own way may make it difficult for them to adjust to limitations in mobility and range of activities caused by pain, weakness, and fatigue. Further, due to the tendency to adhere to normative regulations, they would be distressed by symptoms, such as urinary incontinence and the inability to act as the expected sexual partner.

Head and Neck Cancer

Head and neck cancers may affect a variety of organs, including the nasal cavity and paranasal sinus, the lip and the oral cavity, the larynx, the hypopharynx (the gullet), the salivary gland, and the oropharynx. Some of these cancers are more common than others, e.g., oral cavity cancer and laryngeal cancer are relatively more common, while salivary gland cancer is less common. The majority are squamous cell carcinomas. Major risk factors for the cancers are smoking, chewing of tobacco, alcohol consumption, HPV infection, and exposure to smoke and to different environmental pollutants, including dust, rubber, and asbestos. A major problem related to these cancers is that they occur in organs involved in major functions, such as eating, swallowing, speaking, and breathing. The medical treatments include surgery, radiation, and chemotherapy, which may seriously impair the basic functioning of the affected organs, in addition to the cancers themselves [80].

The presenting symptoms of these cancers may be distressing, e.g., difficulties in swallowing or breathing, hoarse voice, and ear pain. The persisting side effects of the treatments may be no less distressing, e.g., dry mouth, dysphagia, chronic pain, loss of taste, mucositis, and sometimes even loss of the ability to use one's voice. These results may occur even though every effort is made in treatment to conserve or reconstruct the organs or features essential for the operation of the essential functions. Some treatments may cause serious cosmetic outcomes, such as tracheostoma dependence and facial disfigurement. The long-term persistence of side effects may be responsible for profound negative effects on the patients' general well-being and quality of life in different domains, including social (e.g., social isolation, delay in returning to work) and psychological (e.g., depression) [81, 82].

Head and neck cancer patients have been reported to suffer from anxiety and distress [83, 84]. One cause for their anxiety is the information they have about their disease and the chances for its progression [85]. Information affects negatively their quality of life especially when the disease is judged to be severe and of longer duration [86]. The anxiety is often fueled by the patients' fear that the disease is liable to recur since they have undergone not a full but only an organ-sparing surgical treatment [87].

If the disease or treatments have led to facial disfigurement, the patients' suffering is greatly increased [88]. Facial disfigurement may cause shame, lowered self-esteem, damaged overall body image, limited social contacts and social functioning in general, withdrawal from one's roles in the family, reduced or eliminated sexual activity, and difficulties in functioning at work. These effects may impact negatively relations with one's partner and children, as well as the partner himself or herself. Studies show that the partners of these patients are not always aware of the extent of their suffering [89].

Swallowing problems may constitute another source of distress for head and neck cancer patients. Some of the more frequent symptoms with a socially compromising potential are the food and liquids spilling from the mouth or food getting stuck in the throat or nasal cavity.

In some cases head and neck cancer patients have difficulties in speaking. The degree of difficulty depends on the extent of the damage to the larynx due to the disease and the treatments. Hoarseness and low volume are the low-level disturbances. The more serious ones follow total laryngectomy which involves the need to learn a completely new type of speech production – electrolarynx, esophageal speech, or tracheoesophageal speech. All three methods require a lot of practice on the part of the patient, and the produced voice varies in clarity and naturalness. The changes and difficulties in eating and speaking often bring about changes in social behavior and are liable to cause difficulties in interpersonal and marital relations [82].

It is not rare for head and neck cancer patients to experience rejection and blame for their disease on the part of other people. The stigma is based on assigning to these patients some responsibility for their disease through smoking of tobacco, drinking alcohol, poor oral and dental hygiene, and solar exposure. The explicit and more often implicit accusation enhances the patients' difficulty of taking care of their disease and contributes to lowering their quality of life [90–92].

There is also evidence for different psychopathologies developing in these patients [93]. The rate of suicide in these patients was found to be three times higher than in the general population, especially in patients with hypopharyngeal cancer (12 times higher) or laryngeal cancer (five times higher), probably because these sites are linked to impaired swallowing and speaking [94]. However, there is also evidence that after the major period of diagnosis and treatment, a great number of head and neck cancer patients learn to cope with the difficulties and get good long-term psychosocial adaptation [95].

Head/Brain Cancer

There are more than 120 different types of brain and central nervous system tumors, differing in grade and site, and a large number of metastatic brain tumors [96]. The most frequent ones in adults are meningiomas and gliomas. Most (80%) cancers in other body parts have the potential of producing brain metastases. Brain tumors are one of the most dreaded cancers by patients. Patients are afraid that the brain tumor, regardless of its origin and type, may cause cognitive impairment of different kinds, e.g., loss of memory, limited comprehension, and no ability to decide. Actually they fear most loss of their self and identity. The standard treatments include surgery, chemotherapy, and radiation in different combinations, with side effects that depend on the treatments and on the site of the tumor. The range of side effects is very broad and includes cognition, emotions, behavior, and physical state. The symptoms bothering many patients are mainly cognitive, emotional, and physical. The cognitive changes include loss of consciousness and awareness of one's environment, loss of memory or any of its functions, loss of the ability to decide, impaired understanding, decreased attention and concentration, diminished sense of reality, and slowed verbal expression or loss of speech ability [97, 98]. The emotional changes include loss of emotional control, blunting of affect, and weakened recognition of emotions in oneself and others [99]. The physical changes include loss of control over one's body, loss of different sensory functions, walking difficulties, and impaired bodily balance. Evidently, not all of these and similar symptoms occur in each case or in every stage of the disease. But the symptoms that do occur and those that could occur cause these patients a lot of distress. They get into the habit of monitoring themselves for any signs of functional deterioration, which they expect. Often they claim that they feel that they are losing their personality and identity [99]. The overall state of the patient is likely to evoke anxiety and depression [100].

In addition, fatigue, drowsiness, sleep disturbances, apathy, and sluggishness may occur. In some cases psychiatric symptoms such as aggressiveness, mood disorders including depression and mania, disorientation, delirium, and confusion may appear, depending on the treatment and the location of the tumor.

In view of the load of different symptoms, patients with brain tumors often suffer from limited independence and are in need of rehabilitation and a lot of assistance [101, 102].

The load of symptoms and overall psychological and physiological burden [103–105] cause a lot of suffering and a serious impairment of quality of life [106–108].

However, it needs to be emphasized that the symptoms are neither dominant nor persistent in the brain tumor patients. They depend greatly on the type of tumor and its location. So does survival which for some cancers may be higher than 50% for over 5 years in younger patients. The average survival rate is cited as 34.5% [109].

Skin Cancers

The three major kinds of skin cancer are basal cell, squamous cell, and melanoma. Of these three, melanoma is considered as highest in malignancy. Skin cancers are the most common kind of cancer, and at least the first two are almost completely curable. These two differ in pathology, incidence, and nature but most often do not cause mortality. They are usually detected early because they are externally visible on the skin and the treatment is frequently excision. The major risk factors for basal cell and squamous cell cancers are sun exposure and immunosuppression.

Despite the fact that basal cell and squamous cell carcinomas are treatable and largely curable, their occurrence still evokes psychological distress [110]. Patients worry about recurrence of the cancers and about disfigurement following surgery mostly on the face or neck. They also feel stressed by the fact that they are often blamed for the cancers because others tend to assume that they have been caused by sun tanning. Actually the stigma attached to skin cancers is as high as for smoking in regard to lung cancer [62].

Melanoma poses a special problem for patients. It differs from basal cell and squamous cell carcinomas in prevalence, nature, and prognosis. Survival rates differ by stage of the disease: For 5-year survival it is 97% for IA stage, 81% for stage IIA, and 15–20% for stage IV [111]. However, the malignancy of melanoma is potentially more severe than of the other skin cancers, and if it metastasizes, the 5-year survival drops to lower percentages (i.e., about 60% for regional spread or 15% for distant spread). Thus, the majority of patients face a life-threatening but curable disease, very often without any physical deficits [112]. In recent years a new approach to medical treatment of melanoma holds renewed hope to increase the chances of prolonging survival [113].

Some studies show that early-stage melanoma patients feel distressed [114, 115]. The reasons are mostly the procedures of diagnosis, and sometimes there are lymphedema and visible scars and disfigurement or skin grafting following surgery or lymphatic evidence for possible spread of the disease. Symptoms of anxiety are mostly more prevalent than depression. The frequent risk factors for distress are female sex, younger age, lower education, visibility of the affected body site, absence of social support, and negative appraisal of melanoma [115]. Distress reactions are reported by 10–30% of the patients but often pass after several months [116]. Some studies show that the quality of life of melanoma patients after 1 year or more post diagnosis is similar to that of the general population [116, 117] except for differences in particular domains such as emotional and sexual functioning [112].

However, there is also evidence that up to 75% of melanoma patients express concern about the recurrence of melanoma and live in a state of uncertainty and fear that the disease may overcome them suddenly without any preparation and without any really useful means of combatting the disease at that point [118, 119]. Hence, living with melanoma differs in many cases from living with other cancers: the individual has no physical deficits and does not suffer from any physical symptoms or side effects, does not undergo ay treatment, but is distressed and scared. Notably, this situation is surprisingly in accord with the psychological experience reported by many melanoma patients about differences between their inner life and external behavior [120].

There are several psychoeducational programs that have been developed for melanoma patients [121–123]. There is evidence that interventions of this kind result in increased patient satisfaction with clinical care and the information they get and provide support, improvement in coping, and reduction in distress and anxiety [124].

Some Afterthoughts

The objective of the present chapter was to demonstrate the differences between the cancer diseases, mainly from the patient's experiential perspective. The features shared by most of the cancer diseases are well known and have been amply discussed. They include among other factors the reference to a tumor, diagnosis by means of biopsy and other procedures, the basic kinds of treatments and their expected side effects, and the fear of death. Many patients know these features, often even if they are not sick, from acquaintances and the media. However, they do not usually learn about the idiosyncratic features of the cancer diseases that are rarely discussed and are mostly not given sufficient prominence. This situation underscores, the importance of the present chapter. It is designed to fill in the gap in information and expectation in regard to the unique experiencing of the different cancer diseases or at least to alert patients to the possibility that one cancer disease is not like the other.

It seems that information of this kind may prepare the patient for mobilizing coping means that are specifically designed to improve one's quality of life in the situation defined by a particular kind of cancer disease. For example, in prostate cancer, the issue of maintaining one's sense of masculinity may prevail; in head and neck cancers, a focal problem may be preserving one's cognitive functioning; and in melanoma, the characteristic experience may be living as if everything is normal but may collapse irreparably without any forewarning.

Being aware of the unique experiences of the cancer diseases may be particularly important in view of the fact that the individuals who get these different diseases differ in their psychosocial characteristics and hence in their vulnerabilities to different aspects of the disease, as well as in their abilities and manner of coping with it. For example, prostate cancer patients may be sensitive to limitations on their independent functioning which may be due to excessive weakness, while melanoma patients may be used to dissociation between their different life domains, as may happen in regard to the present and potential physical state. Emphasizing or at least not overlooking the unique aspects of the cancer diseases is necessary in order to understand and promote the right kind of response on the part of the patient with the right kind of requirements for adequately coping with the disease and hopefully overcoming it for the patient's optimal benefit.

Awareness of the unique aspects of the cancer disease is also important from a theoretical point of view because it promotes the conception that although a disease is often referred to by a medical label, in a human individual, it is primarily a complex outcome of interactions between the characteristics of the disease, the treatments, and the individual patient.

References

1. About cancer. National Cancer Institute. Washington DC. Retrieved March 28, 2018.
2. Tait, A. (1996). Psychological aspects of breast cancer. In S. Denton (Ed.), *Breast cancer nursing* (pp. 15–45). Boston: Springer.
3. Kreitler, S., & Chaitchik, S. (1996). Self-diagnosis through breast self-examination. Is it a solution? *Journal of Cancer Education, 11*(Suppl), 22.
4. Azami-Aghdash, S., Ghojazadeh, M., Sheyklo, S. G., Daemi, A., Kolahdouzan, K., Mohseni, M., & Moosavi, A. (2015). Breast cancer screening barriers from the womans perspective: A meta-synthesis. *Asian Pacific Journal of Cancer Prevention, 16*(8), 3463–3471.
5. Kreitler, S., Chaitchik, S., & Kreitler, H. (1990). The psychological profile of women attending breast-screening tests. *Social Science & Medicine, 31*, 1177–1185.
6. Crane, L. A., Kaplan, C. P., Bastani, R., & Scrimshaw, S. C. (1996). Determinants of adherence among health department patients referred for a mammogram. *Women Health, 24*(2), 43–64.

7. Mille, A. M., & Champion, V. L. (1997). Attitudes about breast cancer and mammography: Racial, income, and educational differences. *Women Health, 26*(1), 41–63.
8. Kreitler, S., Chaitchik, S., Kreitler, H., & Weissler, K. (1994). Who will attend tests for the early detection of breast cancer? *Psychology & Health, 9*, 463–483.
9. Kreitler, S., Chaitchik, S., & Kreitler, H. (1993). Repressiveness: A personality trait of cancer patients? *European Journal of Cancer, 29A*(Suppl 6), 214.
10. Kreitler, S., & Kreitler, H. (1990). Repression and the anxiety-defensiveness factor: Psychological correlates and manifestations. *Personality and Individual Differences, 11*, 559–550.
11. Vrinten, C., McGregor, L. M., Heinrich, M., von Wagner, C., Waller, J., Wardle, J., & Black, G. B. (2017). What do people fear about cancer? A systematic review and meta-synthesis. *Psychooncology, 26*(8), 1070–1107.
12. Mehnert, A., Berg, P., Henrich, G., & Herschbach, P. (2009). Fear of cancer progression and cancer-related intrusive cognitions in breast cancer survivors. *Psychooncology, 18*(12), 1273–1280.
13. Helms, R. L., O'Hea, E. L., & Corso, M. (2008). Body image issues in women with breast cancer. *Psychology, Health & Medicine, 13*(3), 313–325.
14. Immink, J. M., Putter, H., Bartelink, H., Cardoso, J. S., Cardoso, M. J., van der Hulst-Vijgen, M. H. V., Noordijk, E. M., Poortmans, P. M., Rodenhuis, C. C., & Struikmans, S. (2012). Long-term cosmetic changes after breast-conserving treatment of patients with stage I–II breast cancer and included in the EORTC 'boost versus no boost' trial. *Annals of Oncology, 23*(10), 2591–2598.
15. Kreitler, S., Kovner, F., Inbar, M., Wigler, N., Lelchuk, S., Chairchik, S., & Kreitler, H. (1993). Quality of life in breast cancer patients with mastectomy and lumpectomy. In J. C. Holland, M. J. Massie, W. S. Breitbart, P. B. Jacobsen, & S. D. Passik (Eds.), *Psycho-oncology V: Psychosocial factors in cancer risk and survival* (p. 219). New York: Memorial Sloan-Kettering Cancer Center.
16. Hart, A. M., Pinell-White, X., Egro, F. M., & Losken, A. (2015). The psychosexual impact of partial and total breast reconstruction: A prospective one-year longitudinal study. *Annals of Plastic Surgery, 75*(3), 281–286.
17. Vrouwe, S. Q., Somogyi, R. B., Snell, L., McMillan, C., Vesprini, D., & Lipa, J. E. (2018). Patient-reported outcomes following breast conservation therapy and barriers to referral for partial breast reconstruction. *Plastic and Reconstructive Surgery, 141*(1), 1–9.
18. Lemieux, J., Maunsell, E., & Provencher, L. (2008). Chemotherapy-induced alopecia and effects on quality of life among women with breast cancer: A literature review. *Psycho-Oncology, 17*, 317–328.
19. Playdon, M. C., Bracken, M. B., Sanft, T. B., Ligibel, J. A., Harrigan, M., & Irwin, M. L. (2015). Weight gain after breast cancer diagnosis and all-cause mortality: Systematic review and meta-analysis. *Journal of the National Cancer Institute, 107*(12), djv275.
20. Cusack, L. (2015). Menopausal symptoms in breast cancer survivors: Management update. *The British Journal of General Practice, 63*(606), 51–52.
21. Oktay, J. S. (1998). Psychosocial aspects of breast cancer. *Lippincott's Primary Care Practice, 2*(2), 149–159.
22. Safarinejad, M. R., Shafiei, N., & Safarinejad, S. (2013). Quality of life and sexual functioning in young women with early-stage breast cancer 1 year after lumpectomy. *Psycho-Oncology, 22*(6), 1242–1248.
23. Patenaude, A. F., Tung, N., Ryan, P. D., Ellisen, L. W., Hewitt, L., Schneider, K. A., Tercyak, K. P., Aldridge, J., & Garber, J. E. (2013). Young adult daughters of BRCA1/2 positive mothers: What do they know about hereditary cancer and how much do they worry? *Psycho-Oncology, 22*(9), 2024–2031.
24. Christensen, S., Zachariae, R., Jensen, A. B., Vaeth, M., Møller, S., Ravnsbaek, J., & von der Maase, H. (2009). Prevalence and risk of depressive symptoms 3–4 months post-surgery in a nationwide cohort study of Danish women treated for early stage breast-cancer. *Breast Cancer Research and Treatment, 113*(2), 339–355.

25. Cvetković, J., & Nenadović, M. (2016). Depression in breast cancer patients. *Psychiatry Research, 240*, 343–347.
26. Hermelink, K. (2015). Chemotherapy and cognitive function in breast cancer patients: The so-called chemo brain. *Journal of the National Cancer Institute. Monographs, 2015*(51), 67–69.
27. Meattini, I., Desideri, I., Francolini, G., Vannini, A., Perna, M., Garlatti, P., Grassi, R., & Livi, L. (2017). Systemic therapies and cognitive impairment for breast cancer: An overview of the current literature. *Medical Oncology, 34*(5), 74.
28. Crouch, A., Von Ah, D., & Storey, S. (2017). Addressing cognitive impairment after breast cancer: What do women want? *Clinical Nurse Specialist, 31*(2), 82–88.
29. Henselmans, I., Helgeson, V. S., Seltman, H., de Vries, J., Sanderman, R., & Ranchor, A. V. (2010). Identification and prediction of distress trajectories in the first year after a breast cancer diagnosis. *Health Psychology, 29*(2), 160–168.
30. Lam, W. W., Shing, Y. T., Bonanno, G. A., Mancini, A. D., & Fielding, R. (2012). Distress trajectories at the first year diagnosis of in relation to 6 years survivorship. *Psychooncology, 21*(1), 90–99.
31. Kreitler, S., & Kreitler, M. M. (2012). Personality correlates of breast cancer patients. 30th International Congress of psychology: Psychology serving humanity, Cape Town, South Africa, July 22–27, 2012.
32. Kreitler, S., Kreitler, M. M., Yaal-Hahoshen, N., & Inbar, M. (2006). Personality correlates of breast cancer patients. [In the framework of the Symposium "Cancer in Women: Personality Correlates and Coping", Conveners S. Kreitler and M. M. Kreitler]. 8th World Congress of Psycho-Oncology, (organized by IPOS: International Psychooncology Society), Venice, Italy, October 18–21, 2006.
33. Wardle, J., Williamson, S., Sutton, S., Biran, A., McCaffery, K., Cuzick, J., & Atkin, W. (2003). Psychological impact of colorectal cancer screening. *Health Psychology, 22*(1), 54–59.
34. Tau, L. T., & Chan, S. W. (2011). Exploring the quality of life and the impact of the disease among patients with colorectal cancer: A systematic review. *JBI (Joanna Briggs Institute) Library Systematic Reviews, 9*(54), 2324–2378.
35. Gall, C. A., Weller, D., Esterman, A., Pilotto, L., McGorm, K., Hammett, Z., & Wattchow, D. (2007). Patient satisfaction and health-related quality of life after treatment for colon cancer. *Diseases of the Colon and Rectum, 50*(6), 801–809.
36. Cotrim, H., & Pereira, G. (2008). Impact of colorectal cancer on patient and family: Implications for care. *European Journal of Oncology Nursing, 12*(3), 217–226.
37. Sun, V., Grant, M., McMullen, C. K., Altschuler, A., Mohler, M. J., Hornbrook, M. C., Herrinton, L. J., Baldwin, C. M., & Krouse, R. S. (2013). Surviving colorectal cancer: Long-term, persistent ostomy-specific concerns and adaptations. *Journal of Wound Ostomy & Continence Nursing, 40*(1), 61–72.
38. Mitchell, K. A., Rawl, S. M., Schmidt, C. M., Grant, M., Ko, C. Y., Baldwin, C. M., Wendel, C., & Krous, R. S. (2007). Demographic, clinical, and quality of life variables related to embarrassment in veterans living with an intestinal stoma. *Journal of Wound Ostomy & Continence Nursing, 34*(5), 524–532.
39. Danielsen, A. K. (2013). Life after stoma creation. *Danish Medical Journal, 60*(10), B4732.
40. Nakamura, M., Hosoya, Y., Yano, M., Doki, Y., Miyashiro, I., Kurashina, K., Morooka, Y., Kishi, K., & Lefor, A. T. (2011). Extent of gastric resection impacts patient quality of life: The dysfunction after upper gastrointestinal surgery for cancer (DAUGS32) scoring system. *Annals of Surgical Oncology, 18*(2), 314–320.
41. Boyd, A. D., Brown, D., Henrickson, C., Hampton, J., Zhu, B., Almani, F., Ben-Josef, E., Zalupski, M., Simeone, D. M., Taylor, J. M. G., Armitage, R., & Riba, M. (2012). Screening for depression, sleep-related disturbances, and anxiety in patients with adenocarcinoma of the pancreas: A preliminary study. *The Scientific World Journal, 2012.*, 6 pages, 650707.

42. Steel, J., Hess, S. A., Tunke, L., Chopra, K., & Carr, B. I. (2005). Sexual functioning in patients with hepatocellular carcinoma. *Cancer, 104*(10), 2234–2243.
43. Kreitler, S., Kreitler, M. M., Len, A., Alkalay, Y., & Barak, F. (2008). Psychological risk factors for colorectal cancer? *Psycho-Oncologie, 2*, 131–145.
44. Kreitler, S., & Kreitler, M. M. (2012). Personality correlates of colorectal cancer. *Supportive Care in Cancer, 20*(Suppl 1), S 138.
45. Zabora, J., Brintzenhofeszoc, K., Curbow, B., Hooker, C., & Piantadosi, S. (2001). The prevalence of psychological distress by cancer site. *Psycho-Oncology, 10*, 19–28.
46. Graves, K. D., Arnold, S. M., Love, C. L., Kirsh, K. L., Moore, P. G., & Passik, S. D. (2007). Distress screening in a multidisciplinary lung cancer clinic: Prevalence and predictors of clinically significant distress. *Lung Cancer, 55*(2), 215–224.
47. Morrison, E. J., Novotny, P. J., Sloan, J. A., Yang, P., Patten, C. A., Ruddy, K. J., & Clark, M. M. (2017). Emotional problems, quality of life, and symptom burden in patients with lung cancer. *Clinical Lung Cancer, 18*(5), 497–503.
48. Hopwood, P., & Stephens, R. J. (2000). Depression in patients with lung cancer: Prevalence and risk factors derived from quality-of-life data. *Journal of Clinical Oncology, 18*(4), 893–903.
49. Wang, B., Hao, N., & Zhang, X. (2017). Factors influencing the psychology and quality of life in lung cancer patients. *Saudi Medical Journal, 38*(9), 948–951.
50. Yang, S. C., Lai, W. W., Hsiue, T. R., Su, W. C., Lin, C. K., Hwang, J. S., & Wang, J. D. (2016). Health-related quality of life after first-line anti-cancer treatments for advanced non-small cell lung cancer in clinical practice. *Quality Of Life Research, 25*(6), 1441–1449.
51. Park, S., Kang, C. H., Hwang, Y., Seong, Y. W., Lee, H. J., Park, I. K., & Kim, Y. T. (2016). Risk factors for postoperative anxiety and depression after surgical treatment for lung cancer. *European Journal of Cardio-Thoracic Surgery, 49*(1), e16–e21.
52. Polanski, J., Jankowska-Polanska, B., Rosinczuk, J., Chabowski, M., & Szymanska-Chabowska, A. (2016). Quality of life of patients with lung cancer. *Onco Targets and Therapy, 9*, 1023–1028.
53. Berman, A. T., DeCesaris, C. M., Simone, C. B., 2nd, Vachani, C., DiLullo, G., Hampshire, M. K., Metz, & Hill-Kayser, C. (2016). Use of survivorship care plans and analysis of patient-reported outcomes in multinational patients with lung cancer. *Journal of Oncology Practice, 12*(5), e527–e535.
54. Banik, A., Schwarzer, R., Pawlowska, I., Boberska, M., Cieslak, R., & Luszczynska, A. (2017). Women with family cancer history are at risk for poorer physical quality of life and lower self-efficacy: A longitudinal study among men and women with non-small cell lung cancer. *Health and Quality of Life Outcomes, 15*(1), 62.
55. Nowicki, A., Graczyk, P., & Lemanowicz, M. (2017). The acceptance of illness in lung cancer patients before and after surgical treatment. *Polski Przeglad Chirurgiczny, 89*(4), 11–15.
56. Wang, Z., Li, Y. S., Zhao, N., Yang, J. J., Tu, H. Y., & Wu, Y. L. (2016). Do-not-resuscitate orders among advanced-stage Chinese lung cancer patients who died in hospital. *Supportive Care in Cancer, 24*(4), 1763–1769.
57. Ginsburg, M. L., Quirt, C., Ginsburg, A. D., & MacKillop, W. J. (1995). Psychiatric illness and psychosocial concerns of patients with newly diagnosed lung cancer. *Canadian Medical Association Journal, 152*(5), 701–708.
58. Hung, M. S., Chen, I. C., Lee, C. P., Huang, R. J., Chen, P. C., Tsai, Y. H., & Yang, Y. H. (2017). Incidence and risk factors of depression after diagnosis of lung cancer: A nationwide population-based study. *Medicine, 96*(19), e6864.
59. Sullivan, D. R., Forsberg, C. W., Ganzini, L., Au, D. H., Gould, M. K., Provenzale, D., & Slatore, C. G. (2016). Longitudinal changes in depression symptoms and survival among patients with lung cancer: A national cohort assessment. *Journal of Clinical Oncology, 34*(33), 3984–3991.
60. Rossi, A., Maione, Colantuoni, G., Ferrara, C., Rossi, E., Guerriero, C., Nicolella, D., Falanga, M., Palazzolo, G., & Gridelli, C. (2009). Recent developments of targeted therapies in the treatment of non-small cell lung cancer. *Current Drug Discovery Technology, 6*(2), 91–102.

61. Criswell, K. R., Owen, J. E., Thornton, A. A., & Stanton, A. L. (2016). 61). Personal responsibility, regret, and medical stigma among individuals living with lung cancer. *Journal of Behavioral Medicine, 39*(2), 241–253.
62. Marlow, L. A., Waller, J., & Wardle, J. (2015). Does lung cancer attract greater stigma than other cancer types? *Lung Cancer, 88*(1), 104–107.
63. Hahn, E. J., Hooper, M., Riker, C., Butler, K. M., Rademacher, K., Wiggins, A., & Rayens, M. K. (2017). Lung cancer worry and home screening for radon and secondhand smoke in renters. *Journal of Environmental Health, 79*(6), 8–13.
64. Farley, A., Aveyard, P., Kerr, A., Naidu, B., & Dowswell, G. (2016). Surgical lung cancer patients' views about smoking and support to quit after diagnosis: A qualitative study. *Journal of Cancer Survivorship: Research and Practice, 10*(2), 312–319.
65. Shen, M. J., Coups, E. J., Li, Y., Holland, J. C., Hamann, H. A., & Ostroff, J. S. (2015). The role of posttraumatic growth and timing of quitting smoking as moderators of the relationship between stigma and psychological distress among lung cancer survivors who are former smokers. *Psycho-Oncology, 24*(6), 683–690.
66. Kreitler, S., Or, B., et al. (In preparation). The cognitive orientation of lung cancer patients.
67. Sparla, A., Flach-Vorgang, S., Villalobos, M., Krug, K., Kamradt, M., Coulibaly, K., Szecsenyi, J., Thomas, M., Gusset-Bährer, S., & Ose, D. (2017). Reflection of illness and strategies for handling advanced lung cancer – a qualitative analysis in patients and their relatives. *BMC Health Services Research, 17*(1), 173.
68. Cooley, M. E., Poghosyan, H., & Sarna, L. (2015). Lung cancer. In J. C. Holland, W. S. Breitbart, P. N. Butow, P. B. Jacobsen, M. J. Loscalzo, & R. McCorcle (Eds.), *Psycho-oncology* (3rd ed., pp. 105–113). New York: Oxford University. 111–112.
69. Schellekens, M. P. J., van den Hurk, D. G. M., Prins, J. B., Donders, A. R. T., Molema, J., Dekhuijzen, R., van der Drift, M. A., & Speckens, A. E. M. (2017). Mindfulness-based stress reduction added to care as usual for lung cancer patients and/or their partners: A multicentre randomized controlled trial. *Psycho-Oncology, 26*(12), 2118–2126.
70. Sun, V., Kim, J. Y., Irish, T. L., Borneman, T., Sidhu, R. K., Klein, L., & Ferrell, B. (2016). Palliative care and spiritual well-being in lung cancer patients and family caregivers. *Psycho-Oncology, 25*(12), 1448–1455.
71. Roth, A., Nelson, C. J., Rosenfeld, B., Warshowski, A., O'Shea, N., Scher, H., Holland, J. C., Slovin, S., Curley-Smart, T., Reynolds, T., & Breitbart, W. (2006). Assessing anxiety in men with prostate cancer: Further data on the reliability and validity of the Memorial Anxiety Scale for Prostate Cancer (MAX-PC). *Psychosomatics, 47*(4), 340–347.
72. Egger, S., Calopedos, R. J., O'Connell, D. L., Chambers, S. K., Woo, H. H., & Smit, D. P. (2018). Long-term psychological and quality-of-life effects of active surveillance and watchful waiting after diagnosis of low-risk localised prostate cancer. *European Urology, 73*, 859–867.
73. Hervouet, S., Savard, J., Ivers, H., & Savard, M.-H. (2013). Depression and androgen deprivation therapy for prostate cancer: A prospective controlled study. *Health Psychology, 32*(6), 675–684.
74. Kotwal, A. A., Schumm, P., Mohile, S. G., & Dale, W. (2012). The influence of stress, depression, and anxiety on PSA screening rates in a nationally-representative sample. *Medical Care, 50*(12), 1037–1044.
75. Katz, A. (2016). Counseling men with prostate cancer and their partners. *Sexual and Relationship Therapy, 31*(4), 473–487.
76. Lee, M., Jim, H., Fishman, M., Zachariah, B., Heysek, R., Biagioli, M., & Jacobsen, P. B. (2015). Depressive symptomatology in men receiving androgen deprivation therapy for prostate cancer: A controlled comparison. *Psycho-Oncology, 24*(4), 472–477.
77. Keating, N. L., O'Malley, A. J., Freedland, S. J., & Smith, M. R. (2010). Diabetes and cardiovascular disease during androgen deprivation therapy: Observational study of veterans with prostate cancer. *Journal of the National Cancer Institute, 102*(1), 39.
78. Nguyen, P. L., Alibhai, S. M., Basaria, S., D'Amico, A. V., Kantoff, P. W., Keating, N. L., Penson, D. F., Rosario, D. J., Tombal, B., & Smith, M. R. (2015). Adverse effects of androgen deprivation therapy and strategies to mitigate them. *European Urology, 67*(5), 825.

79. Kreitler, S., Ariely, Y., et al. (In preparation). The cognitive orientation of prostate cancer.
80. Cognetti, D. M., Weber, R. S., & Lai, S. Y. (2008). Head and neck cancer: An evolving treatment paradigm. *Cancer, 113*(70), 1911–1932.
81. Ojo, B., Genden, E. M., Teng, M. S., Milbury, K., Misiukiewicz, K. J., & Badr, H. (2012). A systematic review of head and neck cancer quality of life assessment instruments. *Oral Oncology, 48*(10), 923–937.
82. Rapoport, Y., Kreitler, S., Chaitchik, S., Algor, R., & Weissler, K. (1990). Medical and psychosocial problems in head-and-neck cancer patients. 17th Israeli Surgical Conference, Haifa, Israel, September 1990.
83. Kreitler, S., Chaitchik, S., Kreitler, H., & Rapoport, Y. (1991). Psychosocial effects of information in head-and-neck cancer patients. Current concepts in psycho-oncology IV. New York: Memorial Sloan-Kettering Cancer Center.
84. Kreitler, S., Chaitchik, S., Rapoport, Y., Kreitler, H., & Algor, R. (1993). Life satisfaction and health in cancer patients, orthopedic patients and healthy individuals. *Social Science and Medicine, 36*, 547–556.
85. Kreitler, S., Chaitchik, S., Kreitler, H., & Rapoport, Y. (1991). Psychosocial effects of information in head and neck cancer patients. In J. C. Holland, L. M. Lesko, & M. J. Massie (Eds.), *Current concepts in psycho-oncology IV* (p. 207). New York: Memorial Sloan-Kettering Cancer Center.
86. Rapoport, Y., Kreitler, S., Chaitchik, S., Algor, R., & Weissle, K. (1993). Psychosocial problems in head-and-neck cancer patients and their change with disease duration. *Annals of Oncology, 4*, 69–73.
87. Kreitler, S., Chaitchik, S., Rapoport, Y., & Algor, R. (1995). Psychosocial effects of information and disease severity in head-and-neck cancer patients. *Journal of Cancer Education, 10*, 144–154.
88. Katz, M. R., Irish, J. C., Devins, G. M., Rodin, G. M., & Gullane, P. J. (2003). Psychosocial adjustment in head and neck cancer: The impact of disfigurement, gender and social support. *Head & Neck Journal, 25*(2), 103–112.
89. Chaitchik, S., Kreitler, S., Rapoport, Y., & Algor, R. (1992). What do cancer patients' spouses know about the patients? *Cancer Nursing, 15*, 353–362.
90. Lebel, S., & Devins, G. M. (2008). Stigma in cancer patients whose behavior may have contributed to their disease. *Future Oncology, 4*(5), 717–733.
91. Devins, G. M., Stam, H., & Koopmans, J. P. (1994). Psychological impact of laryngectomy mediated by perceived stigma and illness intrusiveness. *The Canadian Journal of Psychiatry / La Revue Canadienne de Psychiatrie, 39*(10), 608–616.
92. Onakoya, P. A., Nwaorgu, O. G., Adenipekun, A. O., Aluko, A. A., & Ibekwe, T. S. (2006). Quality of life in patients with head and neck cancers. *Journal of the National Medical Association, 98*(5), 765–770.
93. Kreitler, S. (2008). Psychopathologies in otolaryngology. [ENT or ear, nose and throat]. Conference on otolaryngological medicine and the psyche. Monthly Meeting of the Association of ear, nose and throat physicians, head and neck surgeons in Israel, Wolfson Medical center, Holon, Israel, February 22, 2008.
94. Kam, D., Salib, S., Gorgy, G., Patel, T. D., Carniol, E. T., Eloy, J. A., Baredes, S., & Park, R. C. W. (2015). Incidence of suicide in patients with head and neck cancer. *JAMA Otolaryngology - Head & Neck Surgery, 141*(12), 1075–1081.
95. Østhus, A. A., Aarstad, A. K., Olofsson, J., & Aarstad, H. J. (2013). Prediction of survival by pretreatment health-related quality-of-life scores in a prospective cohort of patients with head and neck squamous cell carcinoma. *JAMA Otolaryngology - Head & Neck Surgery, 139*(1), 14–20.
96. Kleihues, P., Burger, P. C., & Scheithauer, B. W. (1993). The new WHO classification of brain tumours. *Brain Pathology, 3*, 255–268.
97. Giovagnoli, A. R. (2012). Investigation of cognitive impairments in people with brain tumors. *Journal of Neurooncology, 108*(2), 277–283.
98. Peers, P. V., Ludwig, C. J., Rorden, C., Cusack, R., Bonfignoli, C., Bundesen, C., Driver, J., Antoun, N., & Driver, J. (2005). Attentional functions of parietal and frontal cortex. *Cerebral Cortex, 15*(10), 1469–1484.

99. Campanella, F., Shallice, T., Ius, T., Fabbro, F., & Skrap, M. (2014). Impact of brain tumour location on emotion and personality: A voxel-based lesion–symptom mapping study on mentalization processes. *Brain, 137*(9), 2532–2545.
100. Arnold, S. D., Forman, L. M., Brigidi, B. D., Carter, K. E., Schweitzer, H. A., Quinn, H. E., Guill, A. B., Herndon, J. E., 2nd, & Raynor, R. H. (2008). Evaluation and characterization of generalized anxiety and depression in patients with primary brain tumors. *Neuro-Oncology, 10*(2), 171–181.
101. Zucchella, C., Capone, A., Codella, V., De Nunzio, A. M., Vecchion, C., Sandrini, G., Pace, A., Pierelli, F., & Bartolo, M. (2013). Cognitive rehabilitation for early post-surgery inpatients affected by primary brain tumor: A randomized, controlled trial. *Journal of Neurooncology, 114*(91), 93–100.
102. Madsen, K., & Poulsen, H. S. (2011). Needs for everyday life support for brain tumour patients' relatives: Systematic literature review. *Cancer Care, 20*(1), 33–43.
103. Taillibert, S., Laigle-Donadey, F., & Sanson, M. (2004). Palliative care in patients with primary brain tumors. *Current Opinion in Oncology, 16*(6), 587–592.
104. Armstrong, T. S., Vera-Bolanos, E., Acquaye, A. A., Gilbert, M. R., Ladha, H., & Mendoza, T. (2016). The symptom burden of primary brain tumors: Evidence for a core set of tumor- and treatment-related symptoms. *Neuro-Oncology, 18*(2), 252–260.
105. Perkins, A., & Liu, G. (2016). Primary brain tumors in adults: Diagnosis and treatment. *American Family Physician, 93*(3), 211–217.
106. King, S., Exley, J., Parks, S., Ball, S., Bienkowska-Gibbs, T., MacLure, C., Harte, E., Stewart, K., Larkin, J., Bottomley, A., & Marjanovic, S. (2016). The use and impact of quality of life assessment tools in clinical care settings for cancer patients, with a particular emphasis on brain cancer: Insights from a systematic review and stakeholder consultations. *Quality of Life Research, International Journal of Quality of Life Aspects of Treatment, Care and Rehabilitation, 25*(9), 2245–2256.
107. Noll, K. R., Bradshaw, M. E., Weinberg, J., & Wefel, J. S. (2017). Relationships between neurocognitive functioning, mood, and quality of life in patients with temporal lobe glioma. *Psycho-Oncology, 26*(5), 617–624.
108. Thavarajah, N., Bedard, G., Zhang, L., Cella, D., Beaumont, J. L., Tsao, M., Barne, E., Danjoux, C., Sahgal, A., Soliman, H., & Chow, E. (2014). Psychometric validation of the functional assessment of cancer therapy – brain (FACT-Br) for assessing quality of life in patients with brain metastases. *Supportive Care in Cancer, 22*(4), 1017–1028.
109. Surveillance, Epidemiology, and End Results program (SEER) Cancer Statistics Review (CSR). (2011). Brain tumor facts data collected by Central Brain Tumor Registry of the United States (CBTRUS) in CBTRUS statistical facts report of primary brain and other central nervous system tumors diagnosed in the United States in 2010–2014. *Journal of the National Cancer Institute, 103*(2), 117–128.
110. Roberts, N., Czajkowska, Z., Radiotis, G., & Körner, A. (2013). Distress and coping strategies among patients with skin cancer. *Journal of Clinical Psychology in Medical Settings, 20*(2), 209–214.
111. American Cancer Society. Last revised 2016. Accessed 21 Sept 2018.
112. Schlesinger-Raab, A., Schubert-Fritschle, G., Hein, R., Stolz, W., Volkenandt, M., Hölzel, D., & Engel, J. (2010). Quality of life in localised malignant melanoma. *Annals of Oncology, 21*(12), 2428–2435.
113. Atkinson, V. (2017). Recent advances in malignant melanoma. *Internal Medicine Journal, 47*, 1114–1121.
114. Atkinson, T. M., Noce, N. S., Hay, J., Rafferty, B. T., & Brady, M. S. (2013). Illness-related distress in women with clinically localized cutaneous melanoma. *Annals of Surgical Oncology, 20*(2), 675–679.
115. Kasparian, N. A., McLoone, J. K., & Butow, P. N. (2009). Psychological responses and coping strategies among patients with malignant melanoma: A systematic review of the literature. *Archives of Dermatology, 145*(12), 1415–1427.
116. Bergenmar, M., Månsson-Brahme, E., Hansson, J., & Brandberg, Y. (2010). Surgical resection margins do not influence health related quality of life or emotional distress in patients

with cutaneous melanoma: Results of a prospective randomised trial. *Scandinavian Journal of Plastic and Reconstructive Surgery and Hand Surgery, 44*, 146–155.
117. Cornish, D., Holterhues, C., van de Poll-Franse, L. V., Coebergh, J. W., & Nijsten, T. (2009). A systematic review of health-related quality of life in cutaneous melanoma. *Annals of Oncology, 20*(Suppl 6), vi51–vi58.
118. Kasparian, N. A., McLoone, J. K., Meiser, B., Butow, P., Barlow-Stewart, K., Charles, M., Mann, G., & Menzies, S. (2012). "Living beneath the sword of Damocles": Perceptions of risk and fears of cancer recurrence among Australian melanoma survivors at high or moderate risk of developing new primary disease. *Asia Pacific Journal of Clinical Oncology, 8*(Suppl 3), 236.
119. Thewes, B., Butow, P., Zachariae, R., Christensen, S., Simard, S., & Gotay, C. (2012). Fear of cancer recurrence: A systematic literature review of self-report measures. *Psychooncology, 21*(6), 571–585.
120. Kreitler, S., Schechter, J. et al. (In preparation). The cognitive orientation of melanoma patients.
121. Fawzy, F. I., Canada, A. L., & Fawzy, N. W. (2003). Malignant melanoma: Effects of a brief, structured psychiatric intervention on survival and recurrence at 10-year follow-up. *Archives of General Psychiatry, 60*(1), 100–103.
122. Boesen, E. H., Ross, L., Frederiksen, K., Thomsen, B. L., Dahlstrøm, K., Schmidt, G., Naested, J., Krag, C., & Johansen, C. (2005). Psychoeducational intervention for patients with cutaneous malignant melanoma: A replication study. *Journal of Clinical Oncology, 23*(6), 1270–1277.
123. McLoone, J., Menzies, S., Meiser, B., Mann, G. J., & Kasparian, N. A. (2013). Psycho-educational interventions for melanoma survivors: A systematic review. *Psychooncology, 22*(7), 1444–1456.
124. Boesen, E. H., Boesen, S. H., Frederiksen, K., Ross, L., Dahlstrøm, K., Schmidt, G., Naested, J., Krag, C., & Johansen, C. (2007). Survival after a psychoeducational intervention for patients with cutaneous malignant melanoma: A replication study. *Journal of Clinical Oncology, 25*(36), 5698–5703.

Chapter 15
Special Populations of Patients

All or One?

There are at present 12 million newly diagnosed cancer patients worldwide, with prospects of increasing to 19 million in 2024 and 24 million in 2050, and 28 million cancer survivors. In view of the numbers on this scale, it is unlikely that one size (in terms of treatment and approach) fits all. On the other hand, there is evidence for a clear trend toward personalized medicine in cancer, for example, targeted treatments that consider the cancer's specific genes and proteins in applying drugs and pharmacogenomics, taking into account the manner in which the body processes the drugs. However, in between the large bulk of millions of cancer patients and the single case of cancer, which is undoubtedly unique, there is an enormous gap which calls for consideration on the part of cancer clinicians.

Criteria? Which Ones?

Bridging the gap between the whole crowd and the single case can be done only by applying criteria for identifying specific groups from the perspective of cancer. There are multiple actually unlimited possibilities for specifying criteria. Personalized medicine is based on genetic criteria concerning primarily the development of the tumor and the reaction to drugs. It is likely that even from the point of view of genetics there exist several criteria. Examples of criteria affecting both screening and treatment are the existence of hereditary cancer syndromes or specification of the kind of mutations underlying the cancer. However, there are many more identified or known criteria, whose application could result in a great number of groupings and subgrouping.

On the one hand, it is evident that defining groups is desirable and often even necessary. Grouping of patients could help in determining the medical treatment,

S. Kreitler, *Psycho-Oncology for the Clinician*,
https://doi.org/10.1007/978-3-030-06126-5_15

especially when there are options, and over and beyond that – specifying also the psychosocial approach and interventions that could help the patients. However, defining too many groups of cancer patients may result in increasing the difficulties of treatment by enlarging the overload of the health professionals in treatment and tests and heaping barriers on medical decisions that could extend their duration and enhance the involved difficulties.

The conclusion is that criteria are necessary, but in order to be helpful, they should be relevant and easy to apply.

Both specifications seem simpler than they actually are. Both are relative and liable to change as contexts and medicine develop. Relevance is a criterion that takes into consideration the state of medical information and availability of treatments, especially in regard to the specific diagnosis and state of the patient. Ease of application involves limitation in at least three respects: the number of resulting groups, familiarity of the parameters involved in the group differentiation, and ease and relative speed of determining the grouping.

It would be advisable to examine the criteria underlying the existing groups of special populations in the domain of cancer.

Some referents to groups of cancer patients are quite common on the scene of cancer treatment. However, their number seems to be limited to a few salient titles. The most common ones are "vulnerable patients," "underserved groups," "low-income patients," "underinsured," and sometimes also patients from "deprived areas." Needless to mention, these groups of patients do not cover most of the groups of patients that need to be considered. The last four mentioned titles seem to refer mainly to the large set of patients who do not get the required treatment and attention mostly because they are poor financially or of low status. The so-called vulnerable patients are less specified and may include any kind of patients who need special attention for any reason whatsoever. Notably, the mentioned descriptive terms are often dealt with under the heading of health inequity, which includes differences between populations in terms of different factors, such as race and ethnicity that result in restricted or lower availability or accessibility of medical resources and treatments [1]. This general characterization is neither sufficiently comprehensive nor sufficiently specific to represent the major medical and sociopsychological status of the patients. It needs to be complemented by other criteria.

In the scientific literature and lay references to cancer, the following groupings or criteria are often mentioned [2].

Most prominent are distinctions based on age differences. Children and adolescents are often mentioned as a separate group as well as the elderly. This corresponds to a habitual approach in medicine, based on the need to adjust the kind and dosage of drugs to pediatric and geriatric patients.

A further distinction that is sometimes used in medicine concerns gender. Concern for gender is based first on the occurrence of certain diseases only in females or males and on the possibility that symptoms of a disease differ in the genders, e.g., cardiological disease. In some cases it is dealt with under the title of sex minority health, which possibly includes a reference to recent distinctions in the conceptualization of gender, e.g., homosexuality.

A third common distinction is based on differences in the socioeconomic status of patients. Wide disparities in the health status of different social groups have been noted in all countries. Individuals with a low socioeconomic status have restricted access to medical resources – both preventive and therapeutic – which may result in lower health status and higher health risks [3, 4]. Education, employment status, and place of residence may be correlates of low socioeconomic status.

A final common distinction concerns culture. It may appear under the title of ethnic or ethnic-racial minorities and sometimes under the heading of cultural diversity. To our mind, religious affiliation and immigrant status may also be included under this heading.

The four abovementioned classifications appear to be both relevant and relatively easy to apply. The present chapter will be devoted to these four classifications.

However, these four criteria are far from inclusive. To our mind, it would be advisable to expand the list to include further important groups of special populations in regard to cancer treatment. Major among these are groups defined by mental diseases and cognitive disabilities; by physical and medical conditions (multiple diseases other than cancer, multiple cancers, rare cancers, extreme deviations in weight, genetic diseases, or genetic risk factors); by disabilities (e.g., eyesight, hearing); or by special conditions (e.g., patients who are incarcerated, homeless, or lonely having no family or no support).

It is possible that these further groupings are also relevant for cancer treatments, but in view of the fact that the available information about them in the context of cancer treatment is still scant and insufficient, they will not be handled in the present chapter.

Age Differences: The Elderly and the Young

The Elderly Cancer Patient

Senior patients are a large and increasing group in the context of oncology. Advancing age is considered as a risk factor for cancer [5], because of the overall physiological decline characteristic of older individuals, not in the least due to the process of general immunosenescence [6]. The chance of a senior adult to be diagnosed with cancer is one in three for men and one in four for women. Persons over 65 account for 60% of newly diagnosed malignancies and 70% of all cancer deaths [7].

In view of the actual or assumed impacted physiologic state of the elderly, there has been a tendency for undertreatment of elderly cancer patients, with dose reduction of chemotherapy and limitation of surgery over a given age, mostly 70. In parallel, the inclusion of elderly patients in clinical trials has also been restricted [8]. Limitations of this kind have been largely given up and were replaced by considerations of the special conditions of the specific patient. It has become evident that the elderly can be categorized as healthy, vulnerable, or frail [9], in line with standard criteria or physician evaluation. Accordingly, considerations for limiting treatments apply only to the vulnerable and the frail, although it needs to be kept in mind that frailty is an ill-defined concept, liable to changes [10].

Nevertheless, it needs to be kept in mind that elderly individuals often suffer from different geriatric syndromes (e.g., dementia, incontinence), have multiple chronic conditions, and use a great number of medications. These characteristics may limit the possibilities for administering to elderly cancer patients aggressive treatments. The fact that elderly patients may suffer from cognitive deficits, difficulties of managing in daily life, and poor social support may further complicate their response to the oncological treatments and put them at higher risk for chemotherapy-related toxicities [11]. Hence, elderly cancer patients may need special attention and consideration on the part of health carers.

One important factor is the frequent comorbidities occurring in the elderly. For example, comorbidity was found in 68.7% of patients with cancer [12], and six chronic conditions were identified in 25% of cancer patients over 85 [13]. Comorbidity complicates the administration of treatments, reduces survival duration and [14], and increases the physical burden on patients.

Comorbidities and the overall reduced physiological stamina of elderly cancer patients may increase their burden and suffering. Pain, fatigue, and depression are common manifestations [15], as well as dementia [16].

There are few studies that deal with the psychosocial state of elderly cancer patients [17]. Existing reports tend to focus on quality-of-life aspects, demonstrating that they are impacted in the elderly patients [18, 19]. The situation is however far from clear or unequivocal. On the one hand, elderly cancer patients may be expected to suffer from the disease and the therapy which may be more burdensome for them than for younger patients. Other factors likely to contribute to their suffering are limited social support, awareness of the age-conditioned closeness of death, suspicions of undertreatment due to age, difficulties of mobility, and limited accessibility to the health centers and to health management administration in general. Further, elderly cancer patients who are holocaust survivors cope on a lower level than other cancer patients [20]. This finding suggests that the elderly may have weaker coping reserves if they have undergone serious traumata in the past, which is probably not rare. On the other hand, there are factors that may contribute to mitigating the suffering of the elderly cancer patients, for example, the awareness that they have had a long and rich life or that they have coped successfully in the past with serious problems. Both kind of factors may contribute to strengthening their confidence in their ability to overcome the present crises as well.

Pediatric Oncological Patients: Children and Adolescents

The incidence of cancer in children is higher than is generally assumed. Cancer is the leading cause of non-accidental death in children in affluent countries. Approximately 1 in 350 children will develop cancer by adulthood [21]. Further, the incidence of the different pediatric cancers is increasing, at the rate of 1–1.5% per year [22]. The most frequent cancer diseases in children differ from those in adult patients. The most common pediatric cancers are leukemia, brain and spinal cord tumors, neuroblastoma, Wilms' tumor, lymphoma, retinoblastoma, sarcoma, and bone cancer [23]. The oncological treatments administered to children include the standard ones, i.e., surgery, chemotherapy, radiotherapy, and BMT. It is generally acknowledged that survival has improved dramatically in children (0–14) and adolescents (0–19). In the last four decades, the overall survival rate has increased from 10% to almost 90% nowadays, but the survival rate is lower for rare cancers. Mortality rate is still high and encompasses 12% of children who have been diagnosed with cancer [24].

A major concern in regard to pediatric cancer is the short-term and mainly the long-term sequelae of the disease and of the treatments. There are multiple medical sequelae which may affect most of the external and internal organs, including the endocrine, pulmonary, cardiological, orthopedic, neurological, and musculoskeletal systems [25–27]. Approximately three quarters of adult survivors of pediatric cancer treated 30–40 years earlier have an increased risk of early death of 7% at the age of 30 [28] and develop a chronic condition by age 40, and about 50% are diagnosed with a serious health condition [29]. Secondary malignant neoplasm is one of the most salient and adverse sequelae, which may even cause mortality. Solid tumors may occur 10 years after the diagnosis, in leukemia and lymphoma even earlier, often post radiotherapy [30]. Endocrine sequelae are most common, affecting 40–60% of survivors. The frequent ones, affecting especially survivors from CNS tumors, leukemia and lymphoma, are growth failure and gonadal and thyroid diseases [31, 32]. As a result the patients and survivors may suffer from disfigurement in the body image, alopecia, obesity, short stature, and limited mobility. Further, the presence of a chronic health condition increases risk for functional impairments and serious activity deficits at school, in social life, and at work [25, 33].

Fertility issues are a most bothersome problem for the survivors and their families. Since the disease and treatments may affect fertility, patients often worry about whether they will be able to have children in the future. Special attention is devoted to fertility preservation in the victims of pediatric cancer, often even prior to initiating the cancer treatments [34].

Cognitive deficits during treatment and following it are a major arena of concern for the pediatric patients and their family. Risk factors for cognitive dysfunction include young age at diagnosis, radiotherapy for the brain, use of parenteral or intrathecal methotrexate, and pre-existing comorbidities. Major problems have been identified in regard to attention, processing speed, executive function, and working memory [35]. A body of studies shows that after radiotherapy, the pediatric patients have a decline of 5–10 points in IQ [36], as well as in causative thinking, mathematical ability, nonverbal intelligence, and visual-motor coordination and integration [37]. Poor concentration and low motivation may be contributing factors to these cognitive difficulties.

The different difficulties of pediatric cancer patients may lower self-efficacy and strengthen the sense of avoidance and depressive symptoms in the survivors, which in turn are reflected in a decline in health behaviors including tobacco and alcohol use, keeping a diet, exercising, use of sunscreen, safe sexual behavior, and medication adherence [38].

Psychiatric symptoms have also been observed in pediatric cancer survivors, including unstable mood, anxiety, depression, and a high rate of adjustment disorders [39].

In recent years attention has turned also to the psychological sequelae of childhood cancer. The psychosocial effects are not surprising in view of the difficulties to which the children are exposed. The major one which should be kept in mind is that children who become cancer patients are robbed of a significant part of their childhood and possibly of their future too. As pediatric patients, they learn to know fear, pain, and death, if not directly in regard to themselves then in regard to other patients in their vicinity. They learn that there are things in regard to which their parents cannot help them, prevent, or even defend against them. They even learn to defend and protect their parents when they hide their pain and fear from them. It needs also to be considered that children in this situation think about the possibility of their own death and sometimes even prepare for it [40].

The disease represents a serious emotional shock to the patients who are exposed to the fear of imminent death, removal from their familiar environment and daily routine, and necessity to undergo long-term medical treatments, often involving pain, stress, anxiety, uncertainty for them and their parents, and quite often physical changes in posture, weight, and hair [41]. These experiences were found to cause in the children undergoing treatments negative emotions, mainly anxiety, depression, and anger, as well as behavioral difficulties and a decline in the children's quality of life [42, 43]. Moreover, even after the successful completion of treatments, the need for medical follow-ups and for treatment of different medical side effects may reinforce the memories of adverse events in the past and enhance the fear of recurrence and of treatments in the future [44, 45]. As may be expected, as compared to healthy controls, pediatric cancer survivors have a lower quality of life, lower self-concept [46], more depression, anxiety, pain, and insomnia [47]; suffer more from fatigue, emotional symptoms [48], and posttraumatic stress [49]; are less likely to have partners or to be married [50]; and tended at least in the past to be more often rejected from work, study, and military service institutions [51].

There is also evidence about the prevalence of suicide ideation and even suicidal attempts in pediatric cancer survivors [52, 53]. A great variety of psychosocial interventions are offered to pediatric cancer patients, including fantasy, art, humor, and pets [54], cognitive behavioral [55], and interventions for improving cognition [37, 56]. Psychosocial interventions for family reintegration are of great importance [57]. Efforts are also devoted to keep up the children's education, sometimes by establishing special school units or classes in the hospitals, so as to prevent a too large gap after termination of treatments [58].

There is evidence also for positive results in regard to survivors of pediatric cancer. Some studies found that as compared to healthy controls survivors do not manifest more distress [59] and do not report more problems [60]. Moreover, they enjoy good health and well-being [61], score high on quality of life [62], have good psychological health and life satisfaction [63], achieve the major standard life goals [64], and do not have more aggression, antisocial behaviors, and drug abuse [65], and many even reported posttraumatic growth [66, 67]. Findings of this kind may be considered as indicating full recovery following pediatric cancer. However, there are studies suggesting that below the apparent positive surface there may be suffering and pain as indicated by findings about the high scores of the survivors on mental pain [68, 69].

Cancer in Women and Men

As is well known, some cancers are gender specific. These include breast, endometrial, cervical, vulvar, and ovarian cancers in women. Prostate cancer is clearly one cancer specific to males. There is a lot of evidence documenting the unique and negative experiences of women and men when diagnosed with one of these cancers which impact seriously their quality of life during the treatments and as survivors [70, 71]. The patient may experience impairment in her sexual functioning and reproductive ability. Changes in the vagina and hormonal treatments may affect the woman's ability and pleasure of sexual intimacy [72]. Different interventions are being applied for helping these women [73, 74]. The permanent or even temporary loss of fertility due to the disease and treatments may cause feelings of loss, frustration, isolation, anxiety, and depression that often last long after the termination of the treatments [75]. Recent years have seen the development of different fertility-preserving procedures and alternatives that can help many of the survivors [76]. The issues concerning sexuality and fertility may cause impairment in the woman's sense of femininity. Women with gynecologic cancers suffer from a lot of depression [73, 77], which may lead even to suicidal ideation, especially in patients with ovarian cancer [78]. Depression is more intense and lasting in younger women [77, 79]. Anxiety, loss of anger control, and disturbances in body image are also common in this group of patients [75, 77, 79].

Prostate cancer patients have their own load of problems that impact negatively their quality of life during the treatments and later [80]. One of the distressing issues is the decision the patients are often called upon to take concerning their treatment, which may be surgery, hormonal, radiotherapy, or follow-up. Involvement in the decision process may be stressful both because the information patients have is limited and because it implies personal responsibility [81]. Following treatment, prostate cancer patients may suffer from different side effects causing emotional problems, major among which may be some degree of sexual dysfunction that may affect marital relations [82].

However, data from different parts of the world shows major gender differences in cancer in general: men are at increased risk for cancer and also have a poorer prognosis than women in most cancer types [83]. Different kinds of reasons have been suggested and explored for this trend that is consistent for countries, ages, and most cancer kinds. The explanatory models may be divided into intrinsic and extrinsic ones. The intrinsic refer to biological and environmental factors, including hormonal [84], immunological [84], anti-oxidative, metabolic, anatomic [85], and genetic factors [84]. For example, gene mutations in BRAF, MSI-high status, and N-ras differ according to gender among patients with colorectal cancer [86]. The extrinsic factors include acquired oncogenic mutations related to contact with environmental carcinogens [84], such as UV radiation, alcohol, tobacco, chronic infections, toxins, and nutrition [87]. The latter are often characterized as lifestyle factors, more often observed in men than in women. For example, a study with colorectal cancer patients showed that the male patients had a significantly higher rate of alcohol, nicotine abuse, and body mass than women and a worse postoperative outcome in the early phase of colorectal cancer but not later [88].

Some studies suggested that differences between men and women in using screening options for early detection may also be a contributing factor to the gender differences in incidence and mortality. Men and women were found to differ in beliefs, behaviors, and readiness to participate in cancer screening [89]. Men engage less in self-examination, are less aware of early cancer signs, and were more likely to delay reporting cancer symptoms to the physician [90]. These findings correspond largely to the findings of another study which showed that there were no gender differences in illness understanding in a prescan interview, but after the results of the scan arrived, women were more likely than men to recognize that their illness was incurable, know that their cancer was at an advanced stage, and report having had discussions of life expectancy with their oncologist [91]. Gender differences were found in the way of viewing screening and the reasons for avoiding it. The reservations mentioned by women were bodily intrusion, fear of perforation, and embarrassment, whereas men mentioned avoidant procrastination with underlying fatalism, unnecessary healthcare, and uncomfortable vulnerability. In general, women had more consistent physician relationships, were more screening-knowledgeable, and were better able to articulate views on screening than men [92]. Greater readiness to undergo screening and communication with the physician may speed diagnosis and treatment and promote survival.

There are gender differences in the behavior, attitudes, and reactions of the patients undergoing treatment for cancer. Thus, in patients with non-small cell lung cancer, postoperative weight loss predicted worse prognosis only in men but not in women [93]. Women were found to experience significantly greater pain, hesitated more to use analgesics, and had lower adherence and inadequate pain management, as compared to men [94]. There are gender differences in the symptoms of the disease and chemotherapy that impact negatively quality of life. In women these included mainly body image, abdominal pain, and dry mouth, while in men these included mainly cognitive function, fecal inconsistency, and sexual impotence [95]. Female patients are in general more likely than males to report symptoms [96]. Notably, women considered their cancer to be associated closely with more childhood experiences of physical and emotional abuse than males [97].

There are gender differences also in the way the disease is experienced and in its sequelae after treatment termination. Women reported significantly higher levels of treatment intensity, greater numbers and types of treatment, and more interpersonal and relational problems with healthcare professionals, while men were more concerned with effects of the disease on work and finances. Hence, predictors of PTSD for women were perceived intensity of cancer treatment, problems with healthcare professionals, and cognitive avoidant coping style. For men, only behavioral voidance predicted PTSD [98]. Gender differences were found also in the impact of the diagnosis on the tendency of survivors to divorce their partner: in women the major determinants were emotional distress and financial/employment problems associated with the cancer diagnosis, while in men the determinant was fear of cancer recurrence [99].

Gender differences were found also in regard to coping with the disease and in the effects of different coping mechanisms. Women used more bagatellization and wishful thinking and more depressive and less active problem-oriented coping strategies and reported higher mental strain than men. In women religious coping and adaptation were positively correlated more than in men, whereas only in men active problem-oriented coping and mental health were positively correlated [100]. Also in patients in India, it was found that men coped more in terms of problem-focused coping, whereas women preferred emotion-coping [101]. Unmarried men had significantly higher levels of psychological distress and lower levels of fighting spirit than married men, and men with spousal support showed higher levels of fighting spirit than men without spousal support. No similar effects were observed in female patients with or without spousal support [102]. In China, family support is often mentioned as an important resource for patients. Support from family showed a stronger negative correlation with negative affect among males, and support from special others showed a stronger negative correlation with negative affect among females, in China [103]. Concerning emotional expression, the partner's overt anger expression was correlated negatively with the mental quality of life in women but positively in men patients, whereas the patient's own overt anger expressions had a more pronounced negative effect on the quality of life for women as compared to men [104]. Another aspect of emotional expression is demonstrated in the finding that emotional expression was effective in reducing negative adjustment in men, while more internally focused emotional processing helped in promoting adjustment in women [105]. Notably, women patients tend more toward emotional expressivity than men, while men experienced significantly greater distress in association with social constraints from their spouse/partner than did women [106]. Another example concerns gender differences in the determinants of affect regulation. In male patients symptoms such as fatigue and nausea/vomiting correlated with affect regulation efficacy, while in women it was affected by physical functioning [107]. Performance status, e.g., mild physical impairment, is in women a risk factor for negative ways of coping, but not in men [102].

Notably, gender differences in distress were found even in the caretakers of cancer patients: Females scored higher than male caregivers on cancer-related anxiety, future uncertainties, fear of recurrence, and future diagnostic tests [108, 109].

By way of summary, gender differences are relevant in regard to how individuals and families react, experience, and cope with cancer. The existing evidence about gender differences is sufficiently comprehensive and well-founded to justify a more gender-oriented oncology, covering diagnosis, treatment, and survival [110].

The Socioeconomic Perspective

The findings of studies in regard to the socioeconomic impact on cancer are highly repetitive. They all support one clear-cut conclusion which is that the poorer section of society gets a lower deal on cancer. The conclusion neither changes nor is modified in any way by considering cancer types, countries, or any medical aspect that could affect the outcome. A survey of incidence and survival data derived from the National Cancer Institute's (NCI) Surveillance, Epidemiology, and End Results (SEER) Program; mortality data derived from the National Center for Health Statistics (NCHS); and data about risk factors and cancer screening derived from the National Health Interview Survey (NHIS) conducted by NCHS – all of these testify that the death rate from cancer is 13% higher in poor countries (in which at least 20% of the population are below the poverty line) than in more affluent ones (in which less than 10% of the population are below the poverty line) [111]. Poorer people have a lower chance of undergoing early screening (mammography, colorectal screening, Pap test) [112, 113]; they tend less to adhere to basic prevention means (e.g., physical activity, tobacco use, recommended diet to prevent obesity) [114]; if they are diagnosed with lung cancer, they have a lower chance to get early surgery [115]; in case of melanoma, they have a lower chance of getting the standard combination treatment [116]; they have a higher incidence of gastrointestinal cancers [117] and of sinonasal squamous cell carcinoma [118]; and they tend to die sooner or earlier than others [119]. Examples of this kind could be greatly extended concerning any aspect of cancer incidence, treatment, or survival. The effect of socioeconomic status on cancer is sturdy. Studies show that even after adjustment for comorbid conditions, cancer stage, tumor histology, and lifestyle factors, socioeconomic differences in survival persisted [120].

Unclarity persists however concerning the precise reason for the relation between the socioeconomic level and cancer survival. It is a complicated question because it requires clarifying and resolving at least the three following issues: firstly, which of the correlates or components of socioeconomic status is functional in regard to cancer, e.g., employment, education, income, and residential area; secondly, which aspect of addressing cancer is affected significantly by socioeconomic status, e.g., prevention, diagnosis, treatment, and follow-up; and thirdly, through which processes socioeconomic status impacts the cancer situation, e.g., religious beliefs that imply the patients should rely only on God [114], scarcity of health providing services in specific areas, and lifestyle behaviors such as foods promoting obesity. Resolving the persisting unclarities is of great importance for devising means for improving the situation for the benefit of patients.

Culture and Cancer

Culture resembles socioeconomic status in several major respects. Like socioeconomic status it represents a complex of components each of which can impact cancer: genetics, cultural beliefs, traditions, attitudes, and behaviors which interact with one another and may affect cancer directly and indirectly. Additionally, the varied culturally grounded factors may affect any of the aspects involved in cancer (e.g., prevention, follow-up) and through varied processes (e.g., lifestyle, voluntary avoidance of treatment). Be it as it may, the effect of culture on cancer is unmistakably there. As has been stated by Jackie Stacey, "cancer is more than an illness – it is a cultural phenomenon" [121].

There is evidence, for example, about the effects of culture on almost any major aspect of cancer, including prevention, undergoing treatment, adherence to treatment, risk factors, the experience of the disease, the meaning assigned to the disease, the definition of recovery and of well-being, and of facing death.

The following paragraphs provide a few examples of studies illustrating intercultural differences, selected out of the many relevant existing ones. A comparison of Dutch and Japanese women diagnosed with breast cancer showed that Dutch women reported poorer physical, role, emotional, and cognitive functioning than Japanese women, whose quality of life varied more in line with the kind of chemotherapy they got [122]. In Chinese women lower positive affect was more strongly associated with worse emotional well-being than in American women [123]. Fatalistic cancer beliefs may influence treatment avoidance among Asian patients in Singapore [124]. Coping mechanisms depend a lot on culture. It was shown that the mobilization of spirituality may be of great importance in providing relief and combatting despair in many cultures [124]. African American men diagnosed with prostate cancer coped more in terms of their religiosity and future temporal orientation than European American men [125]. Asian patients have stronger barriers against managing cancer pain than Western patients [126].

The issue of information provision and communication is a salient theme in cross-cultural studies. It is a highly important issue because of the great differences between cultures in understanding cancer and in the myths and incorrect beliefs about cancer that may delay or even prevent getting the adequate treatment [127, 128]. There is evidence that cultures differ in the degree to which there is communication about genetic cancer tendencies in families. In some cultures this information is not disclosed for fear of evoking the hidden tendencies [129]. In some regions of China, there is a tendency to avoid telling patients their diagnosis for fear of causing them unnecessary worries [130]. Differences were found in imparted information between the three cultural areas of North-Middle Europe, South Europe, and Taiwan. North-Middle Europe patients received more written information, and South Europe patients received more information on different places of care. European patients differed from Taiwanese ones in getting more information about the disease and medical tests and in considering the information more satisfactory and helpful [131].

Dear Patient: Who Are You?

In taking care of a patient, several basic tendencies are evoked which contribute to defining the situation and shaping the practitioner's behavior. First comes the tendency to view all as equal and as similar, reflected in the statement that often comes to mind “a patient is a patient is a patient above all and beyond all.” Then there is the equally dominant statement “everyone is special, no patient is like any other one.” And then there is also the self-bias, reflected in the assumption that may creep into the situation that “all are like me.” None of these common tendencies is based on an explicit bias supporting discrimination. But each is dangerous in its own way because it may bring about overlooking particular features of the patient that may play a role in regard to the efficacy of the proffered treatment. Not all of these features are equally evident and easily detectable, like the female gender in case of breast cancer or the potential risks of cognitive sequelae of whole brain radiation in pediatric patients. Some are less evident, such as genetic mutations that could affect responses to particular chemotherapies in lung cancer patients or even phobic reactions of a patient to a particular treatment. Since it is unlikely to recall at the right moment all the potentially relevant aspects characterizing the individual patient, the cautionary implication resulting from the descriptions of the various classifications of patients is simply to let oneself be guided by respect for the individual patient, whoever he or she may be, and to whatever already identified or not yet identified group that she or he may belong.

References

1. Kawachi, I., Subramanian, S., & Almeida-Filho, N. (2002). A glossary for health inequalities. *Journal of Epidemiology & Community Health, 56*, 647–652.
2. MacKenzie, A. R., & Parker, I. (2015). Introduction to quality issues in vulnerable populations. *Journal of Oncology Practice, 11*(3), 185–186.
3. Lago, S., Cantarero, D., Rivera, B., Pascual, M., Blazquez-Fernandez, B. C., & Reyes, F. (2018). Socioeconomic status, health inequalities and non-communicable diseases: A systematic review. *Zeitschrift fuer Gesundheit Wissenscaft, 26*(1), 1–14.
4. Musterd, S. (2005). Social and ethnic segregation in Europe: Levels, causes, and effects. *Journal of Urban Affairs, 27*(3), 331–348.
5. Velkoff, K. K. (2001). *An aging world* (U.S. Census Bureau P95/01–1). Washington, DC: U.S. Government Printing Office.
6. Solana, R., Alonso, M. C., & Pena, J. (1999). Natural killer cells in healthy aging. *Experimental Gerontology, 34*, 435–443.
7. Ries, L. A. G., Eisner, M. P., Kosary, C. L., Hankey, B. F., Miller, B. A., Clegg, L. X., & Edwards, B. K. (2000). *SEER cancer statistics review, 1973–1998* (2000 NIH publication 00-2789). Bethesda: National Institute of Health.
8. Shenoy, P., & Harugeri, A. (2015). Elderly patients’ participation in clinical trials. *Perspectives in Clinical Research, 6*(4), 184–189.
9. Ferrucci, L., Guralnik, J. M., Cavazzini, C., Bandinelli, S., Lauretani, F., Bartali, B., et al. (2003). The frailty syndrome: A critical issue in geriatric oncology. *Critical Reviews in Oncology/Hematology, 46*, 127–137.
10. Buckinx, F., Rolland, Y., Reginste, J.-Y., Ricour, C., Petermns, J., & Bruyere, O. (2015). Burden of frailty in the elderly population: Perspectives for a public health challenge. *Archives of Public Health, 73*(1), 19.
11. Gillison, T. L., & Chatta, G. S. (2010). Cancer chemotherapy in the elderly patient. *Oncology (Williston Park, N.Y.), 24*(1), 76–85.
12. Ogle, K. S., Swanson, G. M., Woods, N., et al. (2000). Cancer and comorbidity. *Cancer, 88*, 653–663.

13. US Department of Health and Human Services, Centers for Medicare and Medicaid Services, Chartbook. (2012). *Chronic conditions among Medicare beneficiaries*. Baltimore: Centers for Medicare and Medicaid Services.
14. Søgaard, M., Thomsen, R. W., Bossen, K. S., et al. (2013). The impact of comorbidity on cancer survival: A review. *Clinical Epidemiology, 5*(3), 29. suppl 1.
15. Rao, A., & Cohen, H. J. (2004). Symptom management in the elderly cancer patient: Fatigue, pain, and depression. *JNCI Monographs, 32*(1), 150–157.
16. Stiefel, F., & Holland, J. (1991). Delirium in cancer patients. *International Psychogeriatrics, 3*(2), 333–336.
17. Puts, M., et al. (2012). A systematic review of unmet needs of newly diagnosed older cancer patients undergoing active cancer treatment. *Supportive Care in Cancer, 20*(7), 1377–1394.
18. Pasetto, L. M., Falci, Compostella, A., Sinigaglia, G., Rossi, E., & Monfardini, S. (2007). Quality of life in elderly cancer patients. *European Journal of Cancer, 43*(10), 1508–1513.
19. Reimer, T., & Gerber, B. (2010). Quality-of-life considerations in the treatment of early-stage breast cancer in the elderly. *Drugs & Aging, 27*(10), 791–800.
20. Sarell, M., & Baider, L. (1984). Coping with cancer among holocaust survivors in Israel: An exploratory study. *Journal of Human Stress, 10*(3), 121–127.
21. Izraeli, S., & Rechavi, G. (2012). Cancer in children: An overview. In S. Kreitler, W. Ben-Arush, & A. Martin (Eds.), *Pediatric psycho-oncology: Psychosocial aspects and clinical interventions* (2nd ed., pp. 3–6). Chichester: Wiley-Blackwell.
22. Steliarova-Foucher, E., Stiller, C., Kaatsch, P., Berrino, F., Coebergh, J. W., Lacour, B., & Parkin, M. (2004). Geographical patterns and time trends of cancer incidence and survival among children and adolescents in Europe since the 1970s (the ACCIS project): An epidemiological study. *Lancet, 364*(9451), 2097–2105.
23. American Cancer Society. 2016. Risk factors and causes of childhood cancer. Last Medical Review: August 22, 2016. Accessed 11 Aug 2018.
24. O'Leary, M., Krailo, M., Anderson, J. R., & Reaman, G. H. (2008). Progress in childhood cancer: 50 years of research collaboration, a report from the Children's Oncology Group. *Seminars in Oncology, 35*(5), 484–493.
25. Wilson, C. L., Gawade, P. L., & Ness, K. K. (2015). Impairments that influence physical function among survivors of childhood cancer. *Children, 2*, 1–36.
26. Mulhern, R., White, H., & Phipps, S. (2004). Neuropsychological aspects of medical treatments in pediatric oncology. In S. Kreitler & M. W. Ben-Arush (Eds.), *Psychosocial aspects of pediatric oncology* (pp. 9–44). Oxford: Wiley.
27. Scholz-Kreisel, P., Spix, C., Blettner, M., Eckerle, S., Faber, J., Wild, P., Merzenich, H., & Hennewig, U. (2017). Prevalence of cardiovascular late sequelae in long-term survivors of childhood cancer: A systematic review and meta-analysis. *Pediatric Blood & Cancer, 64*(7), e26428.
28. Krivoy, E., Jenney, M. E. M., Mahajan, A., & Peretz-Nahum, M. (2012). Survivorship in childhood cancer. In S. Kreitler, W. Ben-Arush, & A. Martin (Eds.), *Pediatric psycho-oncology: Psychosocial aspects and clinical interventions* (2nd ed., pp. 187–193). Chichester: Wiley-Blackwell.
29. Oeffinger, K. C., Mertens, A. C., Sklar, C. A., Kawashima, T., Hudson, M. M., Meadows, A. T., Friedman, D. L., Marina, N., Hobbie, W., Kadan-Lottick, N. S., Schwartz, C. L., Leisenring, W., Robison, L. L., & for the Childhood Cancer Survivor Study. (2006). Chronic health conditions in adult survivors of childhood cancer. *New England Journal of Medicine, 355*, 1572–1582.
30. Bomken, S., & Skinner, R. (2015). Secondary malignant neoplasms following haematopoietic stem cell transplantation in childhood. *Children, 2*(2), 146–173.
31. Rutter, M. M., & Rose, S. R. (2007). Long-term endocrine sequelae of childhood cancer. *Current Opinion in Pediatrics, 19*(4), 480–487.
32. Sancho, C. P. (2017). Endocrine sequelae in childhood cancer survivors. *Endocrinology Diabetes and Nutrition, 64*(9), 498–505.

33. Hudson, M. M., Ness, K. K., Gurney, J. G., Mulrooney, D. A., Chemaitilly, W., Krull, K. R., Green, D. M., Armstrong, G. T., Nottage, K. A., Jones, K. E., et al. (2013). Clinical ascertainment of health outcomes among adults treated for childhood cancer. *JAMA, 309*, 2371–2381.
34. Levine, J. M. (2014). Preserving fertility in children and adolescents with cancer. *Children, 1*, 166–185.
35. Conklin, H. M., Krull, K. R., Reddick, W. E., Pei, D., Cheng, C., & Pui, C. H. (2012). Cognitive outcomes following contemporary treatment without cranial irradiation for childhood acute lymphoblastic leukemia. *Journal of the National Cancer Institute, 104*(18), 1386–1395.
36. Kreitler, S., Ben-Arush, M., Kriboy, E., Golan, H., Kreitler, H., & Toren, A. (2010). Psychosocial aspects of radiotherapy for the child and family with cancer. In E. C. Halperin, L. S. Constine, N. J. Tarbell, & L. E. Kun (Eds.), *Handbook of pediatric radiation oncology* (5th ed., pp. 449–457). Philadelphia: Lippincott, Williams & Wilkin.
37. Kreitler, S., Krivoy, E., & Toren, A. (2012). Psychosocial aspects of radiotherapy in pediatric cancer patients. In S. Kreitler, M. W. Ben-Arush, & A. Martin (Eds.), *Pediatric psycho-oncology: Psychosocial aspects and clinical interventions* (2nd ed., pp. 62–70). Oxford: Wiley-Blackwell.
38. Vuotto, S. C., Procidano, M. E., & Annunziato, R. A. (2015). Understanding the health behaviors of survivors of childhood and young-adult cancer: Preliminary analysis and model development. *Children, 2*, 174–190.
39. Stuber, M. I. (2012). Psychiatric impact of childhood cancer. In S. Kreitler, M. W. Ben-Arush, & A. Martin (Eds.), *Pediatric psycho-oncology: Psychosocial aspects and clinical interventions* (2nd ed., pp. 43–51). Oxford: Wiley-Blackwell.
40. Kreitler, S., & Krivoy, E. (2012). Psychological intervention with the dying child. In S. Kreitler, M. W. Ben-Arush, & A. Martin (Eds.), *Pediatric psycho-oncology: Psychosocial aspects and clinical interventions* (2nd ed., pp. 209–222). Oxford: Wiley-Blackwell.
41. Oppenheim, D. (2004). The child's subjective experience of cancer and the relationship with parents and caregivers. In S. Kreitler & M. W. Ben Arush (Eds.), *Psychosocial aspects of pediatric oncology* (pp. 111–138). Oxford: Wiley.
42. Kreitler, S., & Kreitler, M. M. (2012). Quality of life in children with cancer. In S. Kreitler, M. W. Ben-Arush, & A. Martin (Eds.), *Pediatric psycho-oncology: Psychosocial aspects and clinical interventions* (2nd ed., pp. 18–31). Oxford: Wiley-Blackwell.
43. Kreitler, S., Kreitler, M. M., & Alkalay, Y. (2015). The children's quality of life questionnaire: A multidimensional measure for the assessment of quality of life in children and adolescents. *Journal of Psychological Sciences, 1*(2), 62–81.
44. Brinkman, T. M., Zhang, N., Recklitis, C. J., Kimberg, C., Zeltzer, L. K., Muriel, A. C., Stovall, M., Srivastava, D. K., Sklar, C. A., Robison, L. L., & Krull, K. R. (2014). Suicide ideation and associated mortality in adult survivors of childhood cancer. *Cancer, 120*(2), 271–277.
45. Kurtz, B. P., & Abrams, A. N. (2010). Psychiatric aspects of pediatric cancer. *Child and Adolescent Psychiatric Clinics of North America, 19*(2), 401–421.
46. Rhee, M. A., Chung, K. M., Lee, Y., Choi, H. K., Han, J. W., Kim, H. S., Shin, Y. J., & Lyu, C. J. (2014). Impact of psychological and cancer-related factors on HRQoL for Korean childhood cancer survivors. *Quality of Life Research, 23*, 2603–2612.
47. Zeller, B., Loge, J. H., Kanellopoulos, A., Hamre, H., Wyller, V. B., & Ruud, E. (2014). Chronic fatigue in long-term survivors of childhood lymphomas and leukemia: Performance and associated clinical factors. *Journal of Pediatric Hematology/Oncology, 36*(6), 438–444.
48. Calaminus, G., Dörffel, W., Baust, K., Carmen, T. M., Riepenhausen, J., Brämswig, H. H., Flechtner, S., Singer, A., & Hinz Günther, S. (2014). *Support Care Cancer, 22*, 1519–1529.
49. Raz, H., Gothelf, D., Yaniv, I., Buchva, L. I., & DeKeyser, G. F. (2010). Post-traumatic stress disorder in Israeli survivors of childhood cancer. *Oncology Nursing Forum, 37*(2), 160–167.
50. Wengenroth, L., Rueegg, C. S., Michel, G., Essig, S., Ammann, R. A., Bergstraesser, E., Kuehni, C. E., & Swiss Pediatric Oncology Group. (2014). Life partnerships in childhood

cancer survivors, their siblings, and the general population. *Pediatric Blood & Cancer, 61*(3), 538–545.

51. Teta, M. J., Del Po, M. C., Kasl, S. V., Meigs, J. W., Myers, M. H., & Mulvihill, J. J. (1986). Psychosocial consequences of childhood and adolescent cancer survival. *Journal of Chronic Diseases, 39*(9), 751–759.
52. Twombly, R. (2006). Decades after cancer, suicide risk remains high. *Journal of the National Cancer Institute, 98*(19), 1356–1358.
53. Recklitis, C. J., Diller, L. R., Li, X., Najita, J., Robison, L. L., & Zeltzer, E. (2010). Suicide ideation in adult survivors of childhood cancer: A report from the Childhood Cancer Survivor Study. *Journal of Clinical Oncology, 28*(4), 655–666.
54. Kreitler, S., Oppenheim, D., & Segev-Shoham, E. (2012). Fantasy, art therapies and other expressive and creative psychosocial interventions. In S. Kreitler, M. W. Ben-Arush, & A. Martin (Eds.), *Pediatric psycho-oncology: Psychosocial aspects and clinical interventions* (2nd ed., pp. 143–159). Oxford: Wiley-Blackwell.
55. Last, B. F., & Grootenhuis, M. A. (2012). Psychosocial interventions: A cognitive behavioral approach. In S. Kreitler, M. W. Ben-Arush, & A. Martin (Eds.), *Pediatric psycho-oncology: Psychosocial aspects and clinical interventions* (2nd ed., pp. 92–103). Oxford: Wiley-Blackwell.
56. Castellino, S. M., Ullrich, N. J., Whelen, M. J., & Lange, B. J. (2014). Developing interventions for cancer-related cognitive dysfunction in childhood cancer survivors. *Journal of the National Cancer Institute, 106*(8). pii:dju186.
57. Peikert, M. L., Inhestern, L., & Bergelt, C. (2018). Psychosocial interventions for rehabilitation and reintegration into daily life of pediatric cancer survivors and their families: A systematic review. *PLoS One, 13*(4), e0196151. https://doi.org/10.1371/journal.pone.0196151.
58. Tadmor, C. S., Rosenkranz, R., & Ben-Arush, M. W. (2012). Education in pediatric oncology: Learning and reintegration into school. In S. Kreitler, M. W. Ben-Arush, & A. Martin (Eds.), *Pediatric psycho-oncology: Psychosocial aspects and clinical interventions* (2nd ed., pp. 104–117). Oxford: Wiley-Blackwell.
59. Gianinazzi, M. E., Rueegg, C. S., Wengenroth, L., Bergstraesser, E., Rischewski, J., Ammann, R. A., Kuehni, C. E., Michel, G., & for Swiss Pediatric Oncology Group (SPOG). (2013). Adolescent survivors of childhood cancer: Are they vulnerable for psychological distress? *Psycho-Oncology, 22*(9), 2051–2058.
60. Chan, C. W., Choi, K. C., Chien, W. T., Cheng, K. K., Goggins, W., So, W. K. W., & Li, C. K. (2014). Health-related quality-of-life and psychological distress of young adult survivors of childhood cancer in Hong Kong. *Psycho-Oncology, 23*(2), 229–236.
61. Mertens, A. C., Brand, S., Ness, K. K., Li, Z., Mitby, P. A., Riley, A., Patenaude, A. F., & Zeltzer, L. (2014). Health and well-being in adolescent survivors of early childhood cancer: A report from the Childhood Cancer Survivor Study. *Psycho-Oncology, 23*(3), 266–275.
62. Kanellopoulos, A., Hamre, H. M., Dahl, A. A., Fosså, S. D., & Ruud, E. (2013). Factors associated with poor quality of life in survivors of childhood acute lymphoblastic leukemia and lymphoma. *Pediatric Blood & Cancer, 60*(5), 849–855.
63. Zeltzer, L. K., Lu, Q., Leisenring, W., Tsao, J. C., Recklitis, C., Armstrong, G., & Ness, K. K. (2008). Psychosocial outcomes and health-related quality of life in adult childhood cancer survivors: A report from the childhood cancer survivor study. *Cancer Epidemiology, Biomarkers & Prevention, 17*(2), 435–446.
64. Green, D. M., Zevon, M. A., & Hall, B. (1991). Achievement of life goals by adult survivors of modern treatment for childhood cancer. *Cancer, 67*(1), 206–213.
65. Verrill, J. R., Schafer, J., Vannatta, K., & Noll, R. B. (2000). Aggression, antisocial behavior and substance abuse in survivors of pediatric cancer: Possible protective effects of cancer and its treatment. *Journal of Pediatric Psychology, 25*, 493–502.
66. Barakat, L. P., Alderfer, M. A., & Kazak, A. (2006). Posttraumatic growth in adolescent survivors of cancer and their mothers and fathers. *Pediatric Psychology, 31*, 413–419.

67. Duran, B. (2013). Posttraumatic growth as experienced by childhood cancer survivors and their families: A narrative synthesis of qualitative and quantitative research. *Journal of Pediatric Oncology Nursing, 30*, 179–197.
68. Raz, H., Tabak, N., & Kreitler, S. (2015). Quality of life and existential anxiety in adult survivors of pediatric cancer. *Psycho-Oncology, 24*(2), 256.
69. Raz, H., Tabak, N., Alkalay, Y., & Kreitler, S. (2016). Mental pain in Israeli adult childhood cancer survivors and its effects on their quality of life. *Journal of Psychology and Psychotherapy, 6*(2), 1–9.
70. Carter, J., Penson, R., Barakat, R., & Wenzel, L. (2012). Contemporary quality of life issues affecting gynecologic cancer survivors. *Hematology/Oncology Clinics of North America, 26*(1), 169–194.
71. Vaz, A., Pinto-Neto, A. M., Conde, D. M., Costa-Paiva, L., Morais, S. S., Pedro, A. O., & Esteves, S. B. (2011). Quality of life and menopausal and sexual symptoms in gynecologic cancer survivors: A cohort study. *Menopause, 18*(6), 662–669.
72. Abbott-Anderson, K., & Kwekkeboom, K. L. (2012). A systematic review of sexual concerns reported by gynecological cancer survivors. *Gynecologic Oncology, 124*(3), 477–489.
73. Chow, K. M., Chan, J. C., Choi, K. K., & Chan, C. W. (2016). A review of psychoeducational interventions to improve sexual functioning, quality of life, and psychological outcomes in gynecological cancer patients. *Cancer Nursing, 39*(1), 20–31.
74. Cook, O., McIntyre, M., Recoche, K., Lee, S., & JBI. (2017). Experiences of gynecological cancer patients receiving care from specialist nurses: A qualitative systematic review. *Database of Systematic Reviews and Implementation Reports, 15*(8), 2087–2112.
75. Yaman, S., & Ayaz, S. (2016). Psychological problems experienced by women with gynecological cancer and how they cope with it: A phenomenological study in Turkey. *Health & Social Work, 41*(3), 173–181.
76. Chhabra, S., & Kutchi, I. (2013). Fertility preservation in gynecological cancers. *Clinical Medicine Insights: Reproductive Health, 7*, 49–59.
77. Jacob, L., Bleicher, L., Kostev, K., & Kalder, M. (2016). Prevalence of depression, anxiety and their risk factors in German women with breast cancer in general and gynecological practices. *Journal of Cancer Research and Clinical Oncology, 142*(2), 447–452.
78. Tang, G. X., Yan, P. P., Yan, C. L., Fu, B., Zhu, S. J., Zhou, L. Q., Huang, X., Wang, Y., & Lei, J. (2016). Determinants of suicidal ideation in gynecological cancer patients. *Psycho-Oncology, 25*(1), 97–103.
79. Gómez-Campelo, P., Bragado-Álvarez, C., & Hernández-Lloreda, M. J. (2014). Psychological distress in women with breast and gynecological cancer treated with radical surgery. *Psycho-Oncology, 23*(4), 459–466.
80. Zajdlewicz, L., Hyde, M. K., Lepore, S. J., Gardiner, R. A., & Chambers, S. K. (2017). Health-related quality of life after the diagnosis of locally advanced or advanced prostate cancer: A longitudinal study. *Cancer Nursing, 40*(5), 412–419.
81. Shirk, J. D., Crespi, C. M., Saucedo, J. D., Lambrechts, S., Dahan, E., Kaplan, R., & Saigal, C. (2017). Does patient preference measurement in decision aids improve decisional conflict? A randomized trial in men with prostate cancer. *The Patient, 10*, 785–798.
82. Albaugh, J. A., Sufrin, N., Lapin, B. R., Petkewicz, J., & Tenfelde, S. (2017). Life after prostate cancer treatment: A mixed methods study of the experiences of men with sexual dysfunction and their partners. *BMC Urology, 17*(1), 45.
83. Cook, M. B., McGlynn, K. A., Devesa, S. S., Freedman, N. D., & Anderson, W. F. (2011). Sex disparities in cancer mortality and survival. *Cancer Epidemiology, Biomarkers & Prevention, 20*(8), 1629–1637.
84. Planchard, D., Loriot, Y., Goubar, A., Commo, F., & Soria, J. C. (2009). Differential expression of biomarkers in men and women. *Seminars in Oncology, 36*(6), 553–565.
85. Tomasetti, C., & Vogelstein, B. (2015). Variation in cancer risk among tissues can be explained by the number of stem cell divisions. *Science, 347*(6217), 78–81.

86. Tsai, Y. J., Huang, S. C., Lin, H. H., Lin, C. C., Lan, Y. T., Wang, H. S., Yang, S. H., Jiang, J. K., Chen, W. S., Lin, T. C., Lin, J. K., & Chang, S. C. (2018). Differences in gene mutations according to gender among patients with colorectal cancer. *World Journal of Surgical Oncology, 16*(1), 128. https://doi.org/10.1186/s12957-018-1431-5.
87. De Martel, C., & Franchesi, S. (2009). Infections and cancer: Established associations and new hypotheses. *Critical Reviews in Oncology/Hematology, 70*(3), 183–194.
88. Katzenstein, J., Steinert, R., Ptok, H., Otto, R., Gastinger, I., Lippert, H., & Meyer, F. (2018). Gender-specific differences of the early postoperative and oncosurgical long-term outcome in rectal cancer-data obtained in a prospective multicenter observational study. Genderspezifische Unterschiede im frühpostoperativen und onkochirurgischen Langzeitoutcome nach Rektumkarzinomresektion. *Der Chirurg, 89*(6), 458–465.
89. Davis, J. L., Buchanan, K. L., Katz, R. V., & Green, B. L. (2012). Gender differences in cancer screening beliefs, behaviors, and willingness to participate: Implications for health promotion. *American Journal of Mental Health, 6*(13), 211–217.
90. Evans, R. E. C., Brotherstone, H., Miles, A., & Wardle, J. (2005). Gender differences in early detection of cancer. *The Journal of Men's Health and Gender, 2*(2), 209–217. Published Online: 3 Jun 2005. https://doi.org/10.1016/j.jmhg.2004.12.012.
91. Fletcher, K., Prigerson, H. G., Paulk, E., Temel, J., Finlay, E., Marr, L., McCorkle, R., Rivera, L., Munoz, F., & Maciejewski, P. K. (2013). Gender differences in the evolution of illness understanding among patients with advanced cancer. *The Journal of Supportive Oncology, 11*(3), 126–132.
92. Ritvo, P., Myers, R. E., Paszat, L., Serenity, M., Perez, D. F., & Rabeneck, L. (2013). Gender differences in attitudes impeding colorectal cancer screening. *BMC Public Health, 13*, 500. https://doi.org/10.1186/1471-2458-13-500.
93. Kawai, H., Saito, Y., & Suzuki, Y. (2017). Gender differences in the correlation between prognosis and postoperative weight loss in patients with non-small cell lung cancer. *Interactive Cardiovascular and Thoracic Surgery, 25*(2), 272–277.
94. Chou, P. L., Fang, S. Y., Sun, J. L., Rau, K. M., & Lee, B. O. (2017). Gender difference in cancer patients' adherence to analgesics and related outcomes of pain management. *Cancer Nursing*. https://doi.org/10.1097/NCC.0000000000000532.
95. Trinquinato, I., da Silva, R. M., Benavente, S. B. T., Antonietti, C. C. L., & Calache, A. L. S. C. (2017). Gender differences in the perception of quality of life of patients with colorectal cancer. *Investigación y Educación en Enfermería, 35*(3), 320–329. (Portugese).
96. Taniguchi, K., Akechi, T., Suzuki, S., Mihara, M., & Uchitomi, Y. (2003). Performance status 1 predicts psychological response in female, but not male, ambulatory cancer patients. *Supportive Care in Cancer, 11*(7), 465–471.
97. Alcalá, H. E., Tomiyama, A. J., & von Ehrenstein, O. S. (2017). Gender differences in the association between adverse childhood experiences and cancer. *Women's Health Issues, 27*(6), 625–631.
98. Hampton, M. R., & Frombach, I. (2000). Women's experience of traumatic stress in cancer treatment. *Health Care for Women, 21*(1), 67–76.
99. Stephens, C., Westmaas, J. L., Kim, J., Cannad, R., & Stein, K. (2016). Gender differences in associations between cancer-related problems and relationship dissolution among cancer survivors. *Journal of Cancer Survivorship, 10*(5), 865–873.
100. Murken, S., Namini, S., Gross, S., & Körber, J. (2010). Gender specific differences in coping with colon cancer – empirical findings with special consideration of religious coping. *Rehabilitation, 49*(2), 95–104. [Article in German].
101. Vidhubala, E., Latha, R. R., Mani, C. S., & Karthikesh, M. (2006). Coping preferences of head and neck cancer patients – Indian context. *Indian Journal of Cancer, 43*(1), 6–11.
102. Taniguchi, K., Akechi, T., Mihara, M., & Uchitomi, Y. (2003). Lack of marital support and poor psychological responses in male cancer patients. *Supportive Care in Cancer, 11*(9), 604–610.

103. You, J., & Lu, Q. (2014). Sources of social support and adjustment among Chinese cancer survivors: Gender and age differences. *Supportive Care in Cancer, 22*(3), 697–704.
104. Julkunen, J., Gustavsson-Lilius, M., & Hietanen, P. (2009). Anger expression, partner support, and quality of life in cancer patients. *Journal of Psychosomatic Research, 66*(3), 235–244.
105. Cho, D., Park, C. L., & Blank, T. (2013). Emotional approach coping: Gender differences on psychological adjustment in young to middle-aged cancer survivors. *Psychology & Health, 28*(8), 874–894.
106. Zakowski, S. G., Harris, C., Krueger, N., Laubmeier, K. K., Garrett, S., Flanigan, R., & Johnson, P. (2003). Social barriers to emotional expression and their relations to distress in male and female cancer patients. *British Journal of Health Psychology, 8*(Pt 3), 271–286.
107. Sato, M., & Sumi, N. (2015). Factors related to self-efficacy among men and women undergoing outpatient chemotherapy in Japan. *Scandinavian Journal of Caring Sciences, 29*(4), 745–750.
108. Matthews, B. A. (2003). Role and gender differences in cancer-related distress: A comparison of survivor and caregiver self-reports. *Oncology Nursing Forum, 30*(3), 493–499.
109. Pitceathly, C., & Maguire, P. (2003). The psychological impact of cancer on patients' partners and other key relatives: A review. *European Journal of Cancer, 39*(11), 1517–1524.
110. Kim, Y., & Loscalzo, M. J. (Eds.). (2018). *Gender in psycho-oncology*. New York: Oxford University Press.
111. Ward, E., Jemal, A., Cokkinides, V., Singh, G. K., & Cardinez, C. (2004). Cancer disparities by race/ethnicity and socioeconomic status. *CA: A Cancer Journal for Clinicians, 54*(2), 78–93.
112. Siegel, R., Ward, E., Brawley, O., Jemal, A., Ghafoor, A., & Thun, M. (2011). The impact of eliminating socioeconomic and racial disparities on premature cancer deaths. *CA: A Cancer Journal for Clinicians, 61*(4), 212–216.
113. Wardle, J., Robb, K., Vernon, S., & Waller, J. (2015). Screening for prevention and early diagnosis of cancer. *American Psychologist, 70*(2), 119–133.
114. Polite, B. N., Cipriano-Steffens, T., Hlubocky, F., Dignam, J., Ray, M., Smith, D., Undevia, S., Sprague, E., Olopade, O., Daugherty, C., Fitchett, G., & Gehlert, S. (2017). An evaluation of psychosocial and religious belief differences in a diverse racial and socioeconomic urban cancer population. *Journal of Racial and Ethnic Health Disparities, 4*(2), 140–148.
115. Belot, A., Fowler, H., Njagi, E. N., Luque-Fernandez, M. A., Maringe, C., Magadi, W., Exarchakou, A., Quaresma, M., Turculet, A., Peake, M. D., Navani, N., & Rachet, B. (2018). Association between age, deprivation and specific comorbid conditions and the receipt of major surgery in patients with non-small cell lung cancer in England: A population-based study. *Thorax.* , pii: thoraxjnl-2017-211395. https://doi.org/10.1136/thoraxjnl-2017-211395.
116. Ibfelt, E. H., Steding-Jessen, M., Dalton, S. O., Lundstrøm, S. L., Osler, M., & Hölmich, L. R. (2018). Influence of socioeconomic factors and region of residence on cancer stage of malignant melanoma: A Danish nationwide population-based study. *Clinical Epidemiology, 10*, 799–807.
117. Weiderpass, E., & Pukkala, E. (2006). Time trends in socioeconomic differences in incidence rates of cancers of gastro-intestinal tract in Finland. *BMC Gastroenterology, 6*, 41.
118. Zhou, A. H., Chung, S. Y., Patel, V. R., Unsal, A. A., Hsueh, W. D., Baredes, S., & Eloy, J. A. (2017). Do geographic differences or socioeconomic disparities affect survival in sinonasal squamous cell carcinoma? *International Forum of Allergy & Rhinology, 7*(12), 1195–1200.
119. Rutherford, M. J., Andersson, T. M., Møller, H., & Lambert, P. C. (2015). Understanding the impact of socioeconomic differences in breast cancer survival in England and Wales: Avoidable deaths and potential gain in expectation of life. *Cancer Epidemiology, 39*(1), 118–125.
120. Ibfelt, E. H., Dalton, S. O., Høgdall, C., Fagö-Olsen, C. L., Steding-Jessen, M., Osler, M., Johansen, C., Frederiksen, K., & Kjær, S. K. (2015). Do stage of disease, comorbidity or access to treatment explain socioeconomic differences in survival after ovarian cancer? –

A cohort study among Danish women diagnosed 2005–2010. *Cancer Epidemiology, 39*(3), 353–359.
121. Stacey, J. (1998). *Teratologies: A cultural study of cancer*. London: Routledge.
122. Fischer, M. J., Inoue, K., Matsuda, A., Kroep, J. R., Nagai, S., Tozuka, K., Momiyama, M., Weijl, N. I., Langemeijer-Bosman, D., Ramai, S. R. S., Nortier, J. W. R., Putter, H., Yamaoka, K., Kubota, K., Kobayashi, K., & Kaptein, A. A. (2017). Cross-cultural comparison of breast cancer patients' Quality of Life in the Netherlands and Research Treatments. *Breast Cancer Research and Treatment, 166*(2), 459–471.
123. Milbury, K., Kavanagh, A., Meng, Z., Chen, Z., Chandwani, K. D., Garcia, K., Perkins, G. H., McQuade, J., Raghuram, N. V., Nagarathna, R., Liao, Z., Nagendra, H. R., Chen, J., Guo, X., Liu, L., Arun, B., & Cohen, L. (2017). Depressive symptoms and positive affect in Chinese and United States breast cancer survivors: A cross-cultural comparison. *Supportive Care in Cancer, 25*(7), 2103–2109.
124. Martsolf, D. S. (1997). Cultural aspects of spirituality in cancer care. *Seminars in Oncology Nursing, 113*(4), 231–236.
125. Hughes Halbert, C., Barg, F. K., Weathers, B., Delmoor, E., Coyne, J., Wileyto, E. P., Arocho, J., Mahler, B., & Malkowicz, S. B. (2007). Differences in cultural beliefs and values among African American and European American men with prostate cancer. *Cancer Control: Journal of The Moffitt Cancer Center, 14*(3), 277–284.
126. Chen, C. H., Tang, S. T., & Chen, C. H. (2012). Meta-analysis of cultural differences in Western and Asian patient-perceived barriers to managing cancer pain. *Palliative Medicine, 26*(3), 206–221.
127. Mitchell, J. L. (1998). Cross-cultural issues in the disclosure of cancer. *Cancer Practice, 6*(3), 153–160.
128. Daher, M. (2012). Cultural beliefs and values in cancer patients. *Annals of Oncology, 23*(suppl 3), 66–69.
129. Etchegary, H., Potter, B., Perrier, C., & Wilson, B. (2013). Cultural differences in family communication about inherited cancer: Implications for cancer genetics research. *Journal of Cultural Diversity, 20*(4), 195–201.
130. Yuxiu, L., Jinhong, Y., Da, H., Honghua, F., & Yufang, G. (2018). Disclosure of cancer diagnosis in China: The incidence, patients' situation, and different preferences between patients and their family members and related influence factors. *Cancer Management and Research, 10*, 2173–2181.
131. Arraras, J. I., Greimel, E., Chie, W. C., Sezer, O., Bergenmar, M., Costantini, A., Young, T., Vlasic, K. K., Velikova, G., & European Organisation for Research and Treatment of Cancer Quality of Life Group. (2013). Cross-cultural differences in information disclosure evaluated through the EORTC questionnaires. *Psycho-Oncology, 22*(2), 268–275.

Chapter 16
The Caretakers

Who Are They?

The caretakers of cancer patients are a varied group, not even completely defined. Originally there have been only the health professionals who included the doctors and the nurses. The doctors included initially the physicians with their specific expertise, mainly oncologists and surgeons. Nowadays the medical health professionals involved in cancer care have become a team including a large number of experts, such as specialist doctors in specific domains of oncology (e.g., gynecology, orthopedics, laryngology, neurology, gastroenterology, bone marrow transplantation) as well as pediatric oncologists, hematologists, geneticists, imaging experts, radiologists, and pain doctors. An emerging field of experts is rehabilitation doctors whose speciality is to help cancer survivors to return to optimal functioning physically and psychologically.

Nurses form a second group of professional cancer caretakers. It is impossible to overrate the importance of oncology nurses in caring for cancer patients [1]. The professional help they provide to cancer patients and their families has become an essential component of cancer care, without which it is impossible to describe or imagine the treatment of a cancer patient in any stage of the disease. As in the domain of physicians, there are nurses with specialization in specific domains, such as gastroenterology (colostomy experts), radiation, breast cancer, or gynecological cancers, or for particular groups of patients, mainly children and patients in palliative care.

A third group of professionals, often called allied health professionals, includes experts in specific domains in which cancer patients need treatment or help for recovery or rehabilitation. Examples are dieticians or nutritionists, pharmaceutical experts, physiotherapists, experts in respiration or kidney functioning, as well as the large group of psychosocial experts including social workers, psychologists and psychooncologists (psychologists who specialize in oncology), art therapists, music therapists, and experts who provide spiritual support in different forms.

S. Kreitler, *Psycho-Oncology for the Clinician*,
https://doi.org/10.1007/978-3-030-06126-5_16

A fourth group includes the informal caretakers. These are primarily family members, joined by friends, acquaintances, neighbors, and a large group of volunteers. The latter are an increasing group of people, often from the community where the patient resides, religious groups or societies, formal registered volunteer groups, and sometimes cancer survivors.

In recent years there has been increasing recognition for an additional group of helpers that may be called patient advocates which nowadays include many national cancer organizations like the National Breast Cancer Coalition, which promotes political lobbying and fund raising for conferences, publications, training, and other activities for the benefit of cancer patients.

There is another large group of experts whose contribution to the advancement of the cancer care cannot be overrated although it does not consist in direct caretaking of cancer patients. These are scientists and researchers in the diverse relevant fields of medicine, biology, immunology, pharmaceuticals, drug development, genetics, epidemiology, and psychosocial aspects of cancer. The present chapter will deal neither with patient advocates nor the scientists because they are not involved directly in caretaking.

Major Characteristics of the Caretakers Groups

The five groups of experts involved in contributing to cancer care differ in major dimensions, mainly goals, expertise, manner of operation, and form of involvement in caretaking. These dimensions determine the kind of difficulties and problems characterizing the members of these groups and the suggested solutions for them.

Goals

In terms of goals, it is evident that the groups share the overarching goal of helping cancer patients but in addition are devoted to goals specific to their primary occupation. It needs barely mentioning that the goal of physicians is to cure. This goal can be formulated more specifically. Doctors strive for identifying the specific problem of a specific patient in medical terms and providing the particular patient the best treatment possible for him or her in view of the established diagnosis and the health state of the patient, considering the existing available treatments. Physicians mostly have a more precise conception of the expected goal of treatment in a particular case, e.g., in the case of chemotherapy, full or partial regression of the tumor; in the case of radiotherapy, relieving symptoms caused by the tumor; and in the case of neoadjuvant chemotherapy, shrinking the tumor so that the next treatment of surgery or radiation can be more effective.

The goals of the nursing personnel may be summarized as assisting the patients in all the issues they confront in the course of their disease, including diagnosis, treatment, recovery, and rehabilitation. Nurses combine medical help with provision of information, support, compassion, and counseling, focusing on the patients' needs while maintaining their optimal quality of life. Their two major goals are medical and supportive. Medically they monitor the patients' state of health, administration of the medical treatments, and their reactions to the treatments, often informing doctors of the developments and other changes and coordinating help of different medical experts when necessary. In terms of support, nurses guide the patients and their families through the emerging issues, explain, counsel, and help by providing support and empathy [2].

The allied health professionals have definite specified goals. Those with expertise in a specific domain, such as diet or breathing or mobility, are approached mainly by patients who are in need of help specifically in those defined domains. The patients may be referred directly to these experts or the experts approach the needy patients on their own. The goals are defined mainly by the professional expertise. The experts provide guidance in the specific domains. However mostly neither the aspired or determined goal nor the attained goal represents perfect resolution of the problem. For example, if the patient suffers from difficulties in mobility or in losing weight, the attained goal often represents merely improvement in mobility or weight control rather than achievement of full mobility or the desired weight. The situation in regard to goals is similar in the case of the psychosocial experts. Their goals too are defined by their expertise but less precisely because of the nature of psychological goals. These are mostly more vague and refer to more diverse aspects of the personality, e.g., emotions, cognitions, behavior, and aspirations, than those defined for experts in diet, physiotherapy, breathing, etc.

The goals of the non-expert or informal caretakers who include family members and volunteers are defined, on the one hand, by their desire to help the patient and, on the other hand, by the state of the patient. Both of these factors are dependent on the available resources of the caretakers, which include time, money, space, stamina, and know-how.

The goals of the fifth group that includes scientists and researchers refer more to cancer and cancer patients in general than to particular patients and caretaking of specific individuals, even if sometimes their interest focuses on particular cases because of their scientific importance.

Special Difficulties of the Caretakers

Difficulties of Oncologists

Each of the groups of caretakers has its own particular difficulties. Studies show that major issues mentioned by oncology physicians focus on communication with patients. One of the most common problems is imparting bad news. This may happen recurrently in the course of various occasions starting with the diagnosis and at later decision points defined by various disease developments. The situation is difficult for a number of reasons: the medical problem is serious and may have connotations concerning the patient's survival; the doctor may not always have a good solution for the problem because there may not exist an adequate treatment; sometimes decisions need to be taken in ethically complex issues; the patient is worried and anxious and may not be able emotionally and sometimes cognitively too to completely comprehend the news but still needs to get from the doctor support and hope. The doctor may be confronted with this complex of issues several times in the course of his or her contact with a particular patient and according to one estimate about 20,000 times in the course of one's career [3]. These encounters are particularly stressful and difficult for oncologists.

In addition, there is evidence about further communication problems between oncologists and patients. Often, doctors and patients have different understanding and perspectives on medical issues without even being aware of the gap. This may lead to serious misunderstandings [4]. For example, despite getting the information, a high percentage of patients – in one study 69% of colorectal cancer patients and 81% of lung cancer patients – did not understand that chemotherapy may not provide perfect recovery. The doctors feel that if they insist on clarifying the situation, the cost may be less satisfaction of the patients with them and maybe even loss of the patients to other doctors [5]. However, there is evidence that it is possible to provide patients the whole truth even in difficult situations without causing them depression and other negative reactions [6]. Efficient communication requires time. Yet doctors are notoriously pressed for time because of the many things to which they need to attend in the setting of their work.

Oncologists are exposed to a lot of pain and suffering in their patients and often experience patient loss. Due to time limitations and missing opportunities for elaborating the pain, the grief remains unprocessed and as such contributes to the doctors' distress, guilt, and even poor clinical decisions [7]. The exposure to the suffering patient may stimulate in the physician identification with the suffering person and often feelings of pain, possibly grounded in mirroring neurons [8–10]. These are enhanced by secondary trauma experiences if the oncologist is aware of the traumatic aspects of the situation [11].

Additionally, oncologists are often faced with the fear, anger, and despair of patients and their families, which are difficult emotions to confront and to respond to. The difficulty is enhanced by the fact that the relations with patients are often of long duration and may extend over months and even years. This intensifies the doctors' emotional reaction to the patients' feelings. Hence, in these situations, the doctors may often feel their own helplessness as doctors and as human beings. Learned helplessness is a reaction that has been observed in individuals repeatedly exposed to painful or aversive stimuli which they cannot escape, avoid, or prevent, so that they feel loss of control and stop trying to do something about them [12]. It is not surprising that after years of caring for many patients who despite the best efforts of the doctors may suffer and eventually die, the oncologists develop a kind of learned helplessness, which is grounded in their feeling responsible for the patient's state and also being considered by the patient as responsible [13]. Learned helplessness in doctors is particularly significant in the palliative phase [14].

Further, doctors try to uphold the patient's hope and to provide as much empathy as possible. Empathy is the ability to experience and understand the feelings of others from their perspective. It plays an important role in the therapeutic situation. Patients expect empathy on the part of their physicians and prefer doctors who are empathic [15]. The doctor's empathy may help in identifying the patient's illness better and faster [16], reduce the patient's anxiety [16], facilitate the healing process [18, 19], and decrease somatoform symptoms [17].

However, empathy is a precious resource. It can be depleted and recovered only slowly, similarly to self-control [20]. Experiencing and manifesting empathy may be difficult for doctors because they may not have the personality tendencies supporting empathy or do not possess the necessary skills for maintaining it for long and replenishing the reservoir as fast as needed [21, 22]. After extended or intense periods of manifesting empathy, the almost unavoidable result is the syndrome of compassion fatigue or emotional exhaustion. It is characterized by hopelessness, a decrease in pleasure experiences, constant stress and anxiety, sleeplessness or nightmares, a pervasive negative attitude, cynicism, a decrease in productivity, difficulty to concentrate, and feelings of incompetency and self-doubt which may evoke thoughts about changing the profession. It includes some symptoms associated with burnout, such as exhaustion, frustration, anger, and depression, and some that are more characteristic of compassion fatigue, such as fear, sleep difficulties, and intrusive thoughts [23]. When doctors try to handle the situation by avoiding empathy manifestations, they may experience distance from patients and misunderstanding of their symptoms, as well as incompetence as a human being and as a health professional [24]. A review of over 50 studies showed that compassion fatigue is highly prevalent in oncology caretakers [25].

However, oncologists are not exempt from other potential problems that are known to pressure clinicians in general. Thus, as may be expected, oncologists suffer from burnout, like doctors in other disciplines, and manifest the common symptoms of exhaustion, depersonalization, feelings of professional incompetence, and desire to withdraw from the work [26]. Thus, it is not uncommon for doctors to suffer from conflicts which may concern, for example, dividing their time adequately between work and family or between taking care of patients and attending to administrative duties or to their career as researchers [27, 28].

Notably, studies showed that when pediatric oncologists were asked about the sources of stress which affect them, they mentioned in the first place stress due to family or to daily life issues rather than to patients and cancer [29]. Similarly, in a study with head and neck surgeons, it was found that while 34% reported feeling burned out, 27% mentioned frustration due to the disease, 67% frustration due to the government, and 58% frustration with the economics of medical practice [30].

Considering the problems of communication, confrontation with difficult emotions in oneself and in patients, dealing with an especially difficult disease, and handling additional profession-dependent conflicts [31, 32], it is not surprising that oncologists suffer from high levels of burnout [33–35]. As noted, they also suffer from more specific work-dependent stresses characterized by learned helplessness and compassion fatigue [36, 37].

Difficulties of Nurses

Nurses are confronted with the pain, the suffering, and the emotional reactions of patients to a no lesser degree than doctors and mostly even more. They spend more time and more continuous time with patients and their families. Through the guidance, accompaniment, and care they provide the patients, they get to know them personally beyond the acquaintance that most doctors have with their patients. Also, nurses accompany patients along their disease journey in better and worse periods, supporting, counseling, and helping medically and psychologically. Nurses do not feel the gap between the medical and psychosocial domains as doctors often do. For them the two domains form parts of the same sphere defining the task of caring for the patient. Nurses do not have to shift between the patient and the human being. What they see is one whole person who may be suffering and in need of help.

Studies reflect the difficulties of nurses in caring for cancer patients. An interesting study with nurses in Turkey reported that caring for terminal patients affected the personal lives of nurses and that they found it difficult to talk to patients about dying, especially those who have had more work experience [38]. Likewise, nurses in Nigeria claimed that their difficulties at work were mainly exhaustion (58.6%), coping with the psychological problems of the patients (25.7%), and frequent deaths of patients (24.3%). Notably, similar to the results obtained with doctors [28], the findings with nurses showed that 28.3% of the difficulties of oncology nursing could be attributed to job-related factors, 30.3% to patient-related factors, and 77% to individual factors [39]. Tasks that are especially draining emotionally for nurses are providing support to needy patients for long periods of time and treating terminal patients [40, 41]. Psychological factors that were found to contribute to the burnout of nurses are psychological inflexibility, self-judgmental attitudes, and perceiving the distress of patients without providing empathy [42, 43].

Therefore it is not surprising that oncology nurses were found to suffer compassion fatigue and burnout to a large extent. A significant number of oncology nurses were found to be suffering from the highest degrees of burnout and emotional exhaustion [44, 45]. On the nurse distress thermometer, nurses scored on the highest levels of distress [46]. High stress levels caused by workload and the death of patients were recorded in nurses [47]. Especially remarkable have been their scores of compassion fatigue [47–49].

Difficulties of Allied Health Professionals

The allied health professionals in oncology represent a varied group of professionals, who differ in the degree to which they are involved in caring directly for cancer patients. The most directly and intensely involved are social workers and psychologists. They more than the other professionals in this group are exposed to the suffering and pain of cancer patients and their families, dealing with them and helping them psychologically. Social workers are concerned with a broad range of issues beyond the strictly psychological, in regard to cancer patients and their families, such as financial problems, traveling to medical centers, and family affairs. Hence, in addition to the psychosocial work with the patients and their families, there may be further difficult issues for the psychosocial experts. Social workers may have a lot of trouble with different government offices, insurance companies, and other agencies that may be involved in supporting cancer patients financially and socially and in integrating their work with one another and with the needs of the patients and the families [50–52].

Psychologists too have their problems with working in the medical system. One study presented in detail some of the more salient issues, such as ambiguity of the role and functioning expected of psychologists, difficulties in cooperating with other professionals in the hospital, barriers in operating liaison work within the hospital, and problems in interacting with different family members [53].

Providing psychological help for psychological problems is a very demanding job. The therapist faces the patients' problems and suffering directly, including their conflicts, doubts, and intense emotions. The therapist is confronted with the patients' fear of death, anxieties, and sometimes aggression, and is bound to react and take a stand that is helpful for the patient. In this work the therapist is alone, and mostly there is no one to consult or provide supervision. Not rarely the therapist responds inwardly with the evocation of one's own fears or conflicts. In contrast to standard psychotherapy that is based on consecutive sessions, psychological help to cancer patients may sometime be discontinuous or limited to one or two compact intense sessions. The stress attending the provision of psychological help to cancer patients is often of the highest degree.

The heavy load of exposure to the suffering of the patients takes its toll on the psychosocial helpers. Several studies report the high levels of burnout and compassion fatigue characterizing these health professionals [53, 54].

Difficulties of Informal Caretakers

An increasing number of cancer patients are being treated outside hospitals both because of the limitation of public health resources and because of the preferences of the patients themselves. Hence, there is a growing reliance on family and other volunteer caregivers to support patients at home [55].

Caretakers of cancer patients share several of the problems they face with other caregivers of these patients, mainly the exposure to a lot of suffering and pain. However, their problems are still different mainly because the cancer patients they help are mostly family members they love or individuals otherwise close to them. The help they provide is usually of long duration, and the caregiving relationship is attended by a lot of difficulty caused by often watching their beloved patient's deterioration, not infrequently into the palliative stage and dying.

The informal caretakers provide help and support to patients in institutions (clinics, nursing homes, hospitals) or at home. Special difficulties of the informal caretakers have been noted in many studies. These include unclarity about their rights, duties, duration of service, and responsibility in case something happens to the patient. Additionally, they often do not get enough information about the patient's medical situation and how to deal with apparent or real emergencies. Not rarely the caretaker is faced with multiple competing priorities none of which can be overlooked. They are expected to provide help of varied kinds, including psychological, emotional, social, informational, and instrumental. They are often responsible directly or indirectly for the patient's nutrition, hygiene, ingestion of medication, clothing, mobility, and even entertainment. In any case, the caretaker is in general forced through the circumstances and relationship with the patient to consider the whole person and most of his or her needs. Considering the whole person may be always difficult, especially when the needs change because the state of the patient may change [56–58].

Sometimes the caretaker is involved in decisions concerning the patient, such as whether to tell or not to tell the patient some medical news. For example, a study in India showed that there may be a collusion between the caretaker and the doctor in hiding information from the patient [59]. Being involved in decisions concerning the patient may be a source of constant stress, doubts, and self-blame for the caretaker. Sometimes the doubts and the guilt continue after the patient's demise [60–63].

Notably studies showed that caretakers are worried more about providing psychological care to the patients than physical and medical care, probably because they get more guidance in regard to the latter [64].

It is not rare that caretakers start the caretaking without proper preparation. In general, many caretakers feel that they were not prepared for the new task and that they lack the competence and skills necessary for performing it and facing up to the challenge [65].

Caretaking may involve radical changes in the role and lifestyle of the caretaker [65]. The patient may be a parent and the caretaker a son or daughter who up to the parent's disease has been dependent on the parent and suddenly had to become the responsible caretaker on whom the parent is dependent. The interviewing of mothers who had lost children to cancer revealed that in some cases, they felt compelled to become their children's main caretakers because they could not fully count on the healthcare professionals. Assuming this role has led to changes in behavior and values of these mothers that persisted after the child's death [66].

The load of work and the conditions under which it is performed often involve for the caretaker a rupture of the daily routine. In some cases, if possible and necessary, the caretakers take a leave of their regular work and spend most of their time with the patient. Sometimes the caretaking involves a financial burden either because of the expenses for medicines or extra help needed for the patient or because the caretaker has to reduce one's regular work [67]. Employed caretakers report adverse impact on their work [55].

Further potential sources of stress for the caretakers are due to the fact that the caretakers and patients are often family relatives. This relation may cause the caretakers anxiety because they are scared they may get cancer due to their genetic background [68, 69].

Another source of stress has to do with the tendency of caretakers to experience high levels of complicated grief pre-death because of their tendency to imagine the death of the patient and preparing themselves inwardly for it ahead of time, partly in order to mitigate the pain when the death actually takes place [70]. The guilt the caregivers may experience after the death of the patient is partly a manifestation of the fairly common survivors' guilt. Yet, it may also reflect specific issues of the caregiver, such as regret about having wished sometimes death for the patient because of one's own fatigue or in order to end the patient's suffering, or because of doubt about whether he or she have given the patient optimal care and attention, and have made the right decisions. Survivor's guilt is enhanced by closeness to the patient and duration of caretaking [61, 62].

The variety of responsibilities, coupled with the involved emotions and frequently lack of adequate preparation or skills, constitute serious sources of stress for caretakers [65]. In addition, review studies showed that caregivers suffered more than controls from high levels of depression, state anxiety, and sleep dysfunctions, as well as systolic and diastolic blood pressure, and in case of caregivers of long duration also of elevated heart rate [71]. There is evidence that they often experience negative health effects, mediated in part by immune and autonomic dysregulation [72]. At the start of the palliative period, caregivers had higher scores of depression and anxiety [55].

Benefits of Treating or Caregiving of Cancer Patients

Despite the many difficulties attending those involved in treating or caretaking of cancer patients, it should not be surprising that there are also benefits to being close to cancer patients and devoting time and energy to helping them in different ways. Many of the caretakers in various specialities (including doctors, nurses, and psychosocial experts) mention the benefits. First in order is the experience of giving. Giving in the sense of helping another person is supported by most religions and social ideologies and is personally attended by a positive feeling, especially if there is no reward expected or presented. More specifically, helping another person in distress is especially rewarding emotionally for many individuals. It provides the feeling of being a good person and thus provides some redress for the guilt many people feel for not being always as good as they would have liked to be. Some people mention also their hope that by helping cancer patients, they may be freed of the fear or phobia of cancer that they have. Feelings of this kind are supported also by scientific evidence. Providing help or support to others, e.g., acquaintances or strangers, was found to be related to positive emotional and physical health results, such as more positive affect [73, 74], reduced stress and increased caregiving activity reflected in specific brain areas [75] and even lower rates of mortality [76], or delayed mortality in older people [77].

Another unexpected aspect is that confronting suffering and distress may have an invigorating impact on at least some people. Facing pain and death may remind many individuals that life is not unlimited so that it is advisable or reasonable to devote their motivation and resources to realizing their goals, repairing different evils or sources of dissatisfaction in their life, or simply to start living and enjoying life.

There is some evidence about development, changes in life, and increase in creativity and satisfaction that caretakers of cancer patients report. Sometimes it takes the form similar to posttraumatic growth [78].

In some cases more personal motives play a role. Some people feel that they may not have behaved as expected with the patient himself or others in the family and experience a kind of drive for compensation for the past in providing help for a specific patient or patients in general. Others may get a mitigation of a general sense of guilt they may have by devoting resources to the help of cancer patents.

Helping the Caretakers

In view of the broad range of difficulties from which the different groups of experts and other caretakers of cancer patients suffer, there is a growing tendency to provide them different interventions and help. This tendency is grounded also in the increasing attention devoted in recent years to helping the caretaker and to an increased awareness of the importance of the cancer experts and caretakers.

The interventions suggested for professionals and for informal caretakers will be presented separately. Concerning doctors, nurses, and psychosocial experts, the major suggested interventions focus on lowering stress and on self-care. Most recommended interventions mention self-care, i.e., activities performed by the individual regularly for maintaining one's well-being [7], for example, getting enough sleep, having regular meals, devoting some time to physical exercise, working fewer hours and making breaks during working time or taking frequent vacations [27], having some fun and entertainment, spending time with family and friends, and getting professional help in case the listed measures provide no help [81]. More specific suggestions are reducing exposure to situations in which empathy is required, for example, by switching to research or administrative work. Somewhat different though more general proposals suggest focusing on self-reflection, identifying what is important for oneself and living in accordance with it [82]. There is barely any evidence about whether suggestions of this kind have been applied or their effects on compassion fatigue tested [83]. Several studies reported significant results on reduced compassion fatigue in participants in several mindfulness sessions [84–86]. The positive results are probably based to some extent on the impact of mindfulness training on diverting one's attention from the stress sensations. Teaching resilience

(Provider Resilience Mobile Application) had no effect on compassion fatigue [87], and the pilot Compassion Fatigue Resiliency Program reduced stress but barely compassion fatigue [88]. Participating in a formalized educational program had only a minimal effect on compassion fatigue [89]. Acquiring specific therapeutic skills [90] or communication skills [91] and participating in different facility interventions [92] were found to have a low effect on reducing burnout and barely any effect on decreasing compassion fatigue. Increasing self-efficacy and support from the environment helped psychosocial workers to some extent to function in the framework of work [91], as well as improved their effort-reward balance in the framework off work [93].

A study with healthcare workers in pediatric oncology found that compassion fatigue as well as other stress contributing factors were decreased by two relief-inducing actions: interacting with people (who are not colleagues or patients) and bodily activities, such as sport [29].

There is one promising program which led to positive results and needs to be tested in further research [21, 79, 80]. This innovative program is called "Empathy without Compassion Fatigue" and is designed for health professionals intended to enable them to apply empathy without suffering compassion fatigue. It is based on the theories of cognitive orientation [94] and of meaning by Kreitler [95]. It includes four parts. One is focused on creating a motivational disposition toward manifesting empathy in a controlled manner. It is based on strengthening attitudes referring to one's goals, norms, self-image, and view of reality that support directly or indirectly the manifestations of empathy in a controlled manner. A second part is focused on producing a mental set oriented toward the interpersonally-shared meaning mode, which helps in orienting oneself to focus on reality and the context-bound situation rather than on one's own subjective internal world. The third part deals with extending in a systematic manner the meaning assignment to the situation and its major aspects and referents. The fourth part orients toward promoting the focusing on the other person, emphasizing the differences between oneself and the other. The program can be employed as one unit or in parts, combined in different sequences. Following its acquisition, it is subjected to a gradual strengthening through its mere application. All four parts of the program together or in different combinations enable the health professional to control one's manifestations of empathy, adjusting the timing, the manner and amount to one's tendencies, the needs of the patients, and the possibilities in the specific situation. The goal is attainment of control of empathy along the scale of minimal to optimal so that compassion fatigue is reduced or does not develop at all. An empirical demonstration of the training of the program and its different parts with health carers showed that the program is operable and easily trained and seems to have the expected effects of reducing compassion fatigue. Notably, the program may be applied outside the context of healthcare and by individuals who are not health professionals. Notably, the components of the program may be adapted as basis of a program for controlling the manifestations of emotions in general.

A large number of interventions have been proposed for the informal caregivers probably because they are in need and get relatively little support [96]. A comprehensive survey of the available interventions between 1980 and 2011 for the informal caregivers led to the identification of a large number which fell into eight categories: psycho education, problem-solving/skills, supportive therapy, family/couples therapy, cognitive-behavioral therapy, interpersonal therapy, complementary and alternative medicine interventions, and existential therapy [97]. The different interventions were applied to a varying number of caregivers caring for cancer patients with different diagnoses in different contexts. On the whole, each of the applied interventions led to positive results in several of the studies. The reviewers concluded that the best and most feasible interventions are those based on structured, goal-oriented, and integrative approaches. The major challenge remains to reach a growing number of caregivers using means of communication such as the Internet, telephone, and Skype that would not overburden them beyond their regular caring activities.

Some Summative Comments

This chapter dealt with the doctors, therapists, and caretakers of cancer patients. The overall message is that it is hard to be a helper. There are many reasons for this conclusion. Some are administrative and have to do with limited resources: insufficient financial resources, too few hospitals and clinics, and too limited teams of doctors and therapists. The shortage is exacerbated in view of the growing numbers of cancer patients of all kinds all over the world and prolonged durations of disease as well as increased numbers of survivors. In addition, applying the improved medical and psychosocial treatments require even more resources than those available or planned. However, there is one recurrent issue that still remains even if resources are increased. This is the issue of being "a true helper." It appears that among the many needs that cancer patients have, there is also the need to be accepted, to experience empathy on the part of the helpers, and to feel that the giver gives naturally, easily, with a truly good intention. A giving of this kind is probably what produces hope and ignites in the patient the desire to cooperate with the therapy and mobilize all one's strength for survival. Survival is a common product of the optimal combined efforts of the therapist/doctor/caretaker and of the patient. This optimal result happens all the time, but it still requires maintaining optimal conditions on the part of both the therapist and the patients. What this chapter showed is that the occurrence of the desired result takes a toll in terms of the resources of the therapists. These resources are psychological – emotional and cognitive. When depleted they reduce the therapists' ability to heal others. But they can and should be recovered through proper psychological therapy. Some positive beginnings for the attainment of this goal have already been done (e.g., "Empathy without Compassion Fatigue"). One dares to hope that when more therapists become skilled in being empathic without suffering burnout and compassion fatigue, they will be able to provide more help to more patients and at the same time advance on the personal road to becoming whole human beings.

References

1. Editorial. (2015). The importance of nurses in cancer care. *The Lancet Oncology, 16*(7), 737.
2. Komatsu, H., & Yagasaki, K. (2014). The power of nursing: Guiding patients through a journey of uncertainty. *European Journal of Oncology Nursing, 18*(4), 419–424.
3. Schmid Mast, M., Kindlimann, A., & Langewitz, W. (2005). Recipients' perspective on breaking bad news: How you put it really makes a difference. *Patient Education and Counseling, 58*(3), 244–251.
4. Elstein, A. S., Chapman, G. B., & Knight, S. J. (2005). Patients' values and clinical substituted judgments: The case of localized prostate cancer. *Health Psychology, 24*(Suppl 4), S85–S92.
5. Weeks, J., Catalano, P. J., Cronin, A., Iman, J. F., Mack, N., Keating, L., & Schrag, D. (2012). Patients expectations for effects of chemotherapy for advanced cancer. *The New England Journal of Medicine, 367*, 1616–1625.
6. Wright, A. A., Zhang, B., Ray, A., Mack, J. W., Trice, E., Balboni, T., Mitchell, S. L., Jackson, V. A., Block, S. D., Maciejewski, P. K., & Prigerson, H. G. (2008). Associations between end-of-life discussions, patient mental health, medical care near death, and caregiver bereavement adjustment. *JAMA, 300*(14), 1665–1673.
7. Sanchez-Reilly, S., Morrison, L. J., Carey, E., Bernacki, R., O'Neill, L., Kapo, J., Periyakoil, V. S., & Thomas, J. L. (2013). Caring for oneself to care for others: Physicians and their self-care. *The Journal of Supportive Oncology, 11*(2), 75–81.
8. Iacoboni, M. (2009). Imitation, empathy, and mirror neurons. *Annual Review of Psychology, 60*, 653–670.
9. Rizzolatti, G., & Craighero, L. (2004). The mirror-neuron system. *Annual Review of Neuroscience, 27*(1), 169–192.
10. Jackson, P. L., Rainville, P., & Decety, J. (2006). To what extent do we share the pain of others? Insight from the neural bases of pain empathy. *Pain, 125*(1), 5–9.
11. Jacob, W., Roden-Foreman, M., Bennett, M., Rainey, E. R., Garrett, J. S., Powers, M. B., & Warren, A. M. (2017). Secondary traumatic stress in emergency medicine clinicians. *Cognitive Behaviour Therapy, 46*(6), 522–532.
12. Seligman, M. E. P. (1972). Learned helplessness. *Annual Review of Medicine, 23*(1), 407–412.
13. Bond, C. (2007). The training of the "helpless" physician. *Medscape General Medicine, 9*(3), 47.
14. Abrahm, J. L. (2012). Integrating palliative care into comprehensive cancer care. *Journal of the National Comprehensive Cancer Network, 10*(10), 1192–1198.
15. Zinn, W. (1993). The empathic physician. *Archives of Internal Medicine, 153*(3), 306–312.
16. Bellet, P. S., & Maloney, M. J. (1991). The importance of empathy as an interviewing skill. *JAMA, 266*(13), 1831–1832.
17. Halpern, J. (2003). What is clinical empathy? *Journal of General Internal Medicine, 18*(8), 670–674.
18. Adler, H. M. (1997). The history of the present illness as treatment: Who's listening, and why does it matter? *The Journal of the American Board of Family Practice, 10*(1), 28–35.
19. Fink, P., Sorensen, L., Engberg, M., Holm, M., & Munk-Jorgensen, P. (1999). Somatization in primary care. Prevalence, health care utilization, and general practitioner recognition. *Psychosomatics, 40*(4), 330–338.
20. Muraven, M., Tice, D. M., & Baumeister, R. F. (1998). Self-control as limited resource: Regulatory depletion patterns. *Journal of Personality and Social Psychology, 74*, 774–789.
21. Kreitler, S. (2018). Empathy without empathic exhaustion. In C. Pracana & M. Wang (Eds.), *Psychological applications and trends (InPact)* (pp. 3–7). Lisboa: InScience Press.
22. Davis, M. H. (1983). Measuring individual differences in empathy: Evidence for a multidimensional approach. *Journal of Personality and Social Psychology, 44*, 113–126.
23. Figley, C. R. (1995). Compassion fatigue as secondary traumatic stress disorder: An overview. In C. R. Figley (Ed.), *Compassion fatigue: Coping with secondary traumatic stress disorder in those who treat the traumatized* (pp. 1–21). New York: Brunner-Routledge.

24. Stamm, B. H. (2002). Measuring compassion satisfaction as well as fatigue: Developmental history of the Compassion Satisfaction and Fatigue Test. In C. R. Figley (Ed.), *Treating compassion fatigue* (pp. 107–119). New York: Brunner-Routledge.
25. Najjar, N., Davis, L. W., Beck-Coon, K., & Doebbeling, C. C. (2009). Compassion fatigue a review of the research to date and relevance to cancer-care providers. *Journal of Health Psychology, 14*(2), 267–277.
26. Maslach, C. (2017). Burnout: A multidimensional perspective. In W. B. Schaufeli, C. Maslach, & T. Marek (Eds.), *Professional burnout: Recent developments in theory and research* (pp. 19–32). New York: Routledge.
27. Nitzsche, A., Neumann, M., Groß, S. E., Ansmann, L., Pfaff, H., Baumann, W., Wirtz, M., Schmitz, S., & Ernstmann, N. (2017). Recovery opportunities, work-home conflict, and emotional exhaustion among hematologists and oncologists in private practice. *Psychology, Health & Medicine, 22*(4), 462–473.
28. Kleiner, S., & Wallace, J. E. (2017). Oncologist burnout and compassion fatigue: Investigating time pressure at work as a predictor and the mediating role of work-family conflict. *Health Services Research, 17*(1), 639.
29. Toren, A., Yalon, M., Golan, H., Goldstein, G., Tamam, V., & Kreitler, S. (2016). Stress or relief of stress—burnout in pediatric oncology health workers. *Journal of Psychological Sciences, 2*(2), 1–13.
30. Johnson, J. T., Wagner, R. L., Rueger, R. M., & Goepfert, H. (1993). Professional burnout among head and neck surgeons: Results of a survey. *Head & Neck, 15*, 557–560.
31. Granek, L., Ben-David, M., Nakash, O., Cohen, M., Barbera, L., Ariad, S., & Krzyzanowska, M. K. (2017). Oncologists' negative attitudes towards expressing emotion over patient death and burnout. *Supportive Care in Cancer, 25*(5), 1607–1614.
32. Bragard, I., Libert, Y., Etienne, A. M., Merckaert, I., Delvaux, N., Marchal, S., Boniver, J., Klastersky, J., Reynaert, C., Scalliet, P., Slachmuylder, J. L., & Razavi, D. (2010). Insight on variables leading to burnout in cancer physicians. *Journal of Cancer Education, 25*(1), 109–115.
33. Hutton, D., Beardmore, C., Patel, I., Massey, J., Wong, H., & Probst, H. (2014). Audit of the job satisfaction levels of the UK radiography and physics workforce in UK radiotherapy centres 2012. *The British Journal of Radiology, 87*(1039), 20130742.
34. Cass, I., Duska, L. R., Blank, S. V., Cheng, G., duPont, N. C., Frederick, P. J., et al. (2016). Stress and burnout among gynecologic oncologists: A Society of Gynecologic Oncology Evidence-based Review and Recommendations. *Gynecologic Oncology, 143*(2), 421–427.
35. Howard, M. (2013). The incidence of burnout or compassion fatigue in medical dosimetrists as a function of various stress and psychologic factors. *Medical Dosimetry, 38*(1), 88–94.
36. Eelen, S., Bauwens, S., Baillon, C., Distelmans, W., Jacobs, E., & Verzelen, A. (2014). The prevalence of burnout among oncology professionals: Oncologists are at risk of developing burnout. *Psycho-Oncology, 23*(12), 1415–1422.
37. Medisauskaite, A., & Kamau, C. (2017). Prevalence of oncologists in distress: Systematic review and meta-analysis. *Psycho-Oncology, 26*(11), 1732–1740.
38. Olfaz, F., Arslan, F., Uzun, S., Ustunsoz, A., Yilmazkol, E., & Unlü, E. (2010). A survey of emotional difficulties of nurses who care for oncology patients. *Psychological Reports, 106*(1), 119–130.
39. Kamisli, S., Yuce, D., Karakilic, B., Kilickap, S., & Hayran, M. (2017). Cancer patients and oncology nursing: Perspectives of oncology nurses in Turkey. *Nigerian Journal of Clinical Practice, 20*(9), 1065–1073.
40. O'Sullivan, D., & Mansour, M. (2015). The nurse's role in managing the psychological and emotional impact on women diagnosed with breast cancer. *Clinical Nursing Studies, 3*(4), 29–35.
41. Tomoyo, S., Mitsunori, M., Masako, K., & Keiko, K. (2003). Difficulties encountered by nurses in the care of terminally ill cancer patients in general hospitals in Japan. *Palliative Medicine, 17*, 520–526.

42. Kutluturka, S., Sozeri, E., Uysal, N., & Bay, F. (2016). Resilience and burnout status among nurses working in oncology. *Annals of General Psychiatry, 15*, 33.
43. Duarte, J., & Pinto-Gouveia, J. (2017). The role of psychological factors in oncology nurses' burnout and compassion fatigue symptoms. *European Journal of Oncology Nursing, 28*, 114–121.
44. De la Fuente-Solana, E. I., Gómez-Urquiza, J. L., Cañadas, G. R., Albendín-García, L., Ortega-Campos, E., & Cañadas-De la Fuente, G. A. (2017). Burnout and its relationship with personality factors in oncology nurses. *European Journal of Oncology Nursing, 30*, 91–96.
45. Cañadas-De la Fuente, G. A., Gómez-Urquiza, G. L., Ortega-Campos, E. M., Cañadas, G. R., Albendín-García, L., & De la Fuente-Solana, E. I. (2018). Prevalence of burnout syndrome in oncology nursing: A meta- analytic study. *Psycho-Oncology, 27*, 1–8.
46. Wahlberg, L., Nirenberg, A., & Capezuti, E. (2016). Distress and coping: Self-efficacy in inpatient oncology nurses. *Oncology Nursing Forum, 43*(6), 738–746.
47. Ko, W., & Kiser-Larson, N. (2016). Stress levels of nurses in oncology outpatient units. *Clinical Journal of Oncology Nursing, 20*(2), 158–164.
48. Emanuel, L., Ferris, F. D., von Gunten, C. F., & Von Roenn, J. H. (2011). Combating compassion fatigue and burnout in cancer care. Excerpted from EPEC-O: Education in palliative and end-of-life care for oncology (Module 15: Cancer Doctors and Burnout). Accessed on 21 Nov 2014 at www.Medscape.com/viewarticle/742941.
49. Yoder, E. A. (2010). Compassion fatigue in nurses. *Applied Nursing Research, 23*, 191–197.
50. Adams, R. E., Boscarino, J. A., & Figley, C. R. (2006). Compassion fatigue and psychological distress among social workers: A validation study. *The American Journal of Orthopedics, 76*(1), 103–108.
51. Yi, Y., Ah Kim, M., Choi, K., Kim, S., & O'Connor, A. (2018). When does compassion fatigue hit social workers? Caring for oncology patients in Korea. *Qualitative Social Work, 17*(3), 337–354.
52. Koocher, G. P. (1979). Adjustment and coping strategies among the caretakers of cancer patients. *Social Work in Health Care, 5*(2), 145–150.
53. Nakajima, K., Iwamitsu, Y., Matsubara, M., Oba, A., Hirai, K., Morita, T., & Kizawa, Y. (2015). Psychologists involved in cancer palliative care in Japan. A nationwide survey. *Palliative & Supportive Care, 13*, 327–334.
54. Wiener, L., Oppenheim, D., Breyer, J., Battles, H., Zadeh, S., & Patenaude, A. F. (2012). A worldview of the professional experiences and training needs of pediatric psycho-oncologists. *Psycho-Oncology, 44*, 123–144.
55. Grunfeld, E., Coyle, D., Whelan, T., Clinch, J., Reyno, L., Earle, C. C., Willan, A., Viola, R., Coristine, M., Janz, T., & Glossop, R. (2004). Family caregiver burden: Results of a longitudinal study of breast cancer patients and their principal caregivers. *Canadian Medical Association Journal, 170*(12), 1795–1801.
56. Ventafridda, V., De Conno, F., Viganò, A., Ripamonti, C., Gallucci, M., & Gamba, A. (1989). Comparison of home and hospital care of advanced cancer patients. *Tumori, 75*(6), 619–625.
57. Bavota, C. (1988). How to coordinate the home care with the hospital care for a better quality of life in cancer patients. *European Journal of Gynaecological Oncology, 9*(1), 17–20.
58. Christ, G., & Siegel, K. (1990). Monitoring quality-of-life needs of cancer patients. *Cancer, 65*(3 Suppl), 760–765.
59. Victor, A., George, C. E., Inbaraj, L. R., & Norman, G. (2018). Not to tell patients: Benefit or harm? A study on impact of collusion on the quality of life among palliative care patients. *Indian Journal of Palliative Care, 24*(1), 61–66.
60. Kreitler, S., Barak, F., & Siegelmann-Danieli, N. (2009). Survivor's guilt: The case of cancer. In D. Cooley, L. Steffen, & R. Fisher (Eds.), *Death and dying*. Oxford: Inter-Disciplinary Press.
61. Kreitler, S., Barak, F., Alkalay, Y., & Siegelman-Danieli, N. (2012). Survivor's guilt in the caretakers of cancer. In A. Kasher & A. Glahn (Eds.), *The presence of the dead in our lives* (Interface/Probing the Boundaries Series) (pp. 77–98). Amsterdam: Rodopi.

62. Kreitler, S., Barak, F., & Siegelman-Danieli, N. (2012). The guilt of the survivors. In S. Kreitler & H. Shanun-Klein (Eds.), *Studies of grief and bereavement* (Book 2 in the Series Death Education). Hauppauge: Nova Publishers.
63. Kreitler, M. M., & Kreitler, S. (2008). Guilt and remorse in family members of patients. The 13th Annual Conference of the Israel Association of Palliative Care (Tmicha): Palliative care – the right for all? Tel-Aviv, Israel, January 23, 2008.
64. Colell Brunet, R., & Limonero, J. T. (2003). What worries the oncology patient's caretaker? [In Spanish: Qué preocupa al cuidador del enfermo oncológico?]. *Revista De Enfermeria, 26*(2), 8–12.
65. Hashemi-Ghasemabadi, M., Taleghani, F., Yousefy, A., & Kohan, S. (2016). Transition to the new role of caregiving for families of patients with breast cancer: A qualitative descriptive exploratory study. *Supportive Care in Cancer, 24*(3), 1269–1276.
66. Saiki-Craighill, S. (2002). The personal development of mothers of terminal cancer patients: How Japanese women change through the experience of caring for and losing their children to cancer. *Qualitative Health Research, 12*(6), 769–779.
67. Warner, E. L., Kirchhoff, A. C., Nam, G. E., & Fluchel, M. (2015). Financial burden of pediatric cancer for patients and their families. *Journal of Oncology Practice/American Society of Clinical Oncology, 11*(1), 12–18.
68. Li, J., Hart, T. L., Aronson, M., Crangle, C., & Govindarajan, A. (2016). Cancer worry, perceived risk and cancer screening in first-degree relatives of patients with familial gastric cancer. *Journal of Genetic Counseling, 25*(3), 520–528.
69. Epstein, S. A., Lin, T. H., Audrain, J., Stefanek, M., Rimer, B., & Lerman, C. (1997). Excessive breast self-examination among first-degree relatives of newly diagnosed breast cancer patients. High-Risk Breast Cancer Consortium. *Psychosomatics, 38*(3), 253–261.
70. Tomarken, A., Holland, J., Schachter, S., Vanderwerker, L., Zuckerman, E., Nelson, C., Coups, E., Ramirez, P. M., & Prigerson, H. (2008). Factors of complicated grief pre-death in caregivers of cancer patients. *Psycho-Oncology, 17*(2), 105–111.
71. Corà, A., Partinico, M., Munafò, M., & Palomba, D. (2012). Health risk factors in caregivers of terminal cancer patients: A pilot study. *Cancer Nursing, 35*(1), 38–47.
72. Bevans, M. F., & Sternberg, E. M. (2012). Caregiving burden, stress, and health effects among family caregivers of adult cancer patients. *JAMA, 307*(4), 398–403.
73. Dulin, P. L., & Hill, R. D. (2003). Relationships between altruistic activity and positive and negative affect among low income older adult service providers. *Aging & Mental Health, 7*, 294–299.
74. Midlarsky, E. (1991). Helping as coping. In M. S. Clark (Ed.), *Prosocial behavior* (pp. 238–264). Thousand Oaks: Sage.
75. Inagaki, T. K., Byrne Halton, K. E., Suzuki, S., Jevtic, I., Hornstein, E., Bower, J. E., & Eisenberger, N. (2016). The neurobiology of giving versus receiving support: The role of stress-related and social reward-related neural activity. *Psychosomatic Medicine, 78*(4), 443–453.
76. Brown, S. L., Nesse, R. M., Vinokur, A. D., & Smith, D. M. (2003). Providing social support may be more beneficial than receiving it results from a prospective study of mortality. *Psychological Science, 14*, 320–327.
77. Harris, A. H. S., & Thoresen, C. E. (2005). Volunteering is associated with delayed mortality in older people: Analysis of the longitudinal study of aging. *Journal of Health Psychology, 10*(6), 739–752.
78. Li, Q., & Loke, A. Y. (2013). The positive aspects of caregiving for cancer patients: A critical review of the literature and directions for future research. *Psycho-Oncology, 22*(11), 2399–2407.
79. Kreitler, S. (2014). How to maintain empathy but avoid empathic exhaustion? Workshop. 1st International Meeting on Wellbeing and Performance in Clinical Practice. Alexandroupolis, Greece, 28 May – 1 June, 2014.
80. Kreitler, S. (2018). Empathy: How much is right? Tools for the management of empathy in the context of healthcare. In C. Pracana & M. Wang (Eds.), *Psychology applications & developments IV*. Lisboa: Science Press.

81. Pfifferling, J.-H., & Gilley, K. (2000). When practicing medicine feels more like labor than a labor of love, take steps to heal the healer. *Family Practice Management, 7*(4), 39–44.
82. Fleurant, M., Lasser, K. E., Quintiliani, L. M., & Liebschutz, J. (2017). Group self-reflection to address burnout: A facilitator's guide. *Med Ed Portal*. 2017, *13*, 10663. https://doi.org/10.15766/mep_2374-8265.10663.
83. Henry, B. J. (2014). Nursing burnout interventions: What is being done? *Clinical Journal of Oncology Nursing, 18*(2), 211–214.
84. Burgess, D. J., Beach, M. C., & Saha, S. (2017). Mindfulness practice: A promising approach to reducing the effects of clinician implicit bias on patients. *Patient Education and Counseling, 100*(2), 372–376.
85. Duarte, J., & Pinto-Gouveia, J. (2016). Effectiveness of a mindfulness-based intervention on oncology nurses' burnout and compassion fatigue symptoms: A non-randomized study. *International Journal of Nursing Studies, 64*, 98–107.
86. Cucarella, S. P., & Giannini, M. C. (2016). Effectiveness of a pilot mindfulness program in volunteers of a breast cancer. *Journal of Evidence-Based Complementary & Alternative Medicine, 21*(4), 291–294.
87. Jakel, P., Kenney, J., Ludan, N., Miller, P. S., McNair, N., & Matesic, E. (2016). Effects of the use of the provider resilience mobile application in reducing compassion fatigue in oncology nursing. *Clinical Journal of Oncology Nursing, 20*(6), 611–616.
88. Pfaff, K. A., Freeman-Gibb, L., Patrick, L. J., DiBiase, R., & Moretti, O. (2017). Reducing the "cost of caring" in cancer care: Evaluation of a pilot interprofessional compassion fatigue resiliency programme. *Journal of Interprofessional Care, 31*(4), 512–519.
89. Klein, C. J., Riggenbach-Hays, J. J., Sollenberger, L. M., Harney, D. M., & McGarvey, J. S. (2018). Quality of life and compassion satisfaction in clinicians: A pilot intervention study for reducing compassion fatigue. *The American Journal of Hospice & Palliative Care, 35*(6), 882–888.
90. Traeger, L., Park, E. R., Sporn, N., Repper-DeLisi, J., Convery, M. S., Jacobo, M., & Pirl, W. F. (2013). Development and evaluation of targeted psychological skills training for oncology nurses in managing stressful patient and family encounters. *Oncology Nursing Forum, 40*(4), E327–E336.
91. Banerjee, S. C., Manna, R., Coyle, N., Johnson Shen, M., Pehrson, C., Zaider, T., Hammonds, S., Krueger, C. A., Parker, P. A., & Bylund, C. L. (2016). Oncology nurses' communication challenges with patients and families: A qualitative study. *Nurse Education in Practice, 16*(1), 193–201.
92. Wentzel, D., & Brysiewicz, P. (2017). Integrative review of facility interventions to manage compassion fatigue in oncology nurses. *Oncology Nursing Forum, 44*(3), E124–E140.
93. Rasmussen, V., Turnell, A., Butow, P., Juraskova, I., Kirsten, L., Wiener, L., Patenaude, A., Hoekstra-Weebers, J., Grassi, L., & IPOS Research Committee. (2016). Burnout among psychosocial oncologists: An application and extension of the effort-reward imbalance model. *Psycho-Oncology, 25*(2), 194–202.
94. Kreitler, S. (2004). The cognitive guidance of behavior. In J. T. Jost, M. R. Banaji, & D. A. Prentice (Eds.), *Perspectivism in social psychology: The Yin and Yang of scientific progress* (pp. 113–126). Washington, DC: American Psychological Association.
95. Kreitler, S. (2014). Meaning and its manifestations: The meaning system. In S. Kreitler & T. Urbanek (Eds.), *Conceptions of meaning* (pp. 3–32). Hauppauge: Nova Publishers.
96. Merckaert, I., Libert, Y., Lieutenant, F., Moucheux, A., Farvacques, C., Slachmuylder, J. L., & Razavi, D. (2013). Desire for formal psychological support among caregivers of patients with cancer: Prevalence and implications for screening their needs. *Psycho-Oncology, 22*(6), 1389–1395.
97. Applebaum, A. J., & Breitbart, W. (2013). Care for the cancer caregiver: A systematic review. *Palliative & Supportive Care, 11*(3), 231–252.

Index

S. Kreitler, *Psycho-Oncology for the Clinician*,
https://doi.org/10.1007/978-3-030-06126-5

MIX
Papier aus verantwortungsvollen Quellen
Paper from responsible sources
FSC® C105338

If you have any concerns about our products,
you can contact us on
ProductSafety@springernature.com

In case Publisher is established outside the EU,
the EU authorized representative is:
Springer Nature Customer Service Center GmbH
Europaplatz 3, 69115 Heidelberg, Germany

Printed by Libri Plureos GmbH
in Hamburg, Germany